YOUR
Yin Yang
BODY TYPE

"*Your Yin Yang Body Type* is a must have. From the very first page you will embark on a journey to optimize your health based on the practice of a unique traditional Korean therapeutic form of medicine called the Sasang medicine. This book is an excellent read for one who is looking for a real-world approach to spiritual, physical, and emotional well-being."

SANDE MCDANIEL, PUBLISHER OF
ORIENTAL MEDICINE JOURNAL

"A one-of-a-kind Sasang medical book that portrays the essence of Lee Je-ma's philosophy in a practical and modern way. I pray that readers in the United States and other English-speaking regions achieve optimum health by its virtue."

JONG YEOL KIM, KMD, PH.D.,
PRINCIPAL RESEARCHER, MEDICAL RESEARCH DIVISION,
KOREA INSTITUTE OF ORIENTAL MEDICINE

"As a practitioner of traditional Chinese medicine, incorporating the perspective of Sasang medicine into the care of my patients has already enhanced my effectiveness. Dr. Wagman clearly lays out all we need to know to begin looking at those we're caring for and ourselves in a unique way according to the principles of Oriental medicine. This book is well written with a great deal of accessible information for the layperson and for the practitioner alike."

JOSHUA SINGER, M.A.O.M., L.AC., DIPL. AC.,
INTEGRATIVE ACUPUNCTURE AND ORIENTAL MEDICINE

YOUR Yin Yang BODY TYPE

The Korean Tradition of Sasang Medicine

GARY WAGMAN, Ph.D., L.Ac.

Healing Arts Press
Rochester, Vermont • Toronto, Canada

Healing Arts Press
One Park Street
Rochester, Vermont 05767
www.HealingArtsPress.com

SUSTAINABLE FORESTRY INITIATIVE Certified Sourcing www.sfiprogram.org SFI-00854

Text stock is SFI certified

Healing Arts Press is a division of Inner Traditions International

Note to the Reader: *This book is intended as an informational guide. The remedies, approaches, and techniques described herein are meant to supplement, and not to be a substitute for, professional medical care or treatment. They should not be used to treat a serious ailment without prior consultation with a qualified health care professional.*

Library of Congress Cataloging-in-Publication Data

Wagman, Gary, 1973–

Your yin yang body type : the Korean tradition of sasang medicine / Gary Wagman.

pages cm

Includes index.

Summary: “Optimize your health by learning the inherent strengths and weaknesses of your body type”— Provided by publisher.

ISBN 978-1-62055-370-1 (paperback) — ISBN 978-1-62055-371-8 (e-book)

1. Medicine, Korean. 2. Somatotypes. 3. Yin-yang. 4. Nutrition. 5. Physical fitness. 6. Self-care, Health. I. Title.

R628.W34 2015

613.2—dc23

2014016304

Printed and bound in the United States by Lake Book Manufacturing, Inc.
The text stock is SFI certified. The Sustainable Forestry Initiative® program promotes sustainable forest management.

10 9 8 7 6 5 4 3 2 1

Text design and layout by Virginia Scott Bowman
This book was typeset in Garamond Premier Pro and Gill Sans with Online and Gill Sans used as display typefaces

To send correspondence to the author of this book, mail a first-class letter to the author c/o Inner Traditions • Bear & Company, One Park Street, Rochester, VT 05767, and we will forward the communication, or contact the author directly at **www.sasangmedicine.com** or **www.harmonyclinics.com**.

Contents

Acknowledgments vii
Introduction 1

PART ONE
Understanding the Yin Yang Body Types

Sasang Medicine and the Yin Yang Body Types 6
Determining Your Yin Yang Body Type 40

PART TWO
Emotional Balance and Your Yin Yang Body Type

The Four Virtues and Emotional Tendencies 72
Yin Type A Emotional Balance 76
Yin Type B Emotional Balance 88
Yang Type A Emotional Balance 97
Yang Type B Emotional Balance 103

PART THREE

Eating and Exercising Right for Your Yin Yang Body Type

Body Type Foods: An Introduction 110

Yin Type A Foods 119

Yin Type B Foods 139

Yang Type A Foods 157

Yang Type B Foods 174

Balancing Your Diet 190

Exercise according to Your Yin Yang Body Type 217

PART FOUR

Addressing Health Issues Based on Your Yin Yang Body Type

Healing with Sasang Medicine: An Introduction 248

Dealing with Stress 254

Reducing High Blood Pressure 263

Getting Rid of Headaches 274

Overcoming Common Colds 286

Getting Better Sleep 298

Maintaining a Healthy Digestive System 307

Shedding Those Extra Pounds 325

Joint Pain 346

Food and Airborne Allergies 360

Visual Challenges 381

Useful Resources 395

Index 398

Acknowledgments

Without the support of so many wonderful people, *Your Yin Yang Body Type* would never have come to fruition. Hour after hour of writing and contemplating would have been inconceivable without the support and patience of my wife, So Young. Perhaps this time could have been spent being a better husband and parent to our daughter, Angelica, who constantly asked Daddy when he would write *her* another book. Their deeply encompassing love surrounded me every step of the way.

My deep gratitude also extends to Karen Christensen, my editor, friend, and, in many ways, my teacher. Her ongoing encouragement, willingness to contribute, and special way with words brought with them a spark that added life to my book. It was this spark that made *Your Yin Yang Body Type* a playful, yet informative introduction to Sasang medicine. Karen's ongoing enthusiasm also enhanced my own appreciation of Sasang medicine and the task involved in writing this book. It was nothing short of a blessing to have worked with her.

A sincere appreciation also goes to my patients, whom I treasure as one would a family. With Sasang medicine as our vehicle, we have witnessed together time and time again the body's ability to heal from within. Not a day goes by in the clinic without my being reminded of how deep our mutually enhancing relationship runs.

I would have never traveled this path in life if it weren't for Lee Je-ma and his profound understanding of Asian philosophy and medicine. As the originator of Sasang medicine, he contributed greatly to the start of a new era of self-empowering medicine. I extend this gratitude to Dr. Kim Man San (Kwan Jung Sonseng Nim) and my mentor No Kyung Mun for capturing the essence of Lee Je-ma's teaching and devoting their lives to preserving and expanding his vision.

My dream of presenting Sasang medicine to the public in an easy-to-read and accessible way never would have come to fruition if it weren't for Inner Traditions publishing and Jon Graham, who first recognized its value. Thanks to the help of Jeanie Levitan (editor in chief), Meghan MacLean (project editor), and other skilled and detail-oriented staff members at Inner Traditions, my book gradually morphed into its present form.

Finally, I would like to thank life itself, for giving me the opportunity to follow my dreams.

Introduction

To stay healthy is no simple task, let alone trying to find our way through the labyrinth of countless new medical discoveries. Conflicting solutions regarding this or that remedy are ubiquitous in the media. Unwanted side effects often outweigh the therapeutic benefits of most pharmaceuticals, and even if they are deemed safe and effective for some, there is no telling what will happen to others. Could there possibly be a way to know which foods, herbs, exercises, and supplements fit our own distinctive physical and emotional needs?

Deeply rooted in the ancient classics of Eastern medicine, the Sasang (Four Body Type) approach provides insight into the particular requirements of our individual body type, serving as a compass to navigate our way toward health and harmony. It takes the guesswork out of discerning where to turn when we are ill, offers us practical ways to maximize our mental and physical well-being, and could even help us figure out why a relationship may have turned sour. Sasang medicine has identified four major body types, based on the relative strength of each bodily organ. Physical and emotional health depends on the harmonious interaction between our stronger and weaker organs. Factors such as stress, trauma, anxiety, and anger disrupt this relationship in different ways, according to our body type. Discovering our own body type gives us the ability to make effective decisions regarding our health and well-being.

Among the first of its kind in Western history, *Your Yin Yang Body Type* reveals the secrets behind the ancient Korean art of Sasang medicine. This user-friendly book contains almost everything you need to know about your Yin Yang body type. It begins with a practical, easy-to-follow introduction to Sasang medicine, offering handy self-analytical tools for determining your body type. Individual sections cover body type–specific foods, herbs, and exercises. "Emotional Balance and Your Yin Yang Body Type" describes the different emotional tendencies of each body type, addressing the mind/body emphasis that is central to Sasang medicine.

My path toward Sasang medicine began at the young age of twelve, when an obsession with Asian culture and philosophy produced an incredible desire to visit Japan. Realizing that there was nothing she could do to sway me, my loving mother reluctantly searched for a way to get me there. Shortly thereafter, I found myself on a plane to Japan thanks to a kind offer from a distant cousin residing in Tokyo. A short visit quickly turned into eight years of living in Asia, where my calling as an Eastern medical doctor slowly began to unfold. While living in South Korea, I became the first foreign student to study Eastern medicine at Daejeon University.

When I was a child, my parents, out of concern for my frail constitution, were always trying to get me to eat more. They could not understand why I ate so little but still had adequate energy to play like other kids. I was such a picky eater that almost all my food wound up being thrown away. Dinnertime was never fun because my sister liked to raid my plate while I couldn't wait to leave the table! Nobody could understand why I was so finicky about food. Many years later, after discovering the Sasang medical approach, I finally realized that this was not a reflection of my mother's cooking; rather it was due to my body type.

According to Sasang medicine, each individual has either a Yin or a Yang body type. My body type, referred to as Yin Type B, is born with a weaker spleen but stronger kidneys. The kidneys, in Sasang medicine, are a major source of energy. They store energy and release it when food sources are insufficient. The spleen is in charge of the digestive system. Thus, a weaker spleen results in a propensity toward digestive issues. As a young child, despite my inability to digest foods well, it was possible for me to tap into the reserve energy of my kidneys. Yet it was only a matter of time until my inability to digest food efficiently started to catch up with me.

"A spleen or not a spleen?" That is the question.

Although the word *bi* (脾) translates as *"spleen"* in most English dictionaries, its function as a digestive organ in Eastern medicine more closely resembles the pancreas. Since Eastern medicine emphasizes the metaphysical rather than physical function of each organ, a direct correlation with Western counterparts is difficult to make. While it is beneficial to keep this difference in mind, I will refer to the formal translation of *bi* as *"spleen"* throughout this book.

While I was attending Eastern medical school, my appetite continued to diminish and my heart constantly pounded strongly in my chest, as if to say, "Where's my food?" I remember consuming various herbs in order to enhance my appetite and calm my heartbeat. Each formula seemed to interfere with my digestive system, only making matters worse. Sure, these herbs were helpful for my digestive system, at least in theory, but they did not seem to match my body and digestive system.

It wasn't until a fateful meeting with Dr. Yun-Kyoung Yim, a visiting professor from Korea, that my interest in Sasang medicine began to flourish. After a discussion about my ongoing health issues, she prescribed for me an herbal formula specifically for my body type. I was quite skeptical, since not a single herb in the formula was indicated for my symptoms. After the first dose, however, my palpitations disappeared, my appetite increased, and I felt an overall sense of balance and well-being. She explained that this herbal formula was focused on balancing and supporting my body, instead of simply eliminating my symptoms. She also pointed out that my symptoms were a mere reflection of innately weak aspects of my body type. This demonstrates a central principle of the Sasang medical system, which promotes and engages the body's natural capacity to overcome illness, pain, and suffering. Simply prescribing herbs for my lack of appetite and palpitations in this case would have been like placing a Band-Aid on a deep wound without letting it heal from the inside out.

Discovering my body type brought me a tremendous sense of relief. For so many years, it had been difficult for my family and me to understand why I felt so insecure around others, why I always wanted to be alone, and why I had such a meager appetite! Close to thirty years later, I finally realized that these were traits associated with my body type. Discovering my body type and connecting with the experiences of other Yin Type B's helped reveal to me that I am not an alien after all! It brought a lot of comfort knowing that I am not alone and that others with the same body type often share similar issues. Over the years Sasang medicine has provided my patients and me with practical tools to overcome our physical and emotional deficiencies and enhance our health. Rather than keeping this information to myself and merely using it with my patients, I feel compelled to share the wisdom and benefits of Sasang medicine with you.

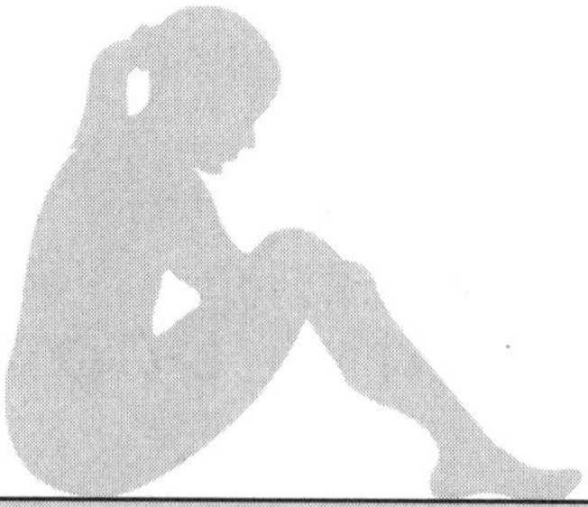

PART ONE

Understanding the Yin Yang Body Types

Sasang Medicine and the Yin Yang Body Types

Have you ever wondered why someone you've known could drink beer like water without getting a hangover? Or how about someone else who blithely chain-smoked into his nineties? Simply thinking that these people were just healthier than you and I would not suffice. Excessive consumption of alcohol eventually leads to cirrhosis of the liver, while chain-smoking is a sure path to emphysema and lung cancer. To avoid these conditions while smoking or drinking excessively throughout one's life may seem almost superhuman. Even though some of us are born healthier than others, genetics alone does not account for these exceptions. According to Sasang medicine, each of us is born with a stronger and a weaker organ, depending on our body type. The state of health of someone who is born with weaker lungs will usually be compromised even after the first cigarette. The person born with a weaker liver often becomes ill even after her first experience with alcohol. However, smoking and drinking may not necessarily adversely affect the health of a person who is born with stronger lungs or or a stronger liver.

WHAT IS SASANG MEDICINE?

The Sasang medical system is based on the theory that each of us is born with particular emotional and physical strengths and weaknesses, depending on our body type. These tendencies have a direct influence on how our minds and bodies react to stress and illness.

Comparing Apples to Apples

Even though Chinese medicine is the most commonly practiced form of Eastern medicine in the world today, other East Asian countries, such as Korea, have established their own traditional medicines. At their core most of these systems share the same basic principle of balancing Yin and Yang and promoting a harmonious flow of energy throughout the body. Yet each approach emphasizes different aspects of Eastern medicine. The Sasang medical system, which was developed in Korea, emphasizes the influence of our emotional and physical strengths and weaknesses on our surroundings. The Chinese medical system focuses on the influence of our surroundings on our health and well-being. When illness strikes, Sasang medical treatment is based primarily on balancing the mind and body, whereas Chinese medicine focuses on chasing away and eliminating the pathogen itself. Despite a difference in emphasis, Chinese and Sasang medicines both take into account the influence of illness, as well as the constitutional needs of the individual.

The Korean word *Sasang* means "Four Types" in English. It signifies the classification of all people into four major body types. This medical system was first established by a Korean doctor named Lee Je-ma (1837–1900), who was well versed in the Eastern medical tradition, a system that focuses on the balance of Yin and Yang energies to treat emotional and/or physical illness. He was puzzled by the fact that certain patients who suffered from the same symptoms improved quickly, while others suffered longer, despite medical treatment. Lee Je-ma developed Sasang medicine based on his ability to address these differences while emphasizing the distinctive constitutional structure of each patient. In a nutshell Sasang medicine is a branch of Eastern medicine that focuses treatment on the individual and our unique differences, rather than the disease.

After getting to know the Sasang approach, you'll be able to:

- Make wiser choices about which foods to eat to promote your health.
- Avoid guessing whether or not this or that supplement works for your body type.
- Choose the right form of exercise and herbs for your constitution type.
- Avoid emotional traps and strengthen your inner self.
- Recognize your innate strengths and weaknesses.

Your Yin Yang Body Type is a book that helps familiarize you with your body type's physical and emotional inclinations. It can serve as a compass to help you achieve optimum health through body type–specific diet, supplements, herbs, exercise, and other beneficial habits. Before jumping into the juicy stuff, however, we'll introduce a few basic concepts. The next section will then provide you with all the information you need to discover your body type and take advantage of everything that Sasang medicine has to offer.

Now that we are ready to proceed, allow me to congratulate you on your journey toward self-discovery and optimum health!

GETTING STARTED

One powerful lesson I have learned during the twelve years of my practice of Eastern medicine is that illness itself does not determine the outcome of treatment. Some patients request treatment for seemingly minor issues that take a substantial amount of time to overcome, while others recover quickly from acute situations. Most of us would be inclined to think that a minor illness, such as a recently occurring muscle ache, would take less time to recover from than a severely injured back, but this simply isn't the case.

From the Clinic

Rebecca is a thirty-four-year-old woman who seems to have it all together, except for one thing. She just can't seem to get over the immense tightness in her neck and shoulders. In great despair she decided to get an MRI before coming to see me. As in many cases involving neck and shoulder tightness, her MRI results did not reveal anything significant. Rebecca is a Yin type who is constantly under a fair amount of stress at work. At the end of the day, like clockwork, her shoulders would tighten up again. Yin types generally have difficulty expressing their emotions. They come across as calm and centered, even if stress is eating away at them. Yang types, on the other hand, cannot hide how they feel. Stress is written all over the face of a stressed-out Yang type. Apparently, Rebecca did not share her feelings about work with anyone, assuming that they wouldn't want to listen—another Yin trait. After discovering her body type during our first session together, Rebecca decided to reflect on her way of thinking and take the steps necessary to release her stress. The discovery of her body type helped her navigate the road to recovery and quickly overcome the tightness in her neck and shoulders. As we will soon discover, our body type plays a significant role in both the onset and the resolution of illness.

If the extent of illness itself does not play a major role in treatment outcome, then what does? There are several other factors beyond the extent of illness that influence our ability to recover. How do you feel about the illness? Is it controlling your every thought? Are you open to trying an alternative approach? Do you take the doctor's word when he gives you a negative prognosis? Do you feel it is possible to overcome this illness, or do you let your mind get in the way of healing? How our mind and body perceive a particular health situation dictates how quickly and how well we will recover from it. Our state of health is not determined by the condition itself. How we react to illness depends on several factors, including our overall outlook on life as well as our innate strengths and weaknesses. A common cold, for example, could take forever to overcome if we are constantly faced with family or work stress. We may also have trouble recovering from colds if we are born with weaker lungs. In either case how our body reacts to illness determines to what extent it affects us.

Symptom ≠ Outcome
Reaction to Symptom = Outcome

WHY SASANG MEDICINE?

At one time almost all medical traditions focused on remedies that support the individual, not just the elimination of a particular disease. By contrast modern medicine has lost its focus on the person; instead, it places emphasis on the illness itself. It is common, even among certain practitioners of Eastern medicine, to get caught up in the endless search for this or that "cure" for a particular illness. Choosing a remedy based on its symptomatic indications has become an intrinsic part of how we approach treatment. I am often asked, "Hey, doc, what do you have for this . . . ?" A remedy that focuses on the illness rather than the person may work for some but could make matters worse for others.

Sasang is not a one-size-fits-all approach. It focuses on supporting and improving health based on each individual's inborn qualities. Some of these qualities naturally contribute to our physical and emotional well-being. Other tendencies have to be modified in order for us to be physically and emotionally well balanced. This set of qualities plays a major role in our day-to-day lives and has a direct effect on how we react to the world around us. Sasang medicine is based on the discovery and balance of these traits through herbal treatment, diet, exercise, and counseling. Our physical and emotional health can be significantly enhanced by eating, exercising, and living according to the particular needs of our minds and bodies.

Overcoming issues such as weight gain or chronic fatigue can be both challenging and frustrating. No matter how much we try, it may seem impossible to shed those extra pounds or gain more energy. Numerous "experts" offer their "solution" to these problems by promoting a special technique or diet plan. It is common for such approaches to work for some but not for others. Advertisements are filled with success stories that motivate us to try this or that approach. Even those who are medically trained seem to bounce from remedy to remedy, based on the latest research. It is easy to get lost in the abundance of research and success claims. We may get excited when scientists suddenly proclaim that coffee or chocolate is high in antioxidants and therefore great for overall health. Before accepting these claims, we need to ask ourselves a number of questions: *Who* may benefit from eating chocolate or coffee? *When* could they benefit from it? And *how* do they benefit from it? Without an understanding of how coffee or chocolate affects our bodies, we could actually be doing ourselves more harm than good. Sasang medicine offers insight into these questions by familiarizing us with our body type. It serves as a compass to help us navigate through current research and make informed decisions based on the needs of our body type.

As mentioned above there are four Sasang body types, each of which is associated with either Yin or Yang. The theory of Yin and Yang forms the basis of Eastern medicine and philosophy. Before delving into the distinctive characteristics of the four body types, let's take a closer look at the theory of Yin and Yang.

YIN AND YANG THEORY

Yin and Yang are opposing forces, or components, into which all existence and natural phenomena can be broken down. If there is day, for example, there will always be night. If there is up, there will always be down. If there is birth, there will always be death. However, Yin and Yang are not always in a state of balance. There is a tendency for one to overshadow the other. Most of us, for example, would choose to avoid death and live forever. This is an example of how Yang (life, in this case) always desires to sustain life and avert death (Yin). It is also difficult to get up and rush out of the house after a deep sleep: Sudden movement (Yang) is difficult to initiate after a deep sleep (Yin). These examples illustrate that Yin and Yang always like to maintain their own momentum. Yin and Yang also reflect the different parts of the human body. The upper body is considered Yang and the lower body Yin. Each organ in the body can also be considered Yin or Yang: The lungs and spleen, situated in the upper body, are considered Yang, and the liver and kidneys, in the lower body, are considered Yin. The goal of Sasang medicine is to enhance health by balancing Yin and Yang within the body.

So what exactly are Yin and Yang? Actually, Yin and Yang have no meaning in and of themselves. Only when they are used in context can we decipher their meaning. If we say the moon is Yin, then we are only comparing it to things that are more Yang, like the sun. If we say the sun is Yang, we are referring to the fact that it is relatively more Yang than the moon. However, our sun may actually be more Yin compared to the central star of a different galaxy. Hence at its core Asian philosophy is based on the theory of relativity and the symbolic relationship between Yin and Yang. Table 1.1 shows a few things that Yin and Yang represent.

TABLE 1.1. YIN YANG NATURAL PHENOMENA

Yin	Yang
Moon	Sun
Dark	Light
Night	Day
Cold	Hot
Down	Up
Moist	Dry
Back	Front
Slow	Fast

THE YIN AND YANG BODY TYPES

Similar to Sasang medicine, numerous other popular theories focus on four major body types, such as the blood type diet (O, A, AB, B) and Dr. Elliot Abravanel's body type diet. Sasang medicine separates the body types into four categories based on Yin and Yang. This book would be only a few pages long if the difference between Yin and Yang were simply black and white! The picture becomes more clouded when we talk about the relative differences of Yin and Yang. Yin may also be mixed with Yang, just as Yang may be mixed with Yin. The Yin and Yang body types of Sasang medicine all have differing degrees of Yin and Yang. The two Yang types share more Yang traits, while the two Yin types share more Yin traits. However, the Yin types always have certain Yang traits, while the Yang types always have Yin traits. This makes it challenging at times to conclude which body type you are. By now you may be asking yourself, what exactly are Yin and Yang traits? Table 1.2 examines different Yin and Yang traits.

TABLE 1.2. YIN YANG TRAITS

Yin	Yang
Complacent	Active
Gets Cold More Easily	Gets Hot More Easily
Stronger Lower Body	Stronger Upper Body
Relaxed	Tense
Night Owl	Morning Person
Slow Metabolism	Fast Metabolism
Slow Motion	Quick Motion
Follower	Leader

WHAT DETERMINES OUR BODY TYPE?

Yang types are born with more Yang, while Yin types are born with more Yin. The lungs and spleen of Yang types are stronger than those of the Yin types, while the liver and kidneys of Yin types are stronger than those of Yang types. In Sasang medicine there are two Yang body types (Yang Type A and Yang Type B) and two Yin body types (Yin Type A and Yin Type B). The Yang Type A, for example, is born with a stronger spleen and weaker kidneys. The Yang Type B is born with stronger lungs and a weaker liver. The Yin Type A is born with a stronger liver and weaker lungs. Finally, the Yin Type B is born with stronger kidneys and a weaker spleen. The relative strengths and weaknesses of the lungs, spleen, liver, and kidneys determine our body type and also play a major role in our emotional and physical health. See Table 1.3 for a look at how this works.

TABLE 1.3. BODY TYPE AND ORGAN STRENGTH

Body Type	**Strongest Organ**	**Weakest Organ**
Yin Type A	Liver	Lungs
Yin Type B	Kidney	Spleen
Yang Type A	Spleen	Kidneys
Yang Type B	Lungs	Liver

THE FOUR PREDOMINANT TEMPERAMENTS

Modern science is becoming exceedingly close to unraveling the mystery behind DNA, shedding light on how genetic structure plays a significant role in how we act.* Certain common psychological disorders, such as depression and anxiety, for instance, appear to be associated with preexisting markers embedded within strands of our DNA. We do not have

*For more on this see Saudino, Kimberly J., "Behavioral Genetics and Child Temperament" *Journal of Developmental and Behavioral Pediatriacs* 26, no. 3 (Jun 2005): 214–23.

to be scientists to acknowledge that some infants scream bloody murder while others sleep away the day without uttering a sound. I remember that, as a baby, my daughter used to pretend she was having convulsions, only to laugh hysterically as soon as we rushed to her side. Shortly after we stopped rushing madly to her side, the "convulsions" stopped. Where could my daughter have learned such off-the-cuff behavior? The only conceivable answer is that she was born with an innately warped sense of humor, which, as her mom would say, closely resembles her dad's. Yikes! From a psychological perspective, these characteristics would be considered a reflection of my daughter's temperament, a set of inborn personality traits that contribute to her everyday emotional behavior.

TABLE 1.4. WHAT'S IN A NAME?*

Body Type (in English)	Korean Name	Translation	Pronunciation Key
Yang Type A	*So Yang*	Lesser Yang	*So* is pronounced like the English word *so* and the first half of the word *Yang* is pronounced much like *Yacht*
Yang Type B	*Tei Yang*	Greater Yang	*Tei* is pronounced *day* and the first half of the word *Yang* is pronounced much like *Yacht*
Yin Type A	*Tei Eum*	Greater Eum	*Tei* is pronounced *day* and *Eum* rhymes with the word *loom*
Yin Type B	*So Eum*	Lesser Eum	*So* is pronounced like the English word *so* and *Eum* rhymes with the word *loom*

*The name of each body type was modified to help English-speaking readers grasp them more easily. This table expresses the actual Korean name of each type.

History has provided us with a variety of temperament theories, ranging from the ancient Greek idea of four humors to the more recent psychoanalytical theories of Carl Jung. Sasang medicine is based on the theory that each body type is born with one of four predominant temperaments (sorrow, anger, satisfaction, or complacency), which plays a major role in how we think and act in everyday life. Every body type has its own predominant temperament, which may manifest in a balanced or unbalanced way. As a predominant emotion, sadness may lead us to feeling sorry for or showing compassion to others around us. On the contrary it may sink us into the depths of depression and isolation. Many of us are not aware of our predominant temperament lying dormant within the subconscious mind waiting for an opportunity to manifest. The loss of a friend or a relationship gone sour, for instance, may trigger extreme depression in people with sorrow as their predominant temperament.

In Sasang medicine each temperament correlates with and determines the strength of each of the four major organs (lungs, spleen, liver, and kidneys), which, in turn, play an essential role in who we are, our general health, and how we behave. Table 1.5 below illustrates how each body type is derived from the strength of its predominant temperament. Sorrow, the predominant temperament of the Yang Type B, leads to stronger lungs. Anger, the predominant temperament of the Yang Type A, gives rise to a stronger spleen. Complacency, the predominant temperament of the Yin Type A, yields a stronger liver. Finally, satisfaction, the predominant temperament of the Yin Type B, leads to stronger kidneys.

No temperament, in itself, can be classified as being inherently good or bad. Each of the four predominant temperaments can either diminish

TABLE 1.5. OUR TEMPERAMENT DETERMINES OUR STRONGEST ORGAN

Sasang Body Type	Predominant Temperament	Strongest Organ
Yin Type A	Complacency	Liver
Yin Type B	Satisfaction	Kidneys
Yang Type A	Anger	Spleen
Yang Type B	Sorrow	Lungs

or enhance our overall well-being, depending on how it is expressed. Sadness, for example, is not necessarily perceived as a negative emotion, while joy is not an unconditionally positive emotion. Sadness may allow us to slow down, reflect, and think deeply about our life. The emotion of joy gives the body a beneficial jolt while it speeds up the heart rate and circulation. Slowing down to a halt or speeding up excessively can cause serious health issues. We all need to slow down at times, just as we sometimes need a lift.

Predominant temperaments become unbalanced through explosive and uncontrolled responses to one's circumstances. The unbalanced temperament injures its corresponding organ, leading to malfunction and disease. The balanced temperament "feeds" energy to, strengthens, and increases the size of its corresponding organ while it is developing inside the womb. Sadness has the potential of strengthening or injuring its corresponding organ, the lungs. Thus an underlying sense of sadness may be a motivating factor in interacting with others to avoid loneliness. Sadness, in this sense, supports the function of the lungs. Depression, by contrast, will stagnate and congest the energy of the lungs.

TABLE 1.6. THE EFFECT OF THE PREDOMINANT TEMPERAMENT

Body Type	Predominant Temperament	Balanced Temperament Leads to . . .	Unbalanced Temperament Leads to . . .
Yin Type A	Complacency	Calm, relaxed nature	Laziness, addictive behavior, isolation
Yin Type B	Satisfaction	Accomplishment, joy	Compulsive behavior, anxiety, jealousy
Yang Type A	Anger	Standing up for oneself and others	Rage
Yang Type B	Sorrow	Compassion	Severe depression

Complacency and Yin Type A

Complacency is an emotion that is associated with the liver, the Yin Type A's strongest organ. A strong liver contributes to a complacent and relaxed nature. However, when this temperament is taken to the extreme, Yin Type A's may become couch potatoes, never wanting to do anything. Relaxation and calmness feed the liver, assisting with the smooth flow of energy throughout the body. But if a Yin Type A becomes too complacent, the liver energy stagnates and causes health issues related to toxic accumulation within the body.

Satisfaction and Yin Type B

Yin Type B's are born with stronger kidneys, which are an abundant source of joy, satisfaction, and cheerfulness. The harmonious feeling of joy and sense of accomplishment are a reflection of strong kidneys. Yet, getting too excited or attached to the feeling of joy or accomplishment eventually stagnates the energy of the kidneys. Happiness for Yin Type B's comes from accomplishing their goals. While this may seem like a lofty trait, it can lead to obsession if the goal itself is unrealistic or impossible to achieve.

Anger and Yang Type A

Yang Type A's are born with a tendency to feel anger because it is released from their strongest organ, the spleen. Anger may be necessary to initiate positive change, in which case it helps to strengthen the spleen. Excessive anger causes heat to build up inside the spleen of Yang Type A's, causing indigestion, anxiety, dizziness, stomach ulcers, and the like. A strong sense of anger, if channeled in the right direction, can lead to the profound ability among Yang Type A's to stand up and fight for what they and others around them believe in.

Sorrow and Yang Type B

The stronger lungs of the Yang Type B contribute to a powerful and constant sense of sadness. When sadness gets out of control, the lungs sustain injury. Since sadness is such a strong emotion for Yang Type

B's, even the slightest blow can plunge them into the depths of depression. On the other hand, the lungs will stay healthy and strong if sadness leads them to reflection and helping others in need.

Can I Be an Angry Yin Type B?

Even though anger is the predominant temperament of the Yang Type A, it can manifest in each of the other body types as well. The other three temperaments (sadness, complacency, and joy/satisfaction) are often felt no matter which body type we are. Yet even momentary anger has a direct effect on the overall health of the Yang Type A because it cuts so deeply. Since anger is a Yang-based emotion, the Yin types simply don't have enough Yang energy for it to seriously affect them. Yin Type B's actually have difficulty expressing their anger for this reason, so an occasional angry spell may help get their blood flowing. The same concept holds true for the other temperaments and their differentiating levels of influence according to the body type.

THE FOUR PREDOMINANT SENSES

In Sasang medicine the four predominant senses (hearing, sight, smell, and taste) also correspond to the four major organs. Hence, each body type also has a relatively stronger and weaker sense. The senses are more than mere sensations that we register from moment to moment. They are a portal through which we perceive and interact with our environment. Communicating directly and instantaneously with our brain, they conjure up emotions that may or may not be consciously apparent. The smell of chlorine may bring back childhood memories of summertime spent by a pool, while the sight of blood may prompt immense fear or nausea with no apparent source. Each body type uses a predominant sense to absorb and gather information from their surroundings. Table 1.7 spotlights each of the body types and their predominant sense.

TABLE 1.7. PREDOMINANT SENSE AND YOUR BODY TYPE

Body Type	Predominant Sense
Yin Type A	Smell
Yin Type B	Taste
Yang Type A	Vision
Yang Type B	Hearing

Let's take a closer look at each of the four senses and how they affect our health.

Smell and Yin Type A

Yin Type A's smell their way through the world. They can "smell" trouble when it comes their way. My Yin Type A mother, for example, would always hold her nose while passing by the bathroom hours after any of us had used it! Yin Type A's are often acutely sensitive to fragrances and pollutants in the air, developing allergies as a result. They can also get to know others simply by smelling them. The Yin Type A's strongest organ, the liver, brings with it an acute sense of smell.

Taste and Yin Type B

Our sense of taste corresponds to the kidneys. Born with stronger kidneys, Yin Type B's have an exquisite sense of taste, a sense that goes beyond the taste of food. It allows them to "taste" the difference between selfishness and kindness in others. They actually relate to the world around them through the sense of taste. With such sensitive taste buds, they tend to be very picky when it comes to food and can often list the ingredients of a particular recipe simply by placing a bite of the dish in their mouth!

Vision and Yang Type A

Yang Type A's have the ability to see through the clutter and cut right to the point. They can quickly find their target, like an eagle spotting its prey from afar. They can see right through a person at first glance. Sharp vision may give voice to a sharp tongue; they may say, "You look heavier today" to a friend who recently gained weight, or "You look like crap" to someone who woke up on the wrong side of the bed. Acute vision depends on the health of the spleen, the Yang Type A's strongest organ.

Cravings: The Good and the Bad

An old saying in Eastern medicine states, "When the body and mind are in balance, our senses crave more balance. If they are not balanced, they crave imbalance." Have you ever felt the urge to indulge in sugary foods, watch gory movies, catch the scent of deep-fried fast food, or listen to ear-shattering music? These are examples of craving imbalance when our organ energies and senses have trouble finding balance. Sure, some of us may enjoy a gory movie once in a while to distance ourselves from the stresses of daily life, or a juicy hamburger to satiate an occasional desire. This type of craving may also occur directly before a monthly cycle, after getting to sleep late, following a spat with a partner, or in other situations that make us feel vulnerable. If these cravings occur consistently, however, they may be a reflection of a deeper imbalance related to our temperament or organ health. Unbalanced cravings may also lead to weight gain and indigestion. For more information about these topics, refer to "Shedding Those Extra Pounds" (pages 325–45) and "Maintaining a Healthy Digestive System" (pages 307–24).

A craving for pleasant and harmonious sounds, tastes, smells, and sights, by contrast, is a reflection of organ balance and harmony. The natural desire to eat healthy foods or watch an uplifting movie are signs that our organ energies, at least for the most part, are flowing smoothly throughout the body. Even if such feelings do not come naturally, our health depends on making a conscious decision to eat foods, view the world, smell fragrances, and listen to and hear sounds that are beneficial to our well-being. Eating and exercising right for your body type are essential components in converting unbalanced cravings to balanced cravings.

Hearing and Yang Type B

The Yang Type B is said to possess the ability to hear the "sound of the heavens" or the "movement of the Earth rotating around its axis." While I have yet to meet a Yang Type B who has actually heard the sound of the Earth moving, the unique auditory ability of this body type cannot be overestimated. I remember a Yang Type B friend of mine who once yelled, "Are you talking about me?!?" after somehow hearing me whisper in another room with the door closed. Yang Type B's surprise others with their ability to seemingly hear through walls! Not only do those with this body type hear sounds easily; they can also hear "voices" inside their head. These voices may offer guidance by unraveling the mysteries of life or simply drive them crazy. My Yang Type B friend also seemed to have a sixth sense about things, but would often seem a bit distracted and confused. Perhaps, there was too much going on all at once inside his head! The sense of hearing among Yang Type B's corresponds to the lungs, their strongest organ.

WHY ONLY FOUR BODY TYPES?

With over 7 billion people living on our planet, why are there only four body types? To answer this question, let's take a further look at the most basic of Eastern concepts—the theory of Yin and Yang. All things in nature consist of a certain amount of Yin and a certain amount of Yang. This can be compared to an atom, having both positive (Yang) protons and negative (Yin) electrons that energetically oppose one another. There are many different combinations of protons and electrons giving rise to many different types of elements. Hydrogen, for example, only has one electron, while lithium has three electrons in its outer shell. What makes all these elements different is simply a unique combination of the same stuff: electrons and protons. Yin and Yang can also be broken down into many different combinations. Men, for example, are said to be more Yang than women. However, there are certain men who are more feminine than some women. Hence, Yang may have strong Yin attributes while Yin may have strong Yang attributes, giving rise to infinite variations. Despite all the potential combinations, we are left with only two building blocks, Yin and Yang.

In Sasang medicine each body type is also differentiated according to Yin Yang theory. Some Yin types are relatively more Yin, while others tend to be more Yang. Sure, it's possible to have an infinite number of Yin and Yang body types, but this would only cause more confusion. The goal of Sasang medicine is to determine as quickly and efficiently as possible the overall tendencies of Yin and Yang according to the individual. Once this is determined, it is much easier to develop a treatment plan. A compass, for example, may reveal an infinite number of positions, depending on the direction we take. However, no matter which direction we face, the four basic directions (north, south, east, and west) are always used as reference points.

STRONGER VERSUS WEAKER ORGANS

In Sasang medicine the stronger organs send blood and energy to the weaker organs and throughout the body. Each body type has its own source of blood and energy flow. The stronger spleen of the Yang Type A helps circulate blood and energy to the weaker kidneys. The stronger lungs of the Yang Type B circulates blood and energy to the weaker liver. The stronger liver of the Yin Type A sends blood and energy to the weaker lungs. Finally, the kidneys of the Yin Type B send energy and blood upward to the weaker spleen. Health is determined by the ability of the stronger organs to circulate ample energy and blood to the weaker organs.

Strength is not necessarily equated with balance. Our stronger organs may overreact and take advantage of our weaker organs. To illustrate let's consider the role of a king who has tremendous power but also must be responsible for the welfare of his kingdom. If he becomes selfish, the common people will suffer. If he is generous, the kingdom will prosper. Like a king, the stronger organs enjoy extreme power, which, if not shared, leads to a deficiency in the weaker organs. As we saw above, sorrow corresponds to the lungs. Yang Type B's depend on their stronger lungs to circulate blood and energy to the liver and other organs. Too much sorrow will cause the lungs to hoard energy and blood, hindering circulation to the liver. Anger affects the spleen. Too much anger will cause the spleen to hoard the body's energy and obstruct its circulation to the kidneys.

Complacency corresponds to the liver. Too much complacency leads to laziness, causing the liver to hoard the body's energy and hinder its circulation to the lungs. Satisfaction and joy correspond to the kidneys. Taken to the extreme, joy can lead to anxiety, causing the kidneys to hoard the body's energy and delay its circulation to the spleen.

While stronger organs give rise to stronger corresponding energies and emotions, weaker organs result in relatively weaker or undeveloped corresponding energies and emotions. It is important for us to get in touch with and cultivate the energies and emotions of our weaker organs. In order to illustrate this point, let's take a closer look at the weaker liver of Yang Type B's. As noted above the liver corresponds to the temperament of complacency. It also assists in the digestive process by breaking down fat and protein. With so much Yang energy, Yang Type B's have a tendency to push themselves too far and forget to relax. They also tend to develop indigestion after eating fatty or high-protein foods. However, after recognizing such tendencies, they might make a strong effort to relax, become more complacent, and reduce their protein intake, resulting in a healthier liver.

NATURE VERSUS NURTURE

To what extent do our inherently stronger and weaker qualities determine how we react to the world around us? While some may argue that behavior is primarily determined by our genetic structure, others may claim that it is shaped through experience. According to Sasang medicine, both factors play an equally influential role. Accordingly, the four predominant temperaments are viewed as inclinations rather than predictors of how we will behave. When a dark cloud covers the sky, we may be inclined to predict rain. Yet who is to say that the sun won't eventually shine through without the advent of rain? Most of us, regardless of whether or not we know our body type, modify different behaviors based on their effects. Let's take a Yang Type B named Jack, for example, who used to get so angry at his wife over the smallest things. After several years of marriage, his wife simply packed her bags and left him. Alone and in despair, he decided to change his ways and humbly asked her for forgiveness and promised never to get so angry again. After reflecting on and modifying his behavior, not only did he save his marriage, but he also prevented the onset of illness due to an unbalanced spleen, which is the source of anger.

Health primarily depends on whether or not energy can flow smoothly from our strongest organ to our weakest organ. We enhance this flow by making decisions that promote our emotional and physical well-being. Making a sincere effort to stay calm in the face of stress, for example, can help improve the energetic flow to our weaker organ. By contrast the inability to deal with stress causes a blockage of energy around our stronger organ, leaving the weaker organ to fend for itself.

From the Clinic

Amy is a twenty-three-year-old Yang Type A who had suffered from chronic migraine headaches since her early teens. She repeatedly talked about her headaches as if they were the enemy, displaying immense anger in her voice. It turned out that Amy's approach to just about everything seemed to be through the lens of anger. Yang Type A's are prone to anger, and anger tends to interfere with the flow of energy from the Yang Type A's stronger spleen to the weaker kidneys. Anger was eating away at Amy's weaker kidney energy. In treating her headaches, we discussed the need to release anger and replace it with joy, the emotion of the kidneys. I also prescribed a Yang Type A formula that focused on promoting the flow of energy from her stronger spleen to her weaker kidneys. After realizing that anger was causing energy to stagnate around her spleen and taking the steps needed to bring joy back into her life, Amy's headaches quickly disappeared. Since anger is an innate response for Amy, she continues to make an effort to find joy and live in the moment, a challenge for the Yang types. I reminded Amy that on one level or another, she will always need to work on her tendency toward anger. But, in doing so, she will continue to grow and enhance her overall well-being.

How Many of Us Are Out There?

Yin Type A's comprise about 70 percent of the total human population. Why so many Yin Type A's? Because Yin Type A's are born with a stronger liver. The liver, according to Sasang medicine, is in charge of our reproductive health. A stronger liver enhances the chances of fertility. The weaker liver of Yang Type B's results in a weaker reproductive system. Not surprisingly, only 2 percent of the total population is Yang Type B. Yin Type B's comprise about 11 percent and Yang Type A's, 17 percent.

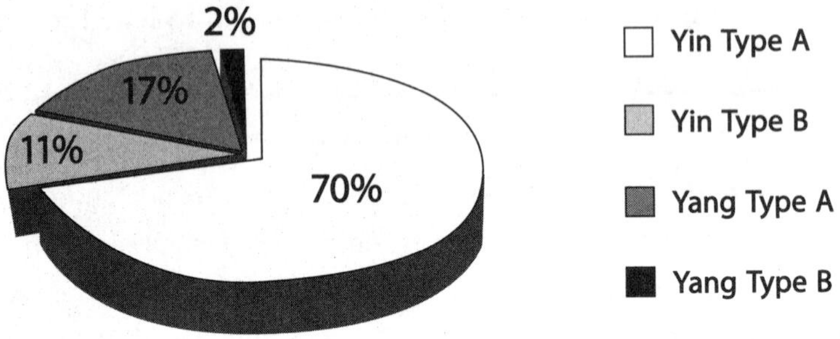

Figure 1.1. Body type population breakdown

While appropriate decision making plays a major role, it is not the only factor involved in staying healthy. Some people need to work harder to keep themselves healthy, while others seem to be healthy no matter what they do. The inherent strengths and weaknesses of our organs play a key role in overall health. The weakest organ for one person may actually be stronger than the strongest organ of another. Some of us are naturally healthier from birth, while others always seem to be plagued with this or that health issue from childhood. No matter how strong our organs are from birth, however, they will eventually weaken if we do not make healthy choices. In order to achieve optimum health, it is critical for us to cultivate our weaker organ energy on one level or another throughout a lifetime.

The concept of *su gi shin* helps further illustrate the Sasang idea of behavior and genetics. This concept, which translates as "polishing one's heart," lies at the core of Confucian theory. It is the ability to reflect on our actions and modify our thinking and behavior when necessary. According to Confucius, the function of the heart is not limited to the circulation of blood; the heart is also our spiritual center and the source of decision making. Healthier decisions result in healthier organs. Hence, the four major organs (lungs, spleen, liver, and kidneys) all depend on the heart's decision-making ability. Reflecting on our actions and making wise decisions will, in turn, promote a healthy heart. The heart itself sits comfortably on its own throne, tucked away from the actions of the four major organs. Yet, as the center of our being, it plays a central role in our health. Thus, each of us has the infinite potential for improving our health by polishing the heart. An unwillingness to reflect on our actions, however, will injure even the strongest of our organs. If the Yang Type A's, for example, do not control their anger, it will eventually destroy their strong spleen, leaving them vulnerable to illness.

THE ENVIRONMENT AND YOU

The practice of self-reflection is definitely helpful in promoting good health, but it's extremely challenging because of the powerful influence of environmental factors. Waking up to the sun shining through our window can surely brighten up our morning. Yet, if a person cuts in front of us while we're waiting in line at the store, this is likely to conjure up a negative emotion. Despite the powerful influence of the environment, it is no match for a strong and sturdy heart. The more we cultivate and balance who we are on the inside, the less swayed we are by our circumstances. If we fail to spend time polishing and improving who we are, we tend to become too excited when things go well and too upset, angry, or anxious when they go wrong. Devoting more time to balancing our energies makes it easier to have an impact on our environment in a positive way. Happiness is as contagious as bitterness. The unspoken word of our inner thoughts dictates how others will feel when they're with us. We can literally transform our world by balancing the flow of energy from our stronger to our weaker organs.

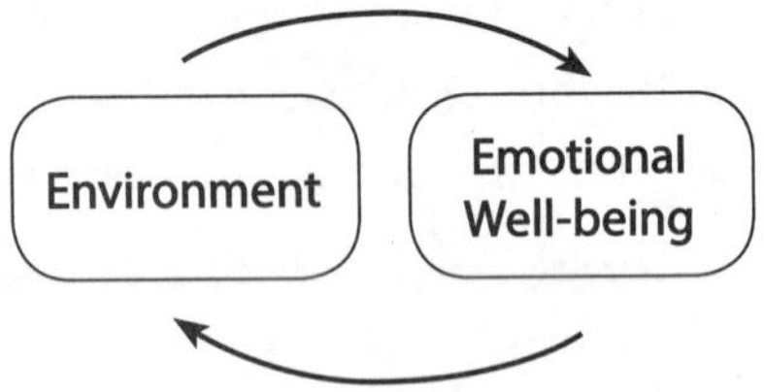

Figure 1.2. Connection between the environment and our emotional well-being

Everything we experience throughout the day is emotionally and physically processed in different ways, depending on several factors. The most basic of these factors is the influence of our body type's predominant temperament (i.e., complacency, satisfaction, anger, and sorrow). To achieve emotional and physical harmony, we need to balance these temperaments, rather than ridding ourselves of them entirely.

The second factor is memory. Everything we experience from moment to moment is interpreted through the memory of events that occurred in our past. Traumatic experiences often conjure up unpleasant emotions when similar experiences occur, while pleasant experiences tend to bring us joy whenever a similar situation arises. It is difficult, for example, to feel excited about going to the dentist, especially if our previous experience caused pain or discomfort. Yet, a fantastic experience while traveling to another country may spark similar emotions every time we are reminded of it.

The third factor, behavior modification, has to do with a combination of the first two—the external influence of the environment and the internal influence of our predominant temperament. By modifying our behavior, we can transform a seemingly negative experience into a positive one. The predominant desire of Yin Type B's for satisfaction, for example, may facilitate the belief that an otherwise dreadful trip to the dentist will improve their health or give them a chance to face their fears and give them a sense of accomplishment. The ability to cultivate and modify our behavior through experience not only makes life more pleasant, but it also improves the flow of energy from our stronger to our weaker organs, thus enhancing our overall health.

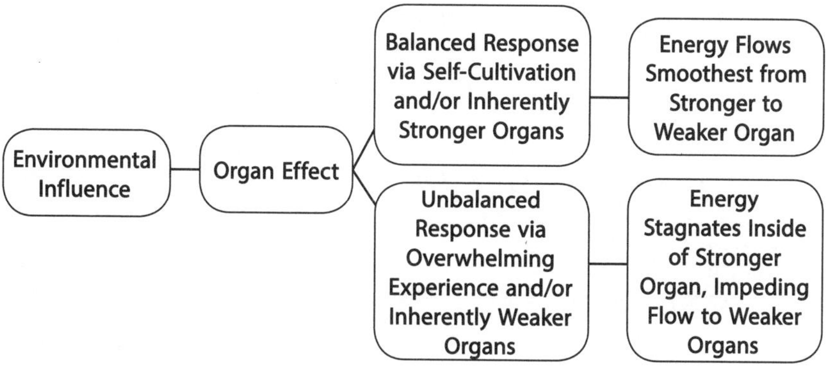

Figure 1.3. Environmental influences on our organs and emotions

A Balanced Response

Energy naturally flows from our stronger organs to our weaker ones, provided that our life is not filled with stress or trauma, which can undermine the health and well-being of even the most well-balanced individual. Yet, according to Sasang medicine, we all have the ability to face stress and trauma with unfaltering inner strength by discovering our body type and making a conscious effort to stay balanced. The strongest organ of each body type is the key player when it comes to how we respond to the environment. Negative experiences may actually enhance the flow from our stronger to our weaker organs if we respond in a balanced way. Positive experience, by contrast, may impede the flow of energy from our stronger to our weaker organs if we do not respond in a balanced way.

Figures 1.4 and 1.5 illustrate how internal balance or imbalance determines the effect of both positive and negative experiences on our health and well-being. While this concept can be applied to all body types, our response and its effect on our health vary according to which of our organs are the strongest. The Yin Type A's stronger liver will respond differently to both positive and negative experience, compared to the Yin Type B's stronger kidneys, while the Yang Type A's stronger spleen will respond differently than the Yang Type B's stronger lungs. For a closer look at what happens when our strongest organs are balanced, see tables 1.8–1.11.

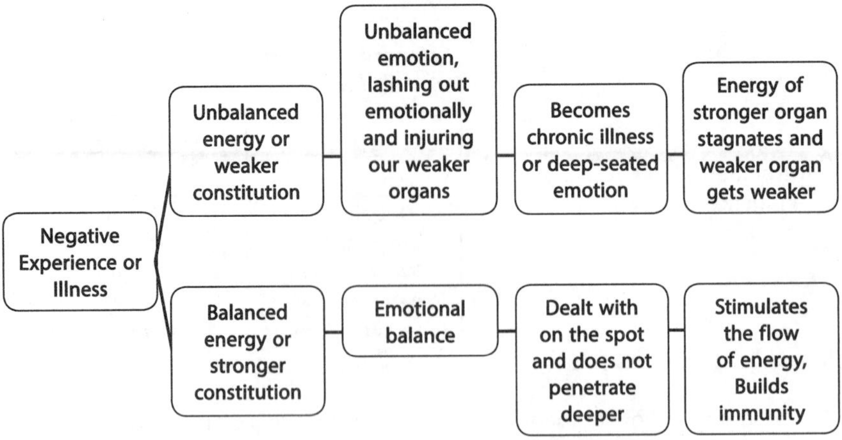

Figure 1.4. The effect of negative experience or illness

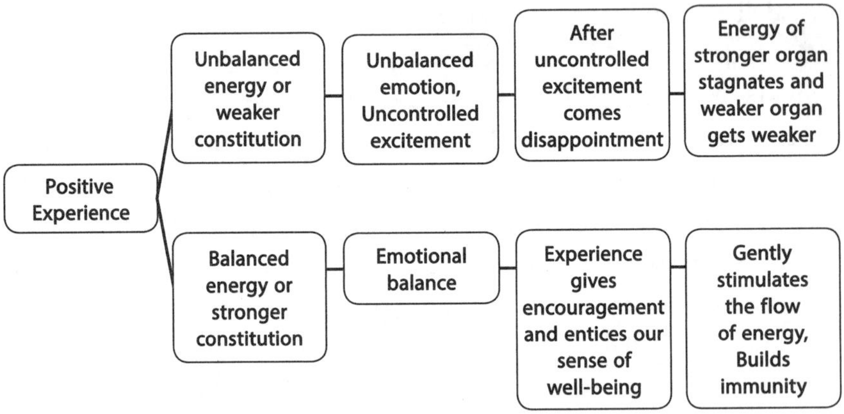

Figure 1.5. The effect of positive experience

TABLE 1.8.
YIN TYPE A—BALANCED LIVER

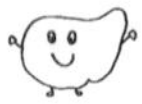

Psychological Effects	Physiological Effects
Helps us stay focused but not obsessed	Helps energy and blood flow to the lungs
Facilitates sleep and dreaming	Controls our sense of smell
Gives us the ability to get along with others and make joint decisions	Filters, absorbs, and eliminates toxins from the bloodstream

TABLE 1.9.
YIN TYPE B—BALANCED KIDNEYS

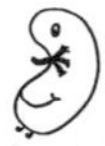

Psychological Effects	Physiological Effects
Help us derive wisdom from experience	Send energy upward from the lower body
Origin of willpower and courage	Control our sense of taste
Correspond to comfort and satisfaction	Regulate water metabolism

TABLE 1.10.
YANG TYPE A—BALANCED SPLEEN

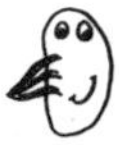

Psychological Effects	Physiological Effects
Controls our ability to understand and relate to others	Controls the digestive system
Tempers anger and hastiness	Sends energy to the kidneys, which, in turn, sends it to the legs
Helps us stay calm and relaxed	Sends energy to the kidneys, which, in turn, sends it to the bones

TABLE 1.11.
YANG TYPE B—BALANCED LUNGS

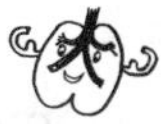

Psychological Effects	Physiological Effects
Origin of the virtues of love and compassion	Send energy and oxygen to the rest of the body
Keep sorrow under control	Send energy from the upper body to the hips
Help us tolerate others without getting too angry	Feed energy to the liver, which releases enzymes that break down meats, oils, and fats

An Unbalanced Response

In an ideal world, the discovery of our body type would be enough to set us on the path to health and longevity. Reality often tells a different story, bringing us unexpected twists and turns that catch us off guard. Factors such as trauma, relationship breakups, the death of a friend, or financial reverses can play a key role in a downward-spiraling health situation, despite our best intentions. Negative situations like these may trigger an imbalance in our predominant temperament. As Pythagoras once said, "No one is free who has not obtained the empire of himself. No man is free who cannot command himself." No matter how difficult a situation may be, introspection helps us overcome our own weaknesses and move onward.

My mentor, Kwan Jong, illustrated this point by recounting a story about an impoverished woman whose husband suddenly left her with five children. He met her while waiting in line at the grocery store and was surprised by how beautiful her skin looked despite other signs of advanced age. Kwan Jong couldn't help but ask how she kept her skin so beautiful. She told him her life story and how she finally accepted the responsibility of raising her children without a husband. At first, this was not an easy task: She had absolutely no money and not even a house to raise them in. She constantly asked herself, "How could I escape this situation?" For months she tried running away from her situation, neglecting her children, and feeling a lack of self-worth. Finally, on the advice of a friend, she went to three counselors who each told her to accept responsibility, for this was her own unique path in life. As soon as she fully accepted this responsibility, a sudden sense of happiness and relief suffused her whole being. Raising her children became a source of joy despite the immense challenges this posed. At the end of the story, she also told him that her children are now all college graduates with successful careers.

Most, if not all of us, would certainly find this woman's situation challenging to deal with. Depending on our body type, however, we would each react in different ways. The elderly woman in the preceding story is likely a Yin Type A because she initially sought to escape her negative situation. The desire to escape reflects the Yin Type A's predominant temperament—complacency. Yet, not all Yin Type A's would respond in the same way. The tendency toward complacency sometimes prompts Yin Type A's to keep a calm demeanor when dealing with troubling circumstances, to the point of helping others stay calm in the face of tragedy. But staying calm and taking appropriate action do not come easily to anyone. These steps are the result of looking inward and showing compassion for others, a challenge for all body types.

How our strongest organ responds to a given situation will eventually determine its effect on our mind and body. For a closer look at what happens when our strongest organs go awry see tables 1.12–1.15.

TABLE 1.12.
YIN TYPE A—UNBALANCED LIVER

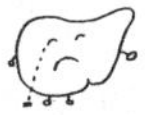

Psychological Effects	Physiological Effects
Lessens cognitive focus	Inhibits the flow of energy and blood to the lungs
Disrupts your dreams, causing restless sleep and/or nightmares	Causes nasal congestion and lack of smell
Causes poor judgment in friendships	Becomes toxic and refuses to cleanse the blood

TABLE 1.13.
YIN TYPE B—UNBALANCED KIDNEYS

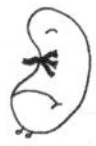

Psychological Effects	Physiological Effects
Cause you to base decisions on selfishness, instead of wisdom	Bring health issues and weakness to the upper body
Cause loss of willpower and courage	Lessen appetite due to an imbalance in the sense of taste
Correspond to fear and social anxiety	Promote water retention

TABLE 1.14. YANG TYPE A—UNBALANCED SPLEEN 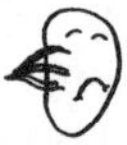

Psychological Effects	Physiological Effects
Unbalanced relationships, causing you to offend and take advantage of others	Refuses to send energy to the kidneys, causing the lower body to get weak
Corresponds to anger and heat (overheating)	Refuses to send energy to the bones, causing pain and weakness of the joints
Heat in the spleen causes hastiness and impatience	Water retention in your lower extremities

TABLE 1.15. YANG TYPE B—UNBALANCED LUNGS 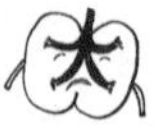

Psychological Effects	Physiological Effects
Block your ability to love and show compassion to others	Refuse to send energy to the liver, making it weaker
Correspond to sadness and depression	Cause you to lose your balance easily because of lack of energy sent to the hips
Lead to rage and bossiness	Make you vomit after eating meat, oils, and fats

The Effects of Illness on Our Temperament

The weakest part of the body is always affected first when it comes to illness. Therefore, each of the body types must keep a cautious eye on their weakest organs in order to maintain good health. Let's take a closer look at how illness tends to affect each body type.

Just because you are a particular body type does not mean that you have to suffer from its associated health issues. Even though Yang Type A's have a tendency toward lower-body weakness, not all of them will have lower-body issues. Moreover, other body types may also suffer from lower-body issues, even if they are not Yang Type A's. How healthy we are depends greatly on the state of our weakest organ. If Yang Type A's do not take care of their weaker organ, lower-body issues will creep in. By exercising and eating according to our body type, we encourage the flow of blood and energy from our stronger to our weaker organs.

An unhealthy liver does not automatically make you a Yang Type B. All other body types could wind up with an unhealthy liver if they drink too much or consistently eat unhealthy foods. However, it does not take long for Yang Type B's to experience liver issues after consuming alcohol or junk food. Consistently eating heavy, oily, or high-protein foods could easily trigger vomiting for Yang Type B's. Interestingly, high-protein and fatty foods rarely cause any other sign of indigestion or discomfort in Yang Type B's because the weaker liver simply rejects them.

Because the lungs are their weakest organ, unhealthy Yin Type A's are prone to frequent colds and other respiratory issues. For this reason, in nine cases out of ten, childhood asthma is an ailment that plagues Yin Type A children, whose lungs are the last of their organs to develop. In the Sasang medical clinic, asthma is often treated with herbs that strengthen and promote the flow of lung energy throughout the body. It is also common for Yin Type A's to have difficulty overcoming colds, which may linger for weeks in one form or another.

According to Sasang medicine, the spleen and stomach are in charge of the digestive process. Born with a weaker spleen, Yin Type B's are prone to digestive issues. The smallest bite of spoiled food could therefore cause major stomachaches, bloating, gas, and the like. As a Yin Type B myself, I recall being rushed to the emergency room several times after eating foods that had been sitting in the refrigerator a bit too long, while others who had eaten the same things escaped unscathed. Stomach pain, vomiting, and diarrhea are common occurrences for the unhealthy Yin Type B. Healthier Yin Type B's keep a cautious eye on what they eat to avoid any major digestive issues.

The Effect of Our Temperament on Illness

It is easy to imagine that an unexpected illness or traumatic event could cause emotional havoc. It is more difficult to fathom how our emotions can prompt the onset of illness. Wouldn't you just hate to hear a doctor say that the source of your pain is "all in your head"? Well, Sasang medicine would at least partially agree with this statement. Before slamming this book shut, read onward and I'll explain.

In this section we will explore how, more often than not, unbalanced temperaments lead to chronic illness, because they obstruct the flow of energy to and from the organs. When slightly unbalanced, they may lead to non-life-threatening issues, such as common colds. At other times we may lose control of our temperament and cause physical injury to our weaker organs. Table 1.16 examines how our predominant temperament may affect our health.

TABLE 1.16. THE EFFECTS OF OUR PREDOMINANT TEMPERAMENT

Body Type	Balanced Temperament	Slightly Unbalanced Temperament	Explosive Temperament May Lead to . . .
Yin Type A	Lack of illness or, if illness/trauma occurs, it is much easier to overcome	Lighter/nonacute symptoms: common cold, general body aches, etc.	Severe colds, frequent colds, lingering colds, pneumonia, stroke, severe asthma and shortness of breath
Yin Type B	Lack of illness or, if illness/trauma occurs, it is much easier to overcome	Lighter/nonacute symptoms: common cold, general body aches, etc.	Severe indigestion (diarrhea, food stagnation, acute stomach pain, etc.), loss of consciousness, extreme cold
Yang Type A	Lack of illness or, if illness/trauma occurs, it is much easier to overcome	Lighter/nonacute symptoms: common cold, general body aches, etc.	Severe kidney and urinary issues, weakness of the lower extremities
Yang Type B	Lack of illness or, if illness/trauma occurs, it is much easier to overcome	Lighter/nonacute symptoms: common cold, general body aches, etc.	Loss of balance, blood toxicity, vomiting after meals

The explosive anger of Yang Type A's predominant temperament causes the body's energy to spiral out of control, further depleting their already weak kidneys. Chronic bouts of explosive anger can cause serious injury to the kidneys, resulting in urinary-tract issues, arthritis, and lower-body weakness. The other body types may certainly experience bouts of rage, but that has no immediate effect on their weaker organs. If the other body types experience explosive emotions, such as rage, those emotions will slowly but surely compromise their weaker organs, but only after causing their own innate temperament to lose control. If Yin Type A's experience rage, for example, there is no immediate effect on their weaker lungs. However, long-term rage will eventually cause their complacent temperament to explode as they attempt to retreat from their circumstances and indulge in unhealthy behavior. Only after the explosion of complacency will their weaker lungs start to feel the effects of rage.

Explosive temperaments often occur when we are faced with a significantly challenging situation, which has a strong effect on how we feel emotionally. The explosion of our temperament strikes a direct blow to the weaker organs, causing immediately damaging effects. The explosive complacency of Yin Type A's makes their body's energy stagnate, further weakening their already weak lungs. A desire to escape from responsibility and/or engage in addictive behavior is a reflection of explosive complacency. Such behaviors prompt the immediate onset of health issues, such as severe/frequent colds, lingering colds, and pneumonia. If the explosion of their predominant emotion is left unaddressed, it could lead to serious health issues, such as high blood pressure, stroke, and serious cardiovascular issues.

The constant desire of Yin Type B's to be satisfied and happy can easily get them in trouble. The inability to accomplish a long-sought goal, for example, often causes them disappointment or grief. The other body types are more inclined to give up or change their strategy, while Yin Type B's have trouble taking no for an answer. They keep striving for the joyful feeling of satisfaction, even at the cost of their own well-being. Dealing with failure is especially difficult for Yin Type B's. It often leads to the explosion of their desire for accomplishment, which further weakens their already weak spleen. An explosive desire for satisfaction may prompt the onset of severe digestive issues, such as uncontrollable diarrhea, plus extreme feelings of cold, unbearable fatigue, and/or potential loss of consciousness. Establishing practical and reachable goals helps to cultivate a deep sense of balance and satisfaction in Yin Type B's. It also helps soothe their weaker digestive system.

Not all illness is a sign of an unbalanced temperament. The common cold, chronic pain, or other illness does not necessarily point to a temperament gone wild. When struck with illness, however, our predominant temperament will make or break the healing process. When we're feeling under the weather, it is crucial to ask ourselves a few important questions, like these:

Am I pushing myself too hard?
Do I need to watch what I'm eating?
Do I need to adjust my sleeping times?
Do I need to balance my predominant temperament?
Do I need to exercise more or less?

If we ask these questions and make the necessary adjustments, our chances of overcoming illness become much greater.

NAVIGATING YOUR WAY TO HEALTH

Common colds and/or indigestion tend to wipe us out, forcing us to slow down and rest. It is sometimes difficult to know, however, when an illness quietly finds its way into our body. When our inherently weaker organ is faced with illness, it may not be able to send a strong enough SOS signal to the brain. Some illnesses may progress very slowly and seem to slip past our internal radar system. In these cases the weaker organ in our body will slowly but surely become even weaker. Chronic issues, such as fatigue, high blood pressure, and heart disease, do not necessarily produce immediate symptoms. In many cases symptoms manifest themselves when illness has already advanced considerably. Such situations can be avoided by recognizing our body type and taking action to balance the energy flow between our weaker and stronger organs.

Health is a two-way interaction between the influence of our external environment and the inherent internal qualities that we each possess. A balanced temperament can provide the ammunition needed to fight off and recover from illness. Sasang medicine can provide us with the appropriate tools to keep our temperament balanced, despite what our environment throws at us. Let's take a closer look at how health is approached the Sasang way.

To stay healthy:

- Eating and exercising right for your body type ensures a consistent flow from your stronger organs to your weaker organs, while enhancing your overall health and preventing illness.
- The awareness of your weaker and your stronger psychological aspects can help you make the right health decisions.
- Supplementing with herbs and foods that are suitable for your body type helps avoid illness and keeps you healthy.

When times get tough:

- Make sure you follow the three approaches above, while giving your mind and body the rest they need.
- Read through "Addressing Health Issues Based on Your Yin Yang Body Type," (beginning on page 247) to see if there is an herb or a combination of herbs that will remedy your situation.
- Check out our website and/or contact the sasangmedicine.com team for further counsel.

Now that you have grasped the theory behind Sasang medicine, it is time to get your feet wet and move onward to discover your body type.

Determining Your Yin Yang Body Type

Everything we do is a reflection of our body type, which is revealed through how we react to pain, illness, joy, love, stress, and the like. In Korea, Sasang medicine continues to evolve as researchers identify new and innovative ways to distinguish each body type from the others. Anything from skin and voice tone to facial features can give you hints as to which body type you may be. However, none of these methods, by themselves, are 100 percent accurate when it comes to determining your body type. Discovering your body type is often a challenging process, which can take a considerable amount of time, because what is expressed outwardly may actually be only a fraction of what is felt deep inside. We also develop traits that are not necessarily associated with our body type. These traits become ingrained over time by observing how others approach life. Acquiring traits from other body types is necessary for our survival and to balance our own weaknesses. The body type is the core matrix of our mind and body; it lurks beneath layer upon layer of who we are on the outside.

Your Yin Yang Body Type utilizes two of the most efficient, time-tested ways to determine your body type. The combination of these different techniques ensures the accuracy of your body type reading. The first method focuses on the size and shape of your bodily features. This method involves close observation of your body features and is approximately 60–70 percent accurate. The second method is the Yin Yang Body Type Test®, a questionnaire that focuses on your daily physical and emotional tendencies; this is approximately 70–80 percent accurate. The former method is generally easier to use because it involves observing external bodily features. The latter method is not as tangible and often requires considerable self-reflection.

In most cases both of these tests will come to the same conclusion about your body type. In some cases, however, they may be at odds with each other. If the two tests each come to a different conclusion about your body type, you might have to do the following:

- Take each test over again to make sure you did not overlook anything.
- Ask someone close to you to go over the results and reflect on them a second time to confirm if your answers were accurate.
- If there is still a discrepancy between the tests after you have tried the above two methods, then the results of the Yin Yang Body Type Test take precedence. Sasang medicine emphasizes internal rather than external aspects of who we are because the shape and size of our body is more easily influenced by environmental factors. The Yin Yang Body Type Test focuses on what underlies our outward appearance by probing our psychological and physiological tendencies, which are usually a stronger indication of our body type.

Discovering your body type opens up a whole new spectrum of relationship and health opportunities. Even with the discovery of your body type, however, the goal of harmony and balance is not always close at hand. There may be aspects of your body type that you wish to change and others that you desire to cling to. Getting to know your body type is a firm step toward navigating through life's challenges and reaching your true potential. Yet, it is also accompanied by the decision to modify and/or accept who each of us is physically and emotionally in order to become a healthier and more balanced person. Identifying your body type is the first step toward revealing the infinite potential that lies deep within you.

METHOD A: OUTWARD APPEARANCE TEST

Have you heard the expression, "A single smile can wipe away a million tears"? Even though a smile is nothing but a momentary contraction of facial muscles, in an instant it can transform the way we and others around us feel. If such a simple expression could do so much, then it goes without saying that our face can also reveal other secrets about who we are. In his book *Conduct of Life,* Ralph Waldo Emerson states, "A man finds room in the few square inches of his face for the traits of all his ancestors; for the expression of all his history." Not only does the face reveal our emotion, but it also provides significant clues about our body type.

In Eastern medicine not just the face, but the entire surface of our body is a direct reflection of what occurs inside. Each organ in our body communicates with the surface in its own way. The lungs, for example, control the opening and closing of the skin pores, the spleen maintains muscle tone, the liver keeps our tendons elastic, and the kidneys uphold the integrity of our hair and skin. If any of these organs begin to fail, its corresponding body part will be affected. As we saw earlier, not only does trauma or illness affect our organs, but our emotions do, too. Anger, which is associated with the spleen, can also have an effect on the contraction of our muscles. Excessive anger, associated with excessive spleen energy, can therefore easily lead to muscle spasms. Weakness of the spleen, on the other hand, can result in a weakened or hunched-over appearance.

The development of different parts of our body is also affected by our major organs. As noted previously, the lungs and spleen are considered Yang organs, while the liver and kidneys are Yin organs. Yang types are born with stronger Yang organs. Since Yang corresponds to the upper body, these organs cause the upper body to be better-developed than the lower body. Yin types, on the contrary, have stronger Yin organs and, hence, are relatively better-developed in their lower body.

Despite these general differences, there are also body type–specific differences in appearance. Yang Type A's, for example, often have protruding cheekbones and broad shoulders. These characteristics also correspond to a stronger spleen. Yet, not all Yang Type A's have protruding cheekbones.

This is where things get a bit tricky. If you're heavyset, your face may look rounded no matter what body type you are. In such cases you might need to look at a childhood picture to see if your face changed as you got older. If so, there may be a Yang Type A lurking within you! Taking a good look in the mirror or asking a friend may also help if you are simply not sure.

Weight often causes confusion when determining your body type. It is common for budding Sasang experts to believe that Yin Type A's are the "heavyset" body type, since their features are often rounded. While most obese people have this body type, there are also many exceptions to this rule. Some of the skinniest people I have met, for example, are Yin Type A's. Don't fret! There are plenty of other clues at your disposal when determining your body type. The lower two to three ribs of skinny Yin Type A's, for example, often flare outward on both sides of the rib cage as if to prepare for the development of a large abdomen, even if there is absolutely no other sign of impending weight gain. This is also because the lowermost ribs cover our liver, which, in the Yin Type A's case, is the largest and strongest organ in the body. This trait, however, is harder to detect in heavyset Yin Type A's, whose abdomen has already protruded outward.

TALLYING UP YOUR OUTWARD APPEARANCE TEST SCORE

Each body type in this section will be assigned a list of eight body type–specific features that count as one point each. Add up the total of the features for each body type that relate to you. The type with the highest score indicates your body type.

Keep in mind the following tips to help ensure the accuracy of your Outward Appearance Test results:

- Observe your body closely and take the time to assess every detail. Use the sample illustrations on pages 46–53 as a guide. Keep in mind that certain body type tendencies are less obvious than others.
- It is often helpful to use a mirror when examining your body type features.

- Some features may not be apparent with clothing on, so you may need to disrobe.
- If you are not sure whether a certain body type feature applies to you, ask a close friend, spouse, or family member.
- We do not always manifest all the features of our body type. Even though most Yin Type B's have a short stature, for example, there may be tall people with this body type, too. Even if you have only two out of seven features under one body type, this may still be your type, especially if you scored less with the other body types.

OUTWARD APPEARANCE CHECKLIST

YIN TYPE A—Body Feature	Points (circle if applies)
Roundish head	1
Roundish eyes	1
Large facial features	1
Thick and/or rough skin	1
Overall calm appearance	1
Last few ribs flare outward	1
Protruding abdomen	1
Larger foot size	1
Total Points:	

YIN TYPE B—Body Feature	Points (circle if applies)
Smaller head	1
Smaller facial features	1
Narrow head	1
Narrow neck	1
Shorter height	1
Narrow chest	1
Developed buttocks	1
Frail appearance	1
Total Points:	

OUTWARD APPEARANCE CHECKLIST (continued)

YANG TYPE A—Body Feature	Points (circle if applies)
Broad forehead	1
Males: Sharp gaze **Females:** Sunrise shaped eyes (bright and radiant, with upper half arching upward)	1
Prominent cheekbones	1
Narrow chin	1
Broad shoulders	1
Well-developed chest and upper body	1
Tapered waist	1
Small buttocks	1
Total Points:	

YANG TYPE B—Body Feature	Points (circle if applies)
Cone shaped head	1
Pointy/large ears	1
Bulging chin	1
Thick neck	1
Well-developed upper body	1
Narrow waist	1
Narrow thighs	1
Overall intense/powerful appearance	1
Total Points:	

Highest Section Score = Your Body Type:

YIN TYPE A FEMALE

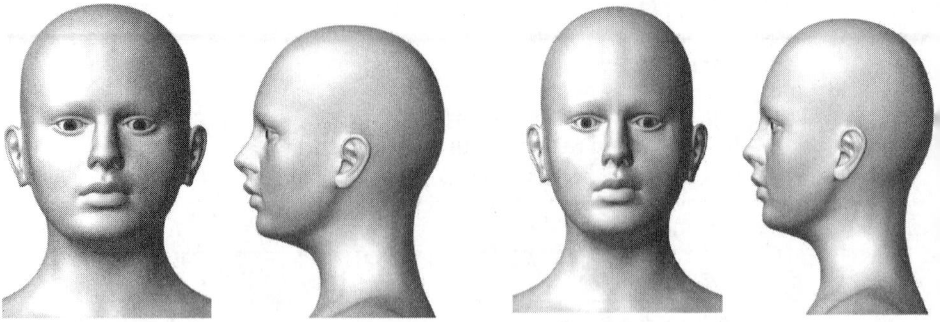

Roundish eyes and head, larger facial features, overall calm/relaxed appearance

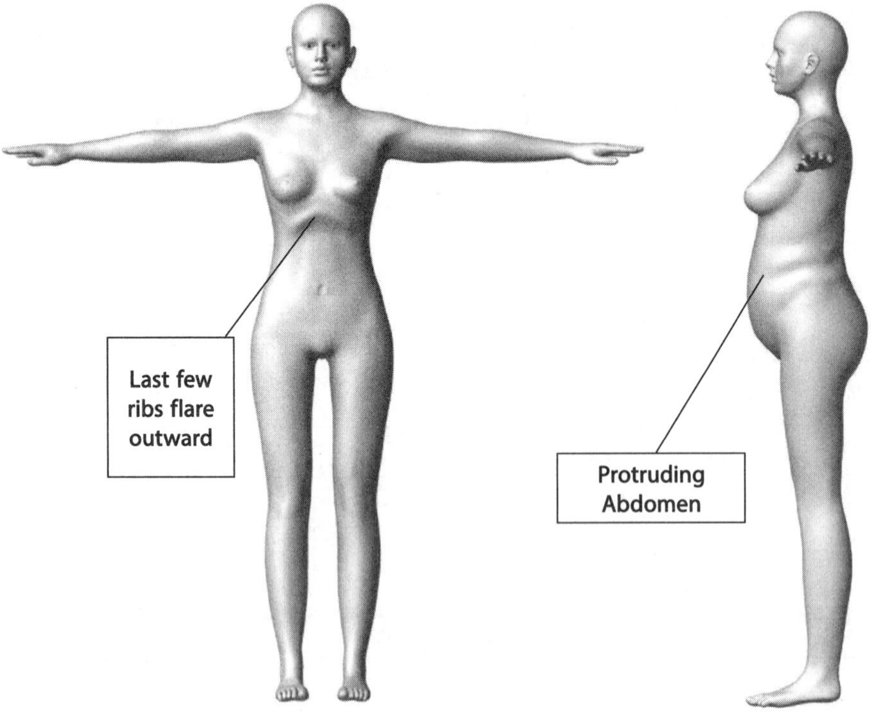

Thick and/or rough skin, large foot size

YIN TYPE A MALE

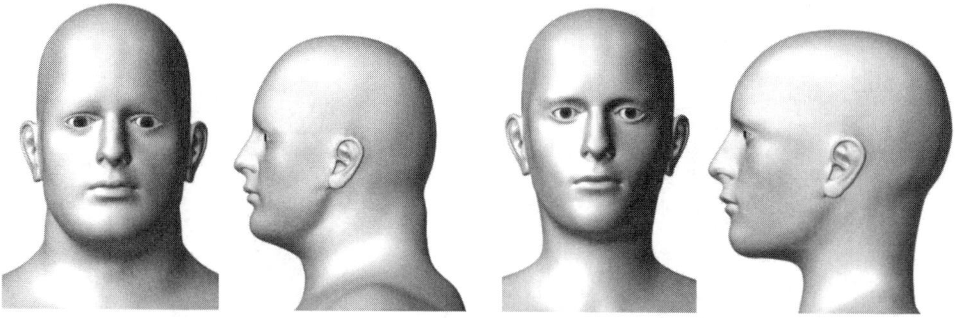

Roundish eyes and head, larger facial features, overall calm/relaxed appearance

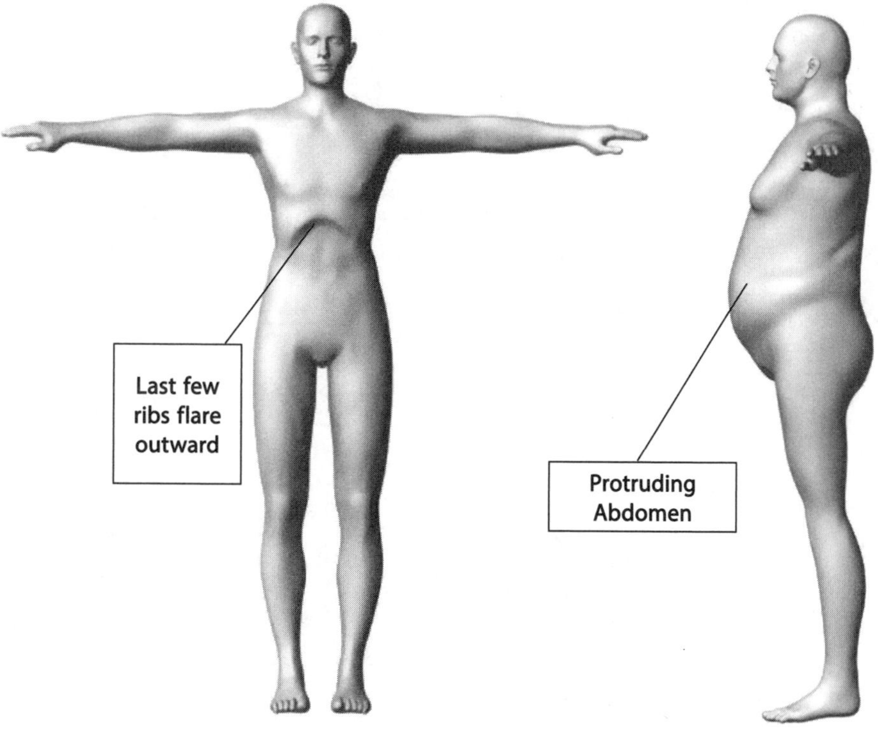

Thick and/or rough skin, large foot size

YIN TYPE B FEMALE

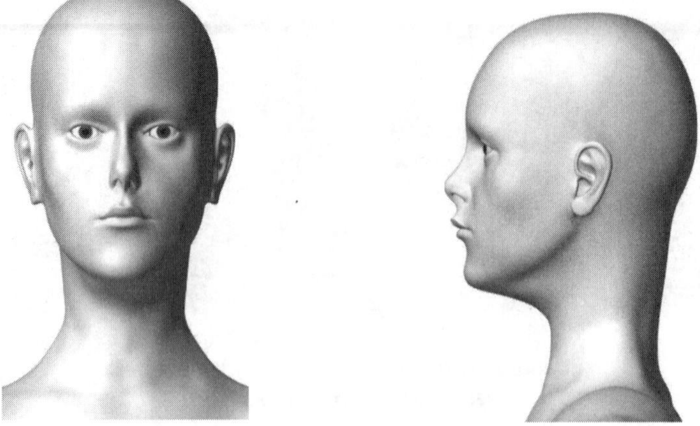

Smaller and narrow-shaped head, narrow neck, smaller facial features

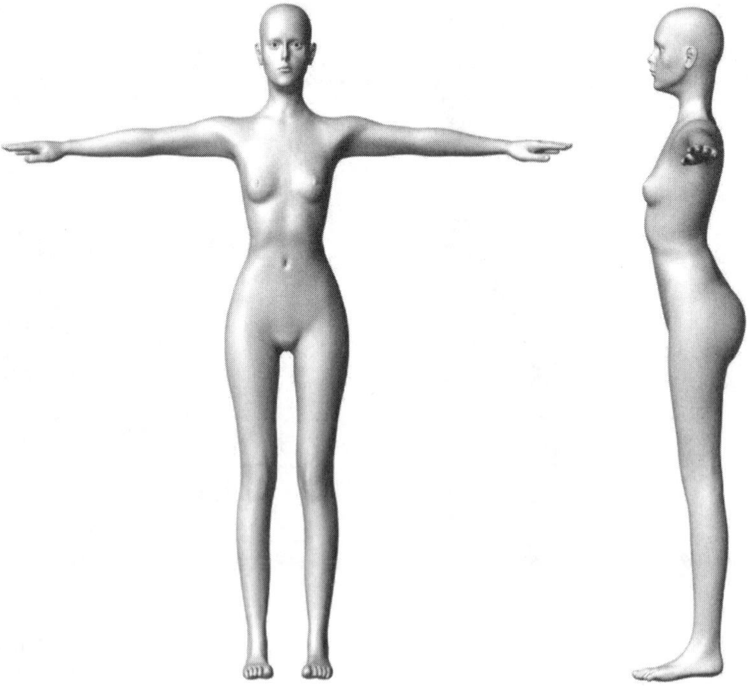

Shorter height, narrow chest, developed buttocks, overall frail appearance

YIN TYPE B MALE

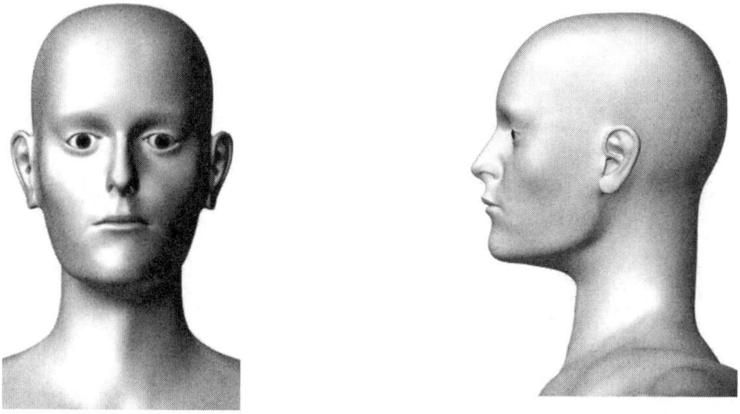

Smaller and narrow-shaped head, narrow neck, smaller facial features

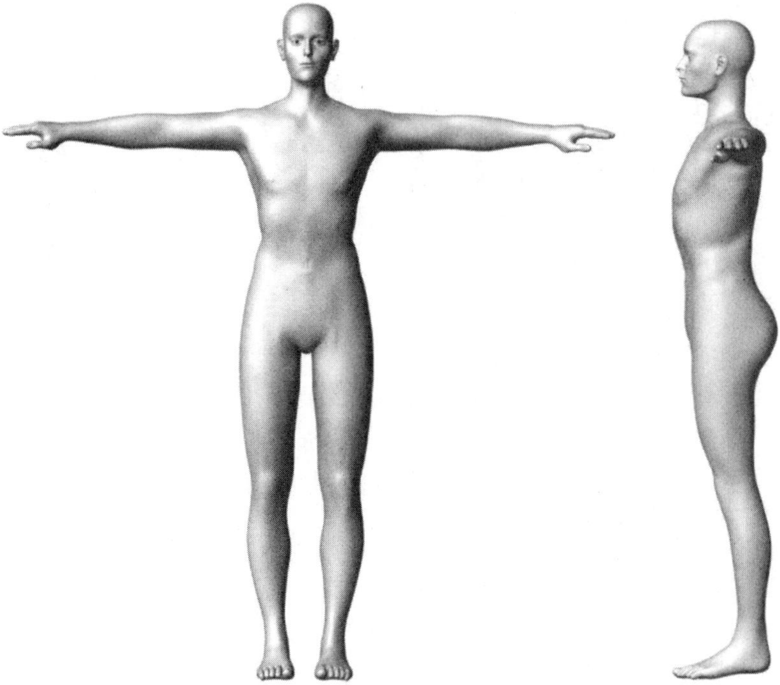

Shorter height, narrow chest, developed buttocks, overall frail appearance

YANG TYPE A FEMALE

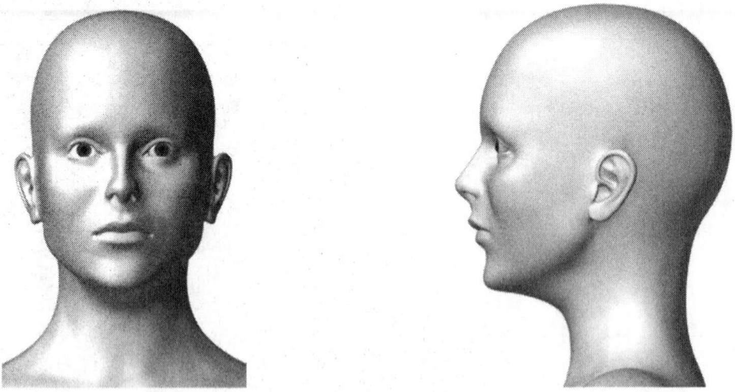

Broad forehead, prominent cheekbones, narrow chin, sunrise-shaped eyes that arch upward like the sun rising above a mountain

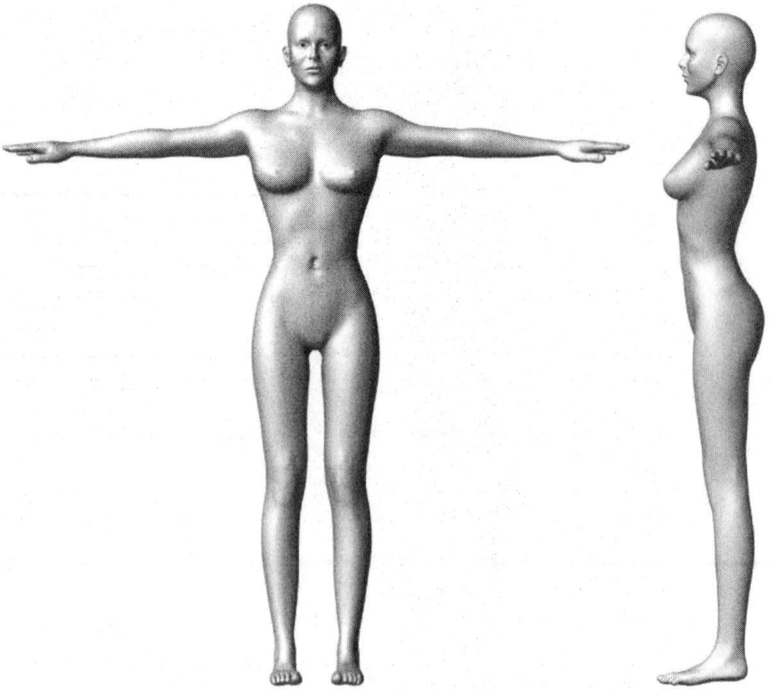

Broad shoulders, developed chest and breast area, tapered waist, smaller buttocks

YANG TYPE A MALE

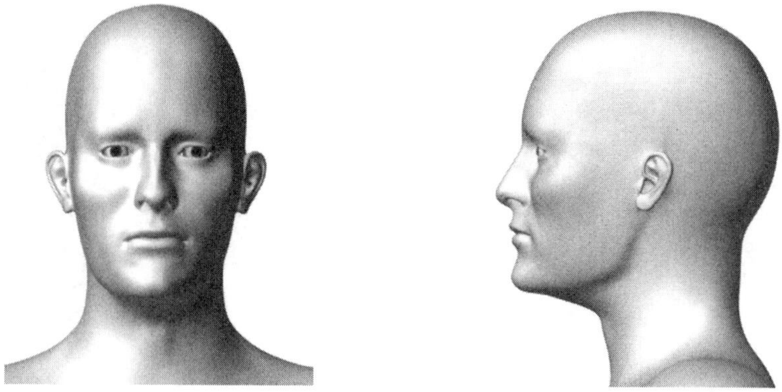

Broad forehead, prominent cheekbones, narrow chin, sharp and piercing gaze

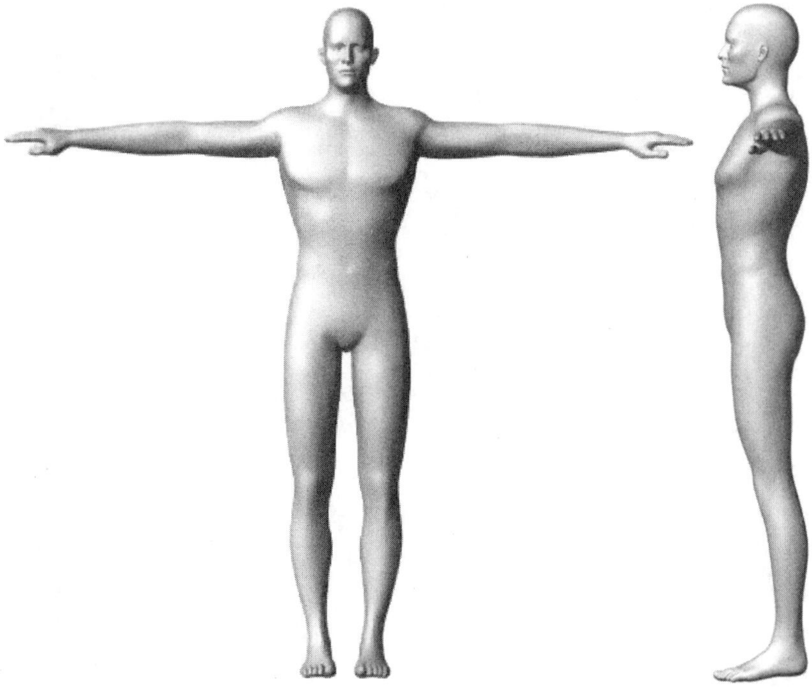

Broad shoulders, developed chest, tapered waist, smaller buttocks

YANG TYPE B FEMALE

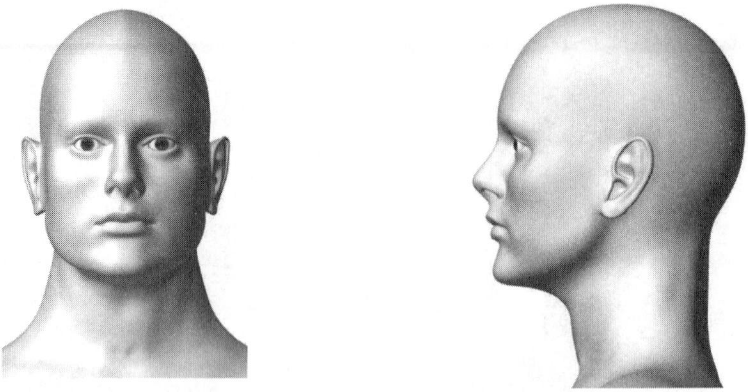

Head has pointy vertex, pointy large ears, bulging chin, thicker neck

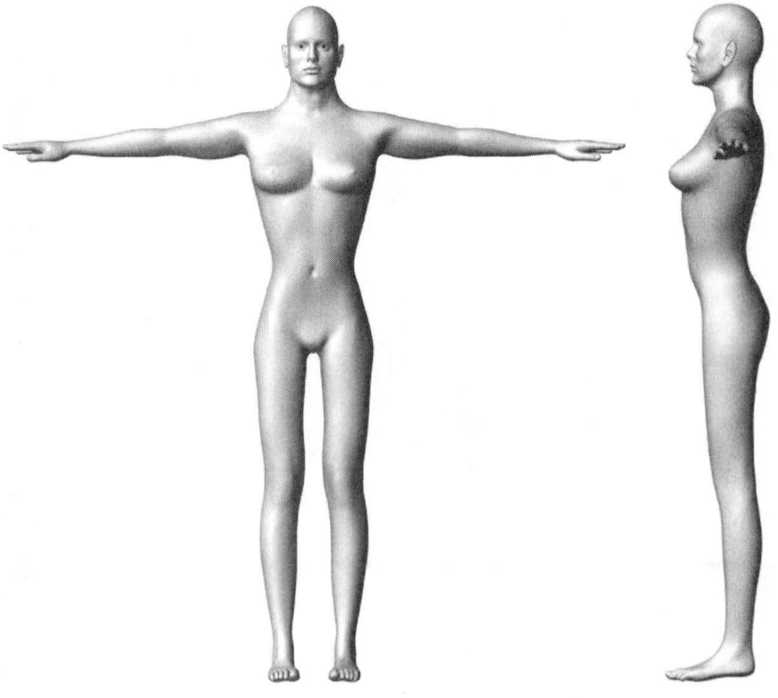

Narrow waist, developed upper body, narrow thighs, overall intense/powerful appearance

YANG TYPE B MALE

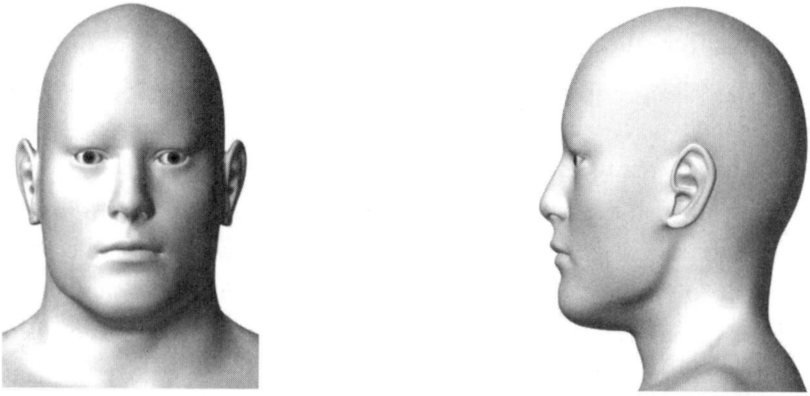

Head has pointy vertex, pointy large ears, bulging chin, thicker neck

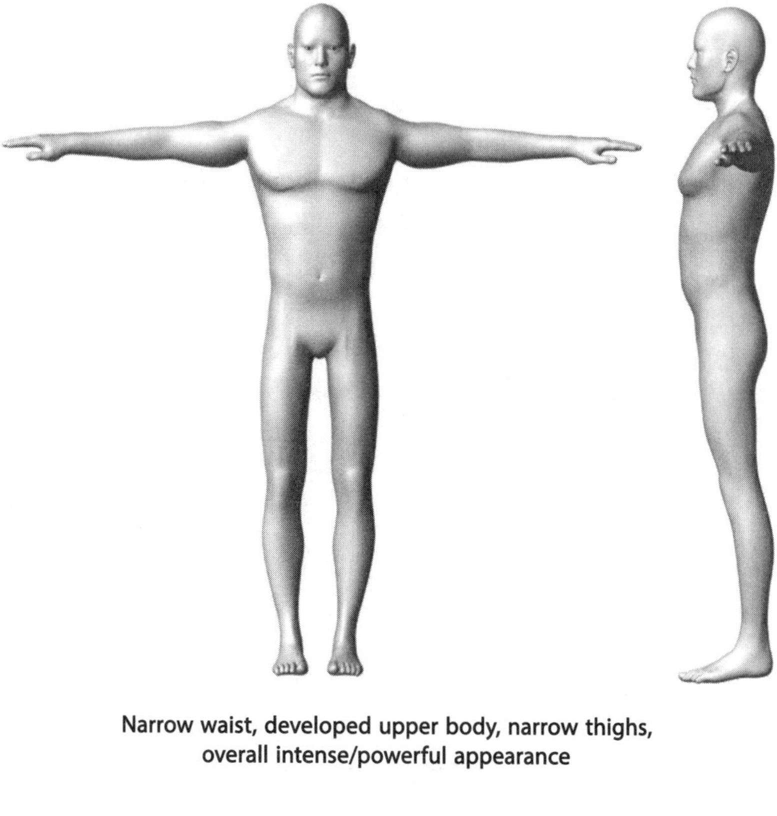

Narrow waist, developed upper body, narrow thighs,
overall intense/powerful appearance

METHOD B: THE YIN YANG BODY TYPE TEST

The Yin Yang Body Type Test is one of several ways to determine your body type based on emotional and psychological tendencies. While some of our tendencies are easy to detect, others may be hidden. Try your best to answer as many questions as possible on the body type test, either by yourself or with the help of a close friend or family member. If you have a chance, try going over this test a second time with a close friend or family member to get another perspective. Others are often able to shed light on aspects of our personality that we may have overlooked. After finishing the body type test, tally up the total score separately under each question group. Refer to the Body Type Key at the end of the questionnaire to determine your body type. An answer key, which explains the significance of each question, is also included in this section. While taking the body type test, keep the following tips in mind:

- If you are not sure of an answer, it may be helpful to consult someone who is close to you, such as your spouse, a parent, a sibling, or a best friend.
- Focus on overall tendencies when taking the body type test. Certain tendencies may change from day to day or throughout the years, making a question difficult to answer. For the sake of the Yin Yang Body Type Test, it is sometimes helpful to reflect on how things used to be when you were a child, or growing up, since our body type never changes.
- Some questions may require you to examine yourself closely. You may have to take a good look in the mirror or examine how you walk when answering certain questions.
- Do not answer the question if, no matter how much you try, an answer does not come to mind. It is better to leave it blank than to obscure the test results.
- If you are not sure how to answer a particular question, refer to the answer key at the end of this section. It offers an explanation for each question, making it easier to answer.

- If you are still unsure of how to answer a particular question or what body type you are, go back to the Outward Appearance section. Your body shape may be enough to help you determine your body type.
- Did you score a tie between two body types? Is the difference between one body type only slightly higher than another? If either of these situations occurs, go over the test again to make sure of your answers. You may also ask for assistance from others who know you well. If, after taking the test again, the difference between two body types remains slight, go with the higher score.
- If you are still in doubt after following these tips, I suggest reviewing the red light foods for each body type in part 3, "Eating and Exercising Right for Your Yin Yang Body Type." Which of the body types have red light foods that cause digestive discomfort or other health issues for you? It is possible that you may be this body type. If you are still not sure, then try eating the green light foods of the body type you scored the highest (or tied) with for three to five days while monitoring your energy levels and digestion. If you feel more energy after a few days, feel lighter, or have more regular bowel movements and urination, it is possible that you are this body type. If you notice any digestive discomfort, lack of energy, or irregular bowel or urination flow, then it is likely you are not this body type and it may benefit you to try the foods of another type. This method can also be applied to the ingestion of supplements, which are listed at the end of each body type section in part 3. I would suggest, however, that foods be explored first. Supplements often have stronger effects on the body than food and could cause significant discomfort if they do not match your type.
- The discovery of your body type often takes a considerable amount of time and self-reflection. A single question of the Yin Yang Body Type Test may take hours, days, or even weeks of careful observation to answer correctly. One of the greatest challenges of discovering your body type is the ability to determine

whether a particular trait is a predominant temperament (a core part of who you are) or simply a fleeting characteristic that does not adequately reflect who you are. It is easy to feel angered, for example, if someone cuts in front of you in line, no matter what body type you are. If you rarely get angry, then this feeling may come as a surprise and you may think, "Wow! I must be an angry natured Yang Type A." Even though anger is a predominant temperament of Yang Type A's, it does not mean that anger makes you a member of this body type. There are often other emotions that lurk beneath our feeling of anger. For Yin Type A's it may be a feeling of "Why can't he be friendly?" since friendship and care are so important to them. Whereas for Yang Type A's, anger in this situation is a result of feeling disrespected and looked down upon as they think "How can they treat ME like this?" Take ample time getting to the root of your emotional and physical characteristics.

- If you are still finding the Yin Yang body type quest to be a challenge, contact our team of Sasang specialists at sasangmedicine.com for additional assistance.

QUESTION GROUP A

	Never (Not True)	Sometimes True (Maybe)	Often True (Likely)	Always True (Definitely)
1. I have difficulty sweating (I sweat less than others around me)	0	2	4	6
2. My abdomen tends to protrude outward AND/OR fat accumulates or begins in my abdomen.	0	2	4	6
3. I tend to walk with one foot OR both feet pointed outward forty-five degrees or more. (Walk a few steps and measure if you are not sure.)	0	2	4	6
4. I have a lazy nature OR relaxation is more appealing for me than physical activity.	0	2	4	6
5. I do not feel well after drinking milk AND/OR eating wheat products.	0	2	4	6
6. I have a very acute sense of smell (when my nose is not congested).	0	2	4	6
7. If I do not take action, common colds tend to last a long time for me.	0	2	4	6
8. I get frequent colds (three or more times a year).	0	2	4	6
9. My body features are roundish, rather than narrow.	0	1	2	3
10. I tend to be a night owl.	0	1	2	3
Total Scores (per column)				
Grand Total Score (all columns combined)				

QUESTION GROUP B

	Never (Not True)	Sometimes True (Maybe)	Often True (Likely)	Always True (Definitely)
1. I have a tendency to develop digestion-related issues.	0	2	4	6
2. Ginger as tea or a condiment helps my digestive system (skip this if you are not sure).	0	2	4	6
3. I am shy.	0	2	4	6
4. I prefer to have only one or two (close) friends.	0	2	4	6
5. I am naturally introverted.	0	2	4	6
6. Fat accumulation usually begins in my buttocks AND/OR hips.	0	2	4	6
7. Chilled foods often cause me indigestion.	0	2	4	6
8. I like to take long, warm baths or showers even on hot summer days.	0	1	2	3
9. I am happiest when I'm alone.	0	1	2	3
10. I have difficulty digesting shellfish (e.g., oysters, clams, crab).	0	1	2	3
11. Excess stress tends to reduce my appetite.	0	1	2	3
Total Scores (per column)				

Grand Total Score (all columns combined)

QUESTION GROUP C

	Never (Not True)	Sometimes True (Maybe)	Often True (Likely)	Always True (Definitely)
1. Skipping a bowel movement for several days causes me other issues (headache, stomachache, bloating, etc.)	0	2	4	6
2. My feet feel hot at night.	0	2	4	6
3. I am very direct with others, offending them as a result.	0	2	4	6
4. I get easily agitated when hungry.	0	2	4	6
5. I tend to be very judgmental of others.	0	2	4	6
6. I am good at multitasking. (If you circled 2 or higher, then answer part 2 of this question.)	0	1	2	3
6b. . . . BUT I have trouble being accurate.	0	1	2	3
7. My anger has a tendency to explode. (If you circled 2 or higher, answer part 2 of this question.)	0	1	2	3
7b. . . . BUT my energy feels drained after getting angry.	0	1	2	3
8. I gain AND lose weight quickly. (Answer "Not True" if only half of this question is true.)	0	1	2	3
9. I am a morning person.	0	1	2	3
10. I usually prefer seafood over chicken.	0	1	2	3
Total Scores (per column)				
Grand Total Score (all columns combined)				

QUESTION GROUP D

	Never (Not True)	Sometimes True (Maybe)	Often True (Likely)	Always True (Definitely)
1. My neck is larger in proportion to the rest of my body.	0	2	4	6
2. The tip of my ears AND/OR my head is/are somewhat pointy.	0	2	4	6
3. Since childhood, I tend to lose my balance.	0	2	4	6
4. I feel the need to be in charge and tell others what to do.	0	2	4	6
5. Fat accumulation usually begins in my upper body (neck, shoulders, AND/OR chest).	0	2	4	6
6. I have OR used to have a tendency to vomit after eating meat.	0	2	4	6
7. I make friends easily but am difficult to get close to.	0	1	2	3
8. I experience episodes of sadness. (If you circled 3, then answer part 2 of this question.)	0	1	2	3
8b. . . . BUT my sadness turns into explosive anger.	0	1	2	3
9. I make it my business to be social and to make as many friends as possible.	0	1	2	3
10. Hearing is my strongest sense (compared to sight, taste, and smell).	0	1	2	3
Total Scores (per column)				

Grand Total Score (all columns combined)

ANSWER KEY

Before we tally up your answers, let's take a look at what body type each question group corresponds to:

Body Type	Highest Score
Yin Type A	Question Group A
Yin Type B	Question Group B
Yang Type A	Question Group C
Yang Type B	Question Group D

Thus, if you score higher in group A than the other four groups, you are likely a Yin Type A. A higher score in group B makes you a Yin Type B. The same theory can be applied to groups C and D.

We are now ready to review your answers to the Yin Yang Body Type Test. The answer key included in this section can help you determine your body type while providing an explanation about why you have this or that tendency. Most of us take for granted why our body and mind react a particular way to a given situation. If you are not sure how to answer a question, make sure to read the answer to the question in the key below before skipping it. Do not feel guilty about cheating on your Yin Yang Body Type Test because reading the answer key beforehand will help clarify each of the questions.

Question Group A—Yin Type A

Question 1: Yin Type A's are born with thicker and/or harder skin, which can be a blessing and a curse. Thicker skin protects their weaker lungs, which are responsible for controlling and supporting immune activity. This trait helps guard against otherwise easily contracted colds and flu. Thicker skin, however, also makes it difficult for sweat to push its way through the pores for weaker Yin Type A's. Sweating is a way to expel unwanted bacteria and toxins from the body. The lack of ability to sweat often results in prolonged colds and other illness. Keep in mind that not all Yin Type A's have trouble sweating. Actually, most healthier Yin Type A's do not have difficulty sweating. They may even sweat abundantly as their bodies rid them of excess heat and toxins.

Question 2: The liver controls the flow of blood and energy through the abdominal area. As the Yin Type A's strongest organ, the liver can easily become congested and stagnant from excessive activity. When this happens, fat has a tendency to accumulate in the abdominal area. Skinnier Yin Type A's will notice that their abdomen is where the skin feels more abundant and full, even if fat has not accumulated there. Heavier Yin Type A's may notice that their abdomen tends to protrude outward. It may be difficult to detect whether or not fat has a tendency to initially accumulate in your abdomen if it has already accumulated in other areas as well.

Question 3: Every body type has its own way of walking. Let's take a look at some of the other body types. Yin Type B's tend to look bashful when they walk. Yang Type A's look confident when they walk as they swing their shoulders from side to side. Yang Type B's have a clumsy walk and often lose their balance. Yin Type A's walk with their feet pointed outward, making them appear relaxed and bottom-heavy.

Question 4: Yin Type A's often have a lazy nature because laziness corresponds to the liver, their strongest organ. Laziness and inactivity are also Yin attributes, while Yang is active and ambitious. Yang body types are usually very active. Yang types may actually become too active and have trouble slowing down. Yin types tend to be less active and face health issues due to an underactive circulatory system. Not all Yin types are lazy, though! Many Yin types choose to challenge themselves and keep themselves busy. If you ask diligent Yin types what they truly desire to do with their time, however, they will most likely say something like this: take it easy, relax, or do nothing.

Question 5: Yin Type A's are generally sensitive to wheat and dairy products because these foods overstimulate their stronger liver. Each body type benefits from eating foods that stimulate their weaker, rather than stronger organ. According to the theory of Yin and Yang, if Yang gets stronger, then Yin will naturally get weaker. Since the strongest and weakest organs form a Yin/Yang relationship, stimulation of the stronger organ will weaken the weaker organ. In the Yin Type A's case, stimulation of the liver will lead to weakness of the lungs. Thus, ingesting dairy and wheat products often lead to the accumulation of phlegm, sinus congestion, fatigue, allergy symptoms, and/or frequent colds.

Question 6: Yin Type A's have an acute sense of smell, thanks to their stronger liver.

Questions 7 and 8: The lungs of Yin Type A's are the weakest organ in their body. Since the lungs regulate and support the immune system, weaker lungs often lead to frequent and/or long-term colds, which seem to last forever. Cardiovascular exercises, which are extremely beneficial for the health of the lungs, help prevent Yin Type A colds.

Question 9: Approximately 80 percent of all Yin Type A's have roundish body features. This is because Yin Type A's have an abundant amount of Yin. According to Asian philosophy, Yin is round while Yang is narrow. Approximately 70–80 percent of all Yin Type A's suffer from obesity as a result of having abundant Yin. Even if they are not overweight, Yin Type A's often have rounder features than the other body types.

Question 10: Yin is associated with nighttime, while Yang is associated with daytime. Yang types tend to have more energy during the day while Yin types have more energy at night. Yin Type A's often say that they have difficulty getting to sleep because they feel like reading a book, writing, or using the computer late into the night.

Question Group B—Yin Type B

Question 1: Yin Type B's are born with a weaker spleen. In Sasang medicine, the spleen helps the stomach metabolize food. Because they have a weaker spleen, it is challenging for the Yin Type B's stomach to break down and digest food, making them very cautious about eating. Issues such as indigestion, stomach flu, or food poisoning could easily and quickly become serious for Yin Type B's, who often compensate for this weakness by becoming picky eaters.

Question 2: Yin represents cold while Yang represents heat. Therefore, excessive coldness tends to affect the digestive system of Yin Type B's. Ginger is a very spicy-tasting vegetable. The warm energy of ginger counters the cold-infested digestive system of Yin Type B's. Actually, ginger is one of the most beneficial foods for Yin Type B's.

Question 3: Yin represents introversion, while Yang represents extroversion. Yin Type B's have an introverted nature and tend to be very shy. They often retreat into their own fantasy world to cope with the stresses of daily life. This behavior tends to isolate them from others.

Question 4: The shy nature of Yin Type B's, discussed in Question 3, makes it challenging for them to open up to strangers. They can often be seen with their head down, as if to avoid talking to others. With close friends, however, they may jabber away, as if to make up for lost time.

Question 5: Refer to the answers to Questions 3 and 4 for an explanation of this trait.

Question 6: Yin represents the lower body, while Yang represents the upper body. The lower body of Yin types is more developed than the upper body. The abdomen of the Yin Type A and the buttocks of the Yin Type B, for example, are the best-developed parts of the body. Fat and muscle tend to accumulate in these areas.

Question 7: Yin body types benefit from and digest Yang (warmer-natured) foods much more easily than Yang types, who benefit from and digest Yin (cooler-natured) foods much more easily than their Yin counterparts. Chicken is one of the most Yang of the Yang foods and is therefore easier to digest for Yin Type B's. Chicken has so much Yang energy that it may cause indigestion or excess heat in Yang Type A's.

Question 8: With so little Yang, Yin Type B's easily get cold and therefore enjoy warming themselves up by taking long, warm baths or showers, which often become a daily ritual needed to kick-start their day. It is very challenging for Yin Type B's to retain heat, and so they often desire to sunbathe or find alternative methods of warming themselves up daily. While other body types may complain of having cold hands and feet, Yin Type B's often feel cold at the core. Cold is what initiates or exacerbates practically every health issue of Yin Type B's.

Question 9: Yin Type B's feel most comfortable when they're alone. They tend to think more clearly and dream away while hiking alone or simply shutting themselves into a locked room. Yin Type B's are the most self-sufficient of all four body types. While the other body types may be independent or need time alone, they will eventually get lonely and need others to comfort them. Yin Type B's may also get lonely at times, but that does not mean being in the presence of others will offer them comfort.

Question 10: Yin represents cold, while Yang represents heat. With so much Yin already lurking in their strong kidneys, cold foods quickly affect the Yin Type B's digestive system. Yin also represents the deeper parts of the ocean, while Yang corresponds to its shallower areas. According to Eastern medicine, shellfish is said to have a very cold nature, since it is often found lurking on the ocean floor, munching on Yin foods. If Yin Type B's eat a substantial amount of shellfish, they will experience symptoms such as stomach pain, lethargy, muscle aches, and/or dark-colored diarrhea. If you like and digest shellfish well, then chances are that you are (a) a very healthy Yin Type B or (b) not a Yin Type B from the get-go.

Question 11: Stress and sickness always affect the constitutionally weaker aspects of each body type. Since Yin Type B's are born with a weaker digestive system, stress and sickness inhibit their appetite. Excessive stress may cause a lack of appetite among the other body types as well. Yin Type B's are so sensitive, however, that even the slightest bit of stress with trigger a reduction of appetite.

Question Group C—Yang Type A

Question 1: According to Sasang medicine, Yin represents the downward movement of energy within the body, while Yang represents the upward movement. Yang types often have trouble taming their Yang energy, as it desires to go up, up, and away. Bowel movements help to release excess Yang from the body. If Yang Type A's skip bowel movements for a few days, pressure starts to accumulate due to blocked Yang energy, eventually leading to a situation referred to as "Yang rebellion" in which energy bursts upward, quickly causing headaches, abdominal pain, or other acute discomfort.

Question 2: Yang types tend to feel hotter and Yin types tend to feel colder because Yang corresponds to heat and Yin corresponds to cold. Sleep is a way to release excess tension and heat from the body. With so much heat already brewing within, Yang types often sweat or otherwise feel hot at night, as they release even more heat. Yang Type A's, therefore, usually sleep without the covers over their feet in order to stay cooler.

Question 3: Yang Type A's are very direct with others as a result of their tendency to be quick-witted and straight to the point without thinking of the consequences. At times this trait may give them the appearance of being tough, as they go straight for the gut. Otherwise, they may seem rash and impolite.

Question 4: Born with a stronger stomach, Yang Type A's need to eat often or consume hardy foods to keep their overactive digestive system busy. Hunger causes a rapid accumulation of stomach acid, or in Eastern medicine "stomach fire," which rebels upward and bombards the heart, leading to agitation and anger. Most of Yang Type A's digestive and emotional issues can be addressed by avoiding long stretches without food and eating body type–compatible foods.

Question 5: Yang Type A's are quick to judge others without truly giving them a chance. However, quick judgment also has its advantages. Quick-witted and wise Yang Type A's are superior at "figuring out" other people, making them often sought after for relationship advice. Yang Type A's appear intuitive to some and harsh to others.

Question 6: Yang also correlates with action, while Yin correlates with inaction. Therefore, Yang body types tend to become hyperactive and have a tendency to take on several tasks at once. While Yang types are good at multitasking, they tend not to focus on detail. Thus, Yang Type A's have a reputation of being too hasty.

Question 6b: Yang Type A's hastiness often leads to inaccuracy and inconsistency.

Question 7: Yang Type A's may easily grow impatient when things do not go their way. As a result Yang Type A's often appear angry. This explosive anger may be expressed toward one person or society at large. Yang Type A's must work to control their anger because, unchecked, it eventually morphs into acute sadness, which could eventually destroy their health.

Question 7b: The energy of Yang Type A's can be compared to a fire that flares up and burns out easily. The kidneys supply the body with consistent energy throughout the day. Since Yang Type A's are born with weaker kidneys, they often burn out in the evenings.

Question 8: Born with weaker kidneys, water retention is an issue for many Yang Type A's, who often gain water weight when fatigued. Excessive weight gain for them, however, is an issue related to urination, rather than fat accumulation. Although fat accumulation is less common for Yang Type A's than for other body types, it may nevertheless pose a challenge for them. The Yang Type A's fat and water accumulation tend to accumulate in areas that are not easily detectable with clothes on, such as the thighs, arms, chest, and ankles.

Question 9: Since Yang Type B's are born with weaker kidneys, they often lose fuel as the day progresses. Hence, they tend to be "morning people," or larks, rather than "evening people," or night owls.

Question 10: Shellfish, which is a cold-natured food, helps to quench the stomach heat of Yang Type A's, making it particularly appetizing for them.

Question Group D—Yang Type B

Question 1: Yang represents the upper body while Yin represents the lower body. The upper body of Yang types is better developed than the lower body, while the lower body of Yin types is better developed than the upper body. Yang Type B's have the most upper-body strength and development, compared to the other three types. Most Yang Type B's have a thicker neck and a larger head, out of proportion with the rest of their body.

Question 2: Yang moves upward, while Yin moves downward. The strong upward movement of Yang in Yang Type B's eventually causes the tips of their ears and head to become pointy.

Question 3: Yang Type B's have a stronger upper body and a weaker lower body. The weakness of the lower body, especially the hip area, causes a loss of balance and clumsiness. Yang Type B's often trip over their own feet!

Question 4: The more Yang you have, the less you are able to take orders from others. This is because Yang is active and ambitious, while Yin is inactive and apathetic. Yang Type B's have to be in charge and make the rules, rather than abiding by them. If they do not assume a leadership position, sickness and/or depression often ensue.

Question 5: Because the upper body of Yang types is more developed than the lower body, the neck and head of the Yang Type B also tend to accumulate more fat and muscle tissue, compared to other parts of the body.

Question 6: Yang Type B's are born with a weaker liver and gallbladder. The liver and gallbladder are in charge of breaking down fat from meat and other high-protein foods. Yang Type B's often vomit after eating meat because of their weak liver, which can easily get overwhelmed. As strange as it may seem, Yang Type B's rarely complain of indigestion, stomach pain, or other symptoms, despite the inability to keep meat down. Their body simply rejects and repels what it cannot handle.

Question 7: As natural-born leaders, Yang Type B's often come across as powerful and charismatic. Yet, they are at a loss when it comes to intimacy. Yang Type B's have trouble being courteous to their close friends or family members; they are often clueless when it comes to sustaining a close relationship, even though they make friends easily. Close friends and/or family members often complain about their domineering habits.

Question 8: Sadness is the predominant emotion of Yang Type B's because it is related to their strongest organ—the lungs. Yang Type B's often look and feel sad about everything.

Question 8b: If the Yang Type B's profound sadness gets out of hand, it will morph into explosive anger, which causes direct injury to their strongest organ, the lungs.

Question 9: Yang Type B's find more comfort being with larger groups than one-on-one with others. The larger the group, the better they feel. Unlike Yin Type A's, however, Yang Type B's prefer being in charge of rather than part of a group.

Question 10: The intuitive and ingenious nature of Yang Type B's is often admired by others. Without much thought, they can whip up a solution or solve a seemingly intractable problem. Sasang medicine equates this talent with their powerful sense of hearing. It is said that Yang Type B's have an almost supernatural ability to hear sounds that other body types cannot pick up on.

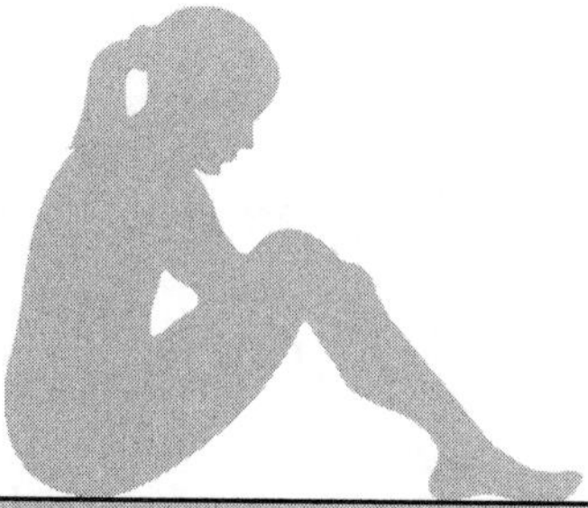

PART TWO

Emotional Balance and Your Yin Yang Body Type

The Four Virtues and Emotional Tendencies

Each body type has both advantageous and disadvantageous tendencies. The disadvantageous tendencies manifest more easily when we are not feeling well or we're in a difficult situation. For example, the tendency to feel angry will emerge in Yang Type A's when they are feeling low or when somebody hurts their feelings. When the going gets tough, Yang Type B's can easily push themselves and others too far. Under stress Yin Type A's tend to ignore their responsibilities and indulge in nonproductive activities. And, finally, Yin Type B's are likely to retreat into their own world, isolating themselves from others when they feel overwhelmed.

Our advantageous tendencies, also referred to as virtues, do not manifest as readily as their non-advantageous counterparts. The ancient Chinese scholar Confucius (550–470 BCE) based his entire philosophy on the concept of virtue. He posited that everyone has the potential to manifest their virtues, or optimal tendencies. However, this is not an easy process. While Yin Type B's have a compassionate nature, not all Yin Type B's are compassionate people. This compassion will simply lie dormant if no attempt is made to bring it to the fore. At the core of Confucian thought is also the idea of *su gi shin,* which translates as "polishing or cultivating one's mind and heart." Sometimes it takes tremendous effort to manifest our innate abilities.

When we are ill or experience trauma, it is even more challenging to reach inside and find our virtue. *Su gi shin* focuses on bringing out our innate strengths and overcoming our weaknesses. By practicing *su gi shin,* each body type is able to show the world its own virtue and pursue its intended path in life.

As we saw in part 1, each body type has a stronger and a weaker organ. These organs may be compared to planets that revolve around the sun. The sun can be compared to the human heart. The health of each organ depends on the heart with its radiant energy. According to Sasang medicine, the heart gives us the ability to make life-changing decisions, and plays a vital role in reaching inward and carrying out our *su gi shin.* The heart can also be likened to a mother who provides food for her children. If the children share willingly, food will be distributed proportionately and every child will stay healthy. However, the younger child will eventually grow weaker if the older or stronger child always snatches his or her food away. So it is with the heart and our stronger/weaker organs. Born with a stronger liver and weaker lung energy, Yin Type A's, through self-cultivation (*su gi shin*) and by overcoming their emotional weaknesses, send ample energy outward from the heart. This is akin to a mother who successfully tempers the excessive behavior of her children. The balanced heart of Yin Type A's encourages the smooth flow of energy from the stronger liver to the weaker lungs. If the heart is cluttered with stress or worry, then the stronger liver will gang up on the weaker lung.

Confucius also conceived the idea of the progressive person as opposed to the narrow-minded person as a model for *su gi shin.* Progressive people challenge their weaknesses by constantly making a sincere effort to become better human beings. Narrow-minded people let their weaknesses take over, finding delight or comfort in suppressing or belittling their humanity. Some of us are naturally gifted at identifying our own faults, while others may have no clue as to how we could improve. It is much easier to carry out *su gi shin* once we understand the various strengths and weaknesses of our body type. If you are not sure of these traits or would like to explore them further, keep reading! The following chapters introduce both the advantageous and non-advantageous aspects of each body type.

Sasang medicine is deeply embedded within Confucian philosophy, which introduces the concept of four virtues: righteousness, wisdom, humility, and compassion. According to Confucius the four virtues signify the highest level of spiritual attainment, which lies dormant in each individual until these virtues are discovered. According to Sasang medicine, balance and harmony are achieved by discovering our innate virtue through persistent self-reflection and mindful action. Lee Je-ma, the founder of Sasang medicine, correlated each of the four virtues with the four major organs—lungs, spleen, liver, and kidneys. Since each of the Yin Yang body types has a stronger organ, they will also have a natural affinity toward one of the four virtues. The discovery of our innate virtue is the ultimate goal of Sasang medicine and Confucian philosophy. Along with virtue, however, is the innate inclination toward unbalanced emotion, which is ignited by stress and trauma. This inclination results in the obstruction and occasional outburst of energy flow, causing injury to the organs. The attainment of virtue is not a momentary accomplishment. Rather, it is an ongoing effort yielding an unshakable state of being that remains untouched by negative experience.

The emotional tendencies of each body type are also related to the relative strengths and weaknesses of their organs. To manifest virtue each body type is faced with the challenge of balancing their innate emotional tendencies. The predominant temperament is the most influential of these emotional tendencies, which can either make or break one's ability to manifest their inner virtue.

The following section is divided into the four body types (Yin Type A, Yin Type B, Yang Type A, and Yang Type B). As virtue does not manifest on its own but is the product of ceaseless sincerity and self-reflection, each body type virtue is followed by the description of a balanced and an unbalanced state. The unbalanced state is when our virtue lies dormant as we fail to recognize and act accordingly. The balanced state is when we recognize our virtue and carry it out through sincere action.

Each emotional tendency also includes both innately positive and innately negative aspects, also referred to below as unbalanced and balanced states. The unbalanced state is when we choose not to act or bring out our positive traits. The balanced state is achieved when we recognize and do our best to bring out our positive traits. The path toward optimum health depends on recognizing our flaws and making an effort to achieve balance in our lives.

Yin Type A
Emotional Balance

KEY TRAITS

Strongest Organ: Liver
Strongest Sense: Smell
Innate/Inborn Virtue: *Eui* (Righteousness)
Inherent Abilities: *In Yun*—the ability to make the right choices and manage things correctly; Yin Type A's can "smell a rat" when things start to go sour

Dang Yo—the ability to associate with others who have similar goals and ideas; this trait is associated with a strong liver.

Predominant Temperament: Complacency

RIGHTEOUSNESS—THE VIRTUE OF *EUI*

Righteousness (or *eui* in Korean) is the strongest virtue of Yin Type A's because it is associated with their strongest organ, the liver. With a strong liver, they have the potential to be extraordinarily righteous. Confucius saw righteousness as the ability to make wise decisions; this ability is called *in yun* in Korean. This virtue, which lies dormant within the liver, is activated through self-cultivation and self-reflection. Even non-virtuous Yin Type A's have a strong sense of whether or not other people are righteous, despite their own shortcomings. *Eui* is the Yin Type A's key to unlocking the door to the other three virtues: wisdom, humility, and compassion.

UNBALANCED STATE Unrighteous Yin Type A's will make decisions and choices based on selfishness. They choose wealth and profit over relationships and spirituality, accumulating wealth and power while becoming more and more arrogant. These individuals may also strive so hard to gain power and wealth that they forget about those close to them. These Yin Type A's take advantage of others through their inherent *in yun,* rather than tapping into *in yun* to make righteous choices.

BALANCED STATE Righteous Yin Type A's are excellent at rationing their belongings. Even though they may enjoy power and luxury, righteous Yin Type A's make it their priority for others to savor the good things in life as well. While becoming prosperous themselves, they give others the same opportunity. Balanced Yin Type A's may not necessarily be affluent or financially powerful, but they believe that empowering others by giving and sharing is the right thing to do.

EMOTIONAL TENDENCIES

Getting Started

Yin Type A's are very reliable but also very set in their ways. Once they put their mind to something, they pursue it to the end. However, Yin Type A's also have a complacent temperament that, if not balanced, can lead to procrastination and choosing the easy way out.

UNBALANCED STATE Yin Type A's may take one of two approaches to get things started. In the first scenario, they launch into a project easily but don't know when to stop. They have a tendency to keep going, becoming addicted to exercise and/or work. In the second scenario, Yin Type A's give in to their lazy nature. They are reluctant to carry out their responsibilities, indulging in leisure rather than working hard. Because they have a strong liver, these individuals may succumb to addictive behavior, such as excessive eating, drinking, and/or smoking.

BALANCED STATE In Korean there is a saying that "by getting started you are already halfway there." The persistent Yin Type A who continuously makes an effort to take the first step will often become successful in life.

Trust Issues

The Yin Type A battles constantly with issues of trust. Can I trust her? Why doesn't he trust me? Such questions constantly prey on the mind of Yin Type A's. In Eastern medicine, relationships are said to be established via lung energy. Since the lungs take in and exhale air, they are also responsible for letting in and letting go of relationships and material possessions.

Did You Know?

In Korean the character for trust, 信, is pronounced as *shin.* On the left side of the character are two lines, one holding up the other. This signifies interdependence. The right side signifies speech. Combined together, this character literally translates as the conversation between two fundamentally connected individuals.

UNBALANCED STATE Since the lungs of Yin Type A's are the weakest organ in the body, relationships are a continuous challenge for them. Yin Type A's find themselves either trusting their partner and/or friends too much or not trusting them at all.

BALANCED STATE Yin Type A's naturally desire harmony and balance in their relationships but often wind up feeling victimized by them. Balanced Yin Type A's challenge themselves not to play the victim in relating to others, as they constantly wonder whether or not to trust them. They realize that by believing in themselves, they can believe in others.

Close Friends

Yin Type A's have a natural inclination to form and join groups of like personalities. In Korean this tendency is referred to as *dang yo.* Yin

Type A's often become active members of religious societies and/or social groups.

The ability to gather and unite others with similar interests is a special talent of Yin Type A's. Large and successful enterprises and corporations are often formed by these individuals. However, if *dang yo* is taken to the extreme, Yin Type A's will come to mistrust others who think differently or do not join their group. Such a Yin Type A is often ridiculed by others for being too narrow-minded.

UNBALANCED STATE Unbalanced Yin Type A's only wish is to meet those who think like them and view other cultures, religions, and ideas with prejudice. These individuals may also try to get others to think and believe just like them, and disdain or act against those with different belief systems. Unbalanced Yin Type A's might also join groups that mirror and promote their own unbalanced views.

BALANCED STATE While Yin Type A's are naturally talented at forming like-minded groups, they benefit from accepting other groups with different ways of thinking. Rather than looking upon these individuals as enemies, balanced Yin Type A's focus on respecting their opinions. Accepting the opinions of others helps to strengthen and broaden the Yin Type A's perspective.

Faith and Commitment

Faith often manifests differently, according to each body type. By nature Yin is embracing while Yang is expanding. Yin types often feel the need to embrace or adopt others' viewpoints while Yang types generally feel the need to spread their own beliefs. Yang body types also emphasize faith in themselves while Yin types tend to place faith in others and/or a higher being. Yin Type A's are usually the most faithful of the four body types. They often choose to follow the guidance of a husband, wife, elder, priest, rabbi, or the like. Balanced Yin Type A's draw on wisdom and skill in choosing where to place their faith. The blind faith of unbalanced Yin Type A's often leads to trouble.

UNBALANCED STATE If they are not careful, Yin Type A's may fall victim to cultlike or radical religious beliefs. The faithful Yin Type A wife or mother may not consider her own feelings when things get out of hand at home. Too much faith in and commitment to others may interfere with the Yin Type A's own well-being. Yang body types, by contrast, have difficulty complying with others, tending to take faith in their own hands.

BALANCED STATE History has proven that a lot can be accomplished through faith. Michelangelo's paintings on the ceiling of the Sistine Chapel most likely resulted from such steadfast faith. Faith, in this sense, is not necessarily related to religion. Michelangelo's magnificent work was said to spring from strong drive and tremendous willpower. The balanced Yin Type A feels a strong sense of responsibility through faith. Like Michelangelo, Yin Type A's may work diligently and tirelessly for their cause. However, balanced Yin Type A's balance faith with wisdom. They often examine their faith and reflect on what they truly believe in. The sincere and devoted Yin Type A neither loses faith easily nor stubbornly clings to it.

Sense of Smell—A Sniff of Trust

Smell is the strongest sense of Yin Type A's. According to Sasang medicine, Yin Type A's smell their way through life. Expressions such as "That smells fishy" or "I can smell him from a mile away" reflect how Yin Type A's relate to others.

UNBALANCED STATE Since Yin Type A's are so sensitive to odor, they often cannot be around or ingest things that smell unappealing or unappetizing. Some Yin Type A's even need to stay away from others or avoid going outdoors to steer clear of disagreeable smells or allergens. According to Sasang medicine, this is a reflection of unbalanced lung energy, the lungs being the Yin Type A's weakest organ.

BALANCED STATE Balanced Yin Type A's are fully aware of having a sensitive sense of smell. Instead of avoiding others and staying indoors, they make every effort to overcome their hypersensitivities. Using their sense of smell to understand more about the world, they don't let weaker lungs inhibit their ability to explore and take chances. Even though it may not seem tempting at first sniff, balanced Yin Type A's may try a not-so-delicious-smelling food if it promises to improve their health.

Did You Know?

A study conducted by Wedekind suggests that we can actually use our sense of smell to find our perfect partner.* In this study women were given T-shirts that were worn by men with a variety of DNA patterns. When asked which smell was most appealing, the women in this study chose the shirt worn by men with DNA patterns that were significantly different from their own. The researchers concluded that this was because more DNA variety between parents results in healthier children. Interestingly, when they performed this test in the same study with women who were taking birth control pills, the opposite result occurred! This suggests that when a woman's body is not prepared to get pregnant, she seeks to be around those with DNA similar to her own (such as her parents or close friends). This study may offer further evidence regarding the Yin Type A's ability to "smell" relationships.

*Wedekind, Claus, Thomas Seebeck, Florence Bettens, and Alexander J. Paepke, "MHC-Dependent Mate Preferences in Humans." *Proceedings: Biological Sciences/The Royal Society* 260, no.1359 (June 1995): 245–49.

Public Affairs

Most Yin Type A's naturally appear relaxed, easygoing, and down-to-earth. This comes with a price, however. When Yin Type A's need to make quick decisions and work with a tight schedule, they end up with the short end of the stick because they are most comfortable working on their own time and schedule. Punctuality is certainly not the Yin Type A's forte.

UNBALANCED STATE Unbalanced Yin Type A's are always late for work. They put the left shoe on the right foot and leave their zipper undone before rushing out of the house. When they are given responsibility, something always seems to get in the way of starting the task. They'd much rather sleep the day away or run away from responsibility than face life's challenges.

BALANCED STATE Yin Type A's are constantly challenging themselves to play by the rules. Waking up early and getting to sleep before 11:00 p.m. are particularly difficult. By challenging themselves to be more punctual and active, Yin Type A's will, without a doubt, live healthier and happier lives. Balanced Yin Type A's may not even be aware of having a lax nature as they make punctuality a priority.

Night Owl

According to Eastern philosophy, Yin represents night while Yang represents day. Yin body types are more active in the evening while Yang body types are more active during the day. Therefore, Yin Type A's tend to enjoy staying up late. In Eastern medicine the energy of the body is said to shift from one organ to the other every two hours. From 11:00 p.m. to 1:00 a.m., the gallbladder is most active. This organ helps facilitate creative thinking and imagination. If we get to sleep before 11:00, creativity and imagination find expression through dreaming. If we stay up past 11:00, creativity and imagination are enhanced during our waking hours. This may make for an all-nighter or at least a very restless evening! For some, this may be the only time they have to themselves. It may be a valuable time devoted to creative thinking and activity. Staying up past 11:00 p.m. now and then does not interfere with the health of Yin Type A's. It may offer them a chance to write, paint, Photoshop, reflect, or simply unwind.

UNBALANCED STATE Unbalanced Yin Type A's are addicted to staying up late. If this becomes a daily habit, their health may be compromised. They may eventually feel tired and sluggish during the day. It is also common for Yin Type A night owls to gain weight. This is because the body's metabolism is most active in the morning and slows down in the evening. Early-morning activity promotes a quicker metabolism, but is often unappealing for those whose energy peaks in the wee hours.

BALANCED STATE Being aware of this tendency and making a firm decision to get to bed early helps promote energy and overall health. Balanced Yin Type A's may occasionally take advantage of enhanced creativity after 11:00 p.m., but they usually aim for an earlier bedtime.

Let It Flow by Letting Go

Yin Type A's have a strong ability to absorb food, fluid, and emotion. According to Yin Yang theory, Yin is associated with absorption while Yang is associated with dispersion. Yang types tend to excrete food, fluid, and emotion much more easily than Yin types. Yin Type A's have a harder time than the other body types letting things go.

UNBALANCED STATE Unbalanced Yin Type A's may gain weight after eating just a few bites of food or drinking a few sips of water. This is because they hold on to every little ounce of food or fluid intake. For this reason constipation is a common occurrence when a Yin Type A's health starts going south. Weight gain is not an issue for all unbalanced Yin Type A's. Other issues, such as difficulty letting emotions go and holding on to the past, may also reflect excess absorption. Thus, Yin Type A's may find it hard to overcome a grudge and/or anger toward someone, or continuously fret over something that has happened to them.

BALANCED STATE Balanced Yin Type A's make a sincere and persistent effort to keep things flowing smoothly. Diet regulation is an important and effective way to keep Yin Type A's balanced and healthy, especially if they eat easily digested and metabolically stimulating foods. Emotionally, they learn to let things go and not get to them. The Yin Type A's powerful absorption is not a bad trait in itself. Balanced Yin Type A's may choose to absorb the love and warmth of others. Stronger absorption may also lead to higher energy levels, allowing the body to hold on to and utilize its energy for longer periods. Healthy Yin Type A's establish a balance between food intake and exercise, while readily absorbing the suffering of others without feeling overwhelmed or distraught as they try to offer help and comfort.

Cheerfulness and Complacency

According to Sasang medicine, each body type has a corresponding predominant temperament, which is often expressed in a subtle way. Occasionally, the predominant temperament may get out of control, leading to an explosive emotional reaction. Complacency, for example, is the predominant temperament of the Yin Type A, and is active pretty much all the time. The ability to remain calm, laid back, and/or relaxed are reflections of complacency. When the Yin Type A's complacency gets out of control, it has a tendency to explode into excessive cheerfulness. Being out of touch, going insane, and/or having a warped sense of joy are examples of excessive cheerfulness. When taken to the extreme, complacency and cheerfulness have a tendency to morph into each other. When this happens Yin Type A's may attempt to escape from their circumstances, finding joy in isolation or in making others suffer instead. However, in the end, explosive complacency is most damaging to none other than Yin Type A's themselves, leading to self-inflicted pain and/or hardship.

UNBALANCED STATE Unbalanced Yin Type A's refuse to acknowledge situations that do not make them feel comfortable and joyful. This refusal is based on selfishness and an unrealistic outlook on life. While unbalanced Yin Type A's rarely lose a total sense of reality, they still tend to brush off difficult situations, refusing to accept responsibility for their actions. Complacency quickly gets out of control for Yin Type A's, and others may lose patience with their nonchalant and sometimes inappropriately cheerful nature.

BALANCED STATE In Eastern medicine each emotion has both positive and negative potential. Complacency, which comes from the strongest organ of Yin Type A's, the liver, can make or break their health. Since complacency comes naturally to them, it cannot be simply ignored. Suppressing complacency could injure the liver. When complacency in Yin Type A's is expressed in a positive way, it gives them a special ability to help others find humor in the face of despair. Humor can be extremely healing and beneficial in situations that make us feel trapped and lost. Balanced Yin Type A's help others laugh off their frustrations and anger. Their relaxed nature also helps others feel calm and at ease in the midst of troubles. Balanced Yin Type A's set these skills in motion to overcome difficult situations, rather than escaping from them. They are aware of their susceptibility to excessive complacency, and therefore make a sincere effort to become more active and responsible.

Habitual and Addictive Behavior

The strength of the hands corresponds to the energy of the liver. Born with a stronger liver, Yin Type A's often have exceptionally well-developed hands, which are a great source of talent and skill. But the hands may also be the culprit behind habitual or addictive behavior. Excessive eating, drinking, and smoking all involve habitual movement of the hands, making addiction a serious issue for Yin Type A's. Habitual behavior may work in favor of or against the well-being of Yin Type A's. This depends on the extent to which Yin Type A's have cultivated their inner potential and virtue.

UNBALANCED STATE If they're stressed, upset, or under the weather, Yin Type A's may resort to unhealthy habits. Most heavy smokers and drinkers, for example, are Yin Type A's. When the body is not in balance, it tends to crave further imbalance. Unbalanced Yin Type A's need to make twice the effort of other body types to overcome self-destructive habits. Many Yin Type A smokers and drinkers often mention that they reach for a drink or cigarette without even being aware of it. This is because the hands of Yin Type A's engage in habitual behavior. The hands can develop incredible skill or, on the contrary, create further imbalance for the Yin Type A. Keep in mind that while not all unbalanced Yin Type A's are addicted to smoking or drinking, they may form other unhealthy habits, such as binge-eating, craving certain unhealthy foods, and/or indulging in self-destructive behaviors.

BALANCED STATE Fully aware of their tendency to engage in addictive behaviors, balanced Yin Type A's habitually pursue productive behaviors, such as waking up early, exercising or meditating daily, and developing their inborn talents.

Addictive Behavior and Yin Type A's

The strongest organ of each body type is often the cause of imbalance, while the weakest organ suffers the effect. This can be compared to a powerful aristocrat who leeches money and resources from the common people. Because the liver is the Yin Type A's strongest organ, it is particularly sensitive to stress. This causes Yin Type A's to become obsessive and engage in habitual behavior.

Since the lungs are the weakest organ of Yin Type A's, they tend to be the scapegoat of obsession and habitual behavior. Hence, smoking addiction is most common among Yin Type A's and will quickly destroy their health. Signs and symptoms, though, may not be present in the early phase of smoking. As time goes on, Yin Type A's may start to notice their blood pressure going up, plus increasing shortness of breath and/or emphysema. If Yin Type A's start to cough or get congested after smoking, this is a sign that they need to stop sooner rather than later.

The susceptibility of Yin Type A's to habitual behavior can contribute considerably to a smoking addiction and this also makes it challenging for them to quit. They may have a strong desire to quit smoking but still have trouble no matter how hard they try. Yin Type A smokers often claim that they automatically reach for a cigarette without even being fully aware of it. Others may claim they hate smoking but just can't seem to kick the habit of placing a cigarette in their mouth. While some Yin Type A's may have the willpower to quit smoking cold turkey, many do not. It can sometimes be effective to work *with* habitual behavior rather than against it by transforming a self-destructive habit into a positive one. Reaching for a healthy low-calorie snack rather than a cigarette, for instance, may help the Yin Type A smoker quit.

Most of us know that excessive alcohol consumption directly affects the health of the liver. The stronger liver of Yin Type A's is not a free pass to drink excessively, however. While most healthy Yin Type A's can drink more alcohol than other body types without suffering a hangover or other adverse side effects, this is not necessarily a good thing. Pain and discomfort are the body's way of signaling the brain that something somewhere in the body is not happy. This signal directs us to health-affirming decisions. Without such signals Yin Type A's often drink until their liver becomes acutely congested. The excessive Yin Type A drinker will eventually wind up with elevated liver enzyme levels or other tangible liver health issues. Breaking the habit of drinking is just as challenging as quitting smoking, both of which are reflections of the Yin Type A's habitual tendencies. It takes courage and conviction to overcome such habits. As mentioned before Yin Type A's are born with a strong sense of *dang yo*—the ability to associate with others who have similar goals and ideas. Since Yin Type A's have a tendency to adapt easily to their social surroundings, they must choose appropriate friends. It is particularly difficult for Yin Type A's to quit drinking if their friends like to drink. Beware, my dear Yin Type A readers, of such friendly but not so healthy friendships!

Yin Type B
Emotional Balance

KEY TRAITS

Strongest Organ: Kidneys
Strongest Sense: Taste
Innate/Inborn Virtue: *Ji* (Wisdom)
Inherent Abilities: *Ji Bang* (Earth + Direction)—this gives Yin Type B's the ability to plan and take appropriate action
Go Cho—strong kidneys enable Yin Type B's to make others feel comfortable, secure, and at home
Predominant Temperament: Cheerfulness

WISDOM—THE VIRTUE OF *JI*

Wisdom, or *ji* in Korean, is the strongest inherent virtue of Yin Type B's, which is associated with their strongest organ, the kidneys. Confucius saw this virtue as signifying the wisdom needed to decipher the appropriate time and place to take action. This ability is called *ji bang* (earth + direction) in Korean. The virtue of *ji* also gives Yin Type B's a strong philosophical foundation, providing a valuable sense of meaning and purpose in their lives. *Ji* contributes to the Yin Type B's superior ability to plan, strategize, and help others navigate out of difficult situations. The wisdom of Yin Type B's, however, does not manifest automatically. It is activated through their sincere effort to express love and compassion, which are the strongest inherent virtues of Yang Type B's. The expression of love and compassion and the manifestation of *ji* are the keys that unlock the door to the other two virtues: humility and righteousness.

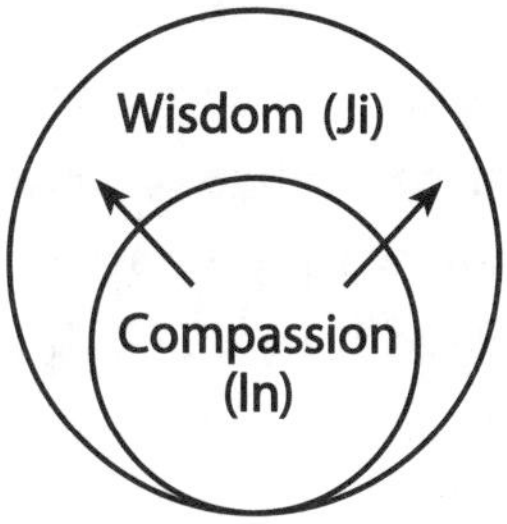

Figure 2.1. Yin Type B's wisdom is activated by compassion

UNBALANCED STATE Unbalanced Yin Type B's do not tap into their innate wisdom and have difficulty making even minor decisions. These poor souls rely heavily on assistance from others, as fear and timidity block their innate wisdom from manifesting.

BALANCED STATE Balanced Yin Type B's make a sincere effort to overcome fear, timidity, and their inherently reclusive nature. They make it a priority to assist others who are going through hard times or have difficulty finding their way. With a profound sense of wisdom and direction from the virtue of *ji,* this almost always results in success.

EMOTIONAL TENDENCIES

Hospitality

In Eastern medicine Yin represents calmness, comfort, and coziness, while Yang signifies anxiety, activity, and a sense of being unsettled. Being comfortable and cozy is always a priority for Yin Type B's, who can be compared to a cat circling its resting place several times before finding the perfect position.

UNBALANCED STATE Unbalanced Yin Type B's think only about their own comfort and security while ignoring the needs of others. They often develop obsessive behaviors, such as excessively washing their hands, or agoraphobia, the fear of leaving their home.

BALANCED STATE Balanced Yin Type B's make it their priority to help others feel comfortable, secure, and at home. This ability is called *go cho* in Korean. *Go cho* depends on the strength of the kidneys. Born with stronger kidneys, Yin Type B's have the capacity to be wonderfully hospitable and comforting. This is because the kidneys are referred to as the mother organ in Eastern medicine, coming to the rescue, and supporting all the other organs when they are in distress. From a biological perspective, cortisol, released from the kidneys, gives us extra strength to escape or plow through challenging situations.

Sense of Taste—Digesting Food and Experience

Yin Type B's strongest organ, the kidneys, corresponds to taste. This sense is so acute that if Yin Type B's place something in their mouth, they will often know right away whether or not it can be digested. This sensitivity is what protects the Yin Type B's weak digestive system. A sensitivity to taste is not always associated with food. Getting into an argument or meeting an unpleasant person may leave a "bad taste" in your mouth. Yin Type B's explore their world through taste, so an unpleasant situation will literally taste terrible to them. Stress immediately affects the digestive system of Yin Type B's, causing a lack of appetite and/or indigestion. The ability to plan and take action, associated with *ji bang,* is also a result of the Yin Type B's sensitive taste.

UNBALANCED STATE With such an acute sense of taste, Yin Type B's may be afraid to eat almost anything! Since they explore their world through the sense of taste, this may lead them to become cowardly and excessively shy as well. Without challenging themselves to overcome this sensitivity, they will also succumb to illness and emaciation. The unbalanced Yin Type B has to realize that not everything has to be done with perfect "taste."

BALANCED STATE Balanced Yin Type B's make an attempt to expand their food intake, becoming more adventuresome. They try different flavors, even if those flavors seem a bit weird at first. As they explore diverse flavors become more and more pleasant. Not only does this help their digestive system, but it also increases their courage and confidence. In this case the sensitivity to taste can be used to their advantage. Those who get acquainted with balanced Yin Type B's often admire their good sense of taste. Taste can also be understood as the ability to discern the appropriate time and place to take action. Choosing appropriate friends, the perfect outfit, or the right partner may be thanks to a good sense of taste. This is the merit of *ji bang.*

Location, Location, Location!

Yin Type B's always like to feel comfortable and at home, a trait also associated with the strength of the kidneys. In Korean this sensitivity is called *go cho,* which literally means "arranging the home." The kidneys are considered the "home" of the body's energy. All energy emerges from the kidneys in order to travel to the other organs. Yin Type B's like to stay close to home, which is where they feel the most energetic. They devote a lot of energy to making their environment comfortable and appealing, often keeping their home beautiful and spotless.

UNBALANCED STATE Because of this sensitivity, Yin Type B's may be afraid to leave home. Home is the only place where they feel comfortable. Leaving home may induce anxiety and fear for unbalanced Yin Type B's. As time goes on, they will likely become less and less social and more isolated from others.

BALANCED STATE It is beneficial for Yin Type B's to associate with others and leave the comfort of their home. This will help them develop courage, strength, and understanding. Yet the desire to stay close to home is not all that bad! A natural sense of home being a place of comfort makes Yin Type B's more family oriented and hospitable. If they learn to balance this sensitivity, Yin Type B's can get the best of both worlds.

Frog Living in a Well

With a shy and timid nature, the Yin Type B often has trouble coping in the real world. While some Yin Type B's challenge themselves to become more social and to succeed in society, others isolate themselves further. The Yin Type B can be compared to a frog living in a well. The frog is content inside the well, surrounded by concrete walls, living on his own small lily pad. But if another frog enters the well, he feels threatened and hops away. Yin Type B's are very content living in their own world, as long as that world is not threatened by outside forces.

UNBALANCED STATE Unbalanced Yin Type B's are surrounded by a fortress of fantasy and fabrication. Lying, or stretching the truth "just a bit," becomes a way to achieve their dreams. In the extreme state, Yin Type B's may eventually experience delusions or hallucinations. Be aware of the Yin Type B liar! They are the best at persuading others because they often believe their own lies.

BALANCED STATE Balanced Yin Type B's are able to turn their fantasy world into reality through writing, painting, and/or other artistic pursuits. With such a tremendous imagination, the Yin Type B can become quite the storyteller! By feeling as if this is their mission, Yin Type B's can promote the imagination and ideals of others around them.

Willpower

The Yin Type B's kidneys are equated with willpower, which they have an abundance of, even with a frail and weak appearance. Once Yin Type B's make up their mind, they are very determined or even obsessed with achieving their goals.

UNBALANCED STATE Extreme willpower leads to stubbornness and narrow-mindedness. Yin Type B's need to be cautious about obstinately proceeding in the wrong direction. Even if things are going the wrong way, it is difficult for Yin Type B's to turn around and start again. Unbalanced Yin Type B's may become so obsessed with accomplishment that they become delusional and detached from reality.

BALANCED STATE For balanced Yin Type B's, the will to succeed runs as deep as the ocean. Once they have their mind set on a goal, Yin Type B's keep going and going, like the Energizer Bunny. Strong willpower, balanced by a deep sense of wisdom, can help Yin Type B's overcome their limitations and become successful in life.

Oh the Cold!

Yin Type B's have the least Yang of all the other body types. Since heat is a Yang trait, Yin Type B's are the most sensitive to cold. Cold weather and foods tend to affect the weak digestive system of Yin Type B's. The winter is the harshest time for many Yin Type B's. During this season they tend to get stomachaches, stomach flu, and diarrhea. They usually dream of traveling to warmer places or hanging out inside a sauna during the wintertime. Spicy foods and warm tea greatly comfort Yin Type B's.

UNBALANCED STATE A strong sensitivity to cold may cause Yin Type B's to huddle indoors during the cold weather. To a certain extent this may help them avoid getting colds and succumbing to indigestion. However, in the long run this leads to further isolation, insecurity, and a weakened immune system.

BALANCED STATE Yin Type B's can benefit from bundling up and getting outdoors in the cold weather. Outdoor sports, such as skiing or sleigh riding, could help improve circulation to the digestive organs. Exercising will also help keep the Yin Type B's body warm in the winter. Warmth helps Yin Type B's feel healthy and balanced.

Fear

In Eastern medicine each organ of the body corresponds to a particular emotion. Fear is associated with the kidneys. Since Yin Type B's have strong kidneys, they also have a strong tendency to be fearful. They fear leaving home and exposing themselves to others and the environment.

UNBALANCED STATE Unbalanced Yin Type B's let fear take over, feeling shy and fearful when interacting with others. They may also be paranoid about others trying to attack or harm them. Staying home, and isolating themselves from others, is the only way unbalanced Yin Type B's can feel somewhat comfortable. In certain situations they may be aware of their fear and try to overcome it by making irrational decisions. They may deliberately put themselves in harm's way just to prove that it is possible to overcome fear. Making extreme decisions like this could cause more harm than good for Yin Type B's, since they are so sensitive. This behavior could set them back and make them even more fearful.

BALANCED STATE Balanced Yin Type B's have the discernment to know when to fear and when not to fear. They are cautious about situations that may actually harm them but still willing to take chances and challenge their fears. Balanced Yin Type B's devote themselves to making new friends, trying new foods, and/or traveling to new places. With their heightened sensitivity, they work to challenge their fears in a gentle and harmonious way without making extreme decisions.

I Am a Delicate Butterfly!

Yin Type B's have a predominantly feminine nature, which manifests itself whether they are male or female. The Female Yin Type B has the most feminine nature, compared to other body types. She exhibits various womanly body and facial features, which bring out her beauty, but also make her look somewhat delicate and frail. A Male Yin Type B often associates more easily with women than with men and rarely enjoys engaging in masculine activities. He may also identify more easily with the viewpoint of female friends and family members. Don't let the Yin Type B's appearance fool you! Both males and females of this body type may look frail on the outside but are often strong on the inside. Frail-looking butterflies may sway left and right as the wind blows, but despite a challenging journey, they usually make it to their destination. With strong willpower, frail-looking Yin Type B's keep plugging along!

UNBALANCED STATE Unbalanced Yin Type B's are extremely feminine, to the point of avoiding anything masculine. The unbalanced female may refuse to hang out with or date men, while the unbalanced male may never engage in or enjoy the company of other males. This reminds me of an interesting conversation that I had with a Yin Type B friend while eating at a restaurant. After just a few bites, she started talking about how all men are "evil, power-hungry monsters!" I felt a bit uncomfortable being a male myself, but was reassured to know that she could confide in me as a fellow Yin Type B.

BALANCED STATE Balanced Yin Type B's utilize their feminine side to offer sympathy and gentle care when it is needed the most. They are soft-spoken, having the capability of soothing even the most extreme emotion. Their feminine nature does not stop them from standing up for themselves when appropriate. Even in a position of authority, they never fail to be gentle in dealing with their subordinates. Approximately five hundred years ago in Korea, there lived a powerful general who helped his country win several battles against an army several times the size of his. It is said that he was a Yin Type B who, instead of using brute strength, mastered the art of war through strategy and wisdom. These are Yin Type B traits that, if brought to the fore through self-reflection, can yield powerful results.

Cheerfulness and Obsession

Occasionally, a body type's predominant temperament may get out of control, leading to an explosive emotional reaction. Cheerfulness, which is associated with their strongest organ, the kidneys, is the predominant temperament of Yin Type B's, and they feel this way almost all the time. Yin Type B's make it a priority to be cheerful and happy-go-lucky. While there is a place for happiness and cheerfulness, these emotions can be taken too far. When the Yin Type B's cheerfulness gets out of control, it can explode into obsession and impracticality. The pursuit of happiness takes control of them as they crave the feeling of accomplishment and satisfaction. If their goals do not come to fruition, the Yin Type B's cheerfulness morphs into mockery and ridicule of others, as they laugh at others' shortcomings. It may also interfere with the Yin Type B's sense of reality, as they escape into their own cheerful fantasy world. In the end explosive complacency is most damaging to Yin Type B's themselves, leading to self-inflicted suffering and/or hardship.

UNBALANCED STATE Unbalanced Yin Type B's refuse to leave the house or to socialize with others. This refusal is based on an obsession with cheerfulness, which is easier for them to feel when they're alone. They may occasionally think about others and desire to spend time with them, but in the end they fail to take action. Unbalanced Yin Type B's have difficulty overcoming a shy and cowardly nature and instead dive into further isolation, making excuse after excuse to be alone. Isolation and comfort quickly get out of control for the reclusive Yin Type B, who finds it easy to lose touch with reality and fall into the abyss of delusion. In a delusional state, Yin Type B's appear excessively cheerful and giggly when they're alone, for they live in their own little world. This world, however, is completely disconnected from their surroundings. Extreme cheerfulness, in this case, eats away at their strongest organ, the kidneys.

BALANCED STATE Balanced Yin Type B's are aware of their excessive desire for cheerfulness, and realize that they do not live in an isolated fantasy world. They make a sincere effort to become more sociable by interacting with others and leaving their safety zone. Striving for success and achievement of their goals becomes a source of pleasure and cheerfulness, rather than focusing on just the outcome itself. Balanced Yin Type B's draw on their kidney energy to help others feel comfortable and cheerful, but do not fall victim to their own inclinations. They also utilize time alone to renew their energy and conduct self-reflection, rather than completely isolating themselves.

Yang Type A Emotional Balance

KEY TRAITS

Strongest Organ: Spleen
Strongest Sense: Sight
Innate/Inborn Virtue: *Ye* (Humility)
Inherent Abilities: *Sei Wei*—inherent social skill; in Sasang medicine social skill is a trait controlled by the spleen
Kyo Wu—the ability to treat others with respect and humility
Predominant Temperament: Anger

HUMILITY—THE VIRTUE OF *YE*

Humility, or *ye* in Korean, is the strongest virtue of Yang Type A's because it is associated with their strongest organ, the spleen. Since Yang Type A's are born with a strong spleen, they have the potential to be extremely humble and courteous to others. According to Confucius humility also signifies the ability to choose our friends and treat them appropriately. This virtue, which lies dormant in the spleen of Yang Type A's, is activated only through self-cultivation and self-reflection. However, even the non-virtuous Yang Type A has a strong sense of whether or not others are humble or courteous. While social skill comes naturally to them, they still need to develop the ability to feel comfortable in a group setting. This ability comes naturally to the Yin Type A, but not to the Yang Type A. Accordingly, the Yin and Yang body types have a lot to offer each other. Cultivating this Yin Type A skill will inevitably bring out the Yang Type A's true colors.

UNBALANCED STATE Without manifesting their humility, Yang Type A's look down on others, treating them as subordinates rather than equals. They become excessively judgmental of others, criticizing them for inappropriate reasons.

BALANCED STATE Balanced Yang Type A's make an effort to treat others with respect and modesty. Once Yang Type A's do this, they are often sought after for friendship and guidance. This is due to their distinctive ability to interact one-on-one with and understand others.

EMOTIONAL TENDENCIES

The Social Type

Yang Type A's have a natural ability to socialize with others and make friends. These skills surpass that of other body types. It is common for others to seek friendship with Yang Type A's because they are gifted at expressing themselves and getting acquainted with others. The social skills of Yang Type A's come from an inborn trait called *sei wei,* in Korean, which refers to the ability to discover one's societal role. Yang Type A's have a keen understanding of friendship and their role as a friend, son, daughter, mother, and so on. In Sasang medicine *sei wei* is a trait that is derived from the strength of the spleen, the Yang Type A's strongest organ. Yang Type A's also have the innate ability to understand and sympathize with others. Compared to the other body types, it is easier for Yang Type A's to meet and socialize with others, even if they have different opinions. This ability, called *kyo wu* in Korean, is also associated with the Yang Type A's strong spleen. However, strength is not necessarily equated with skill. The Yang Type A must foster and cultivate these strengths to manifest them appropriately.

UNBALANCED STATE Unbalanced Yang Type A's use friendship as a means to assert their authority over others. They purposely choose friends they can take advantage of and sway. Others are lured in by the Yang Type A's social savvy. Yet, these friends will eventually feel betrayed once they get close to an unbalanced Yang Type A. Since social skills are the Yang Type A's strength, gossip spreads quickly among them. Unbalanced Yang Type A's have difficulty knowing what to share with others and what to keep to themselves.

BALANCED STATE Balanced Yang Type A's treat others with respect and humility. They are both straightforward and sincere when it comes to friendship. They are careful not to offend others but, at the same time, get their point across. Balanced Yang Type A's look after their friends at all times.

Sense of Sight—External Focus

Yang Type A's tend to be extroverted. They devote most, if not all, of their energy to work and friendship. It is a challenge for them to focus inwardly and on household affairs. Yang Type A's are quite intuitive, often making quick-witted decisions to accomplish their outward-focused goals.

UNBALANCED STATE Unbalanced Yang Type A's lose touch with their inner self. They immerse themselves into everyday life, often collapsing from exhaustion by the end of the day. There is little room for family or household chores when the Yang Type A is unbalanced.

BALANCED STATE Balanced Yang Type A's take time out of their busy life to relax and meditate. They deliberately slow down their thoughts, breathe, and reach inward for guidance. They are devoted mothers, fathers, and caregivers, establishing a healthy balance between work and family. Balanced Yang Type A's also take the time to replenish their energies, exercise, and get enough sleep.

Straightforwardness

Yang Type A's may sometimes seem rude to others because of their straightforwardness. Most people would get offended if an acquaintance told them they looked like they were gaining weight. Yet, the Yang Type A rarely thinks twice about mentioning this to a friend or family member. This trait could be both a blessing and curse. The straightforwardness of the Yang Type A may also help others understand their own *sei wei,* or societal role. The other body types may ignore the fact that a friend is gaining weight, talk about her behind her back, or be overly polite to the point of avoiding a potentially beneficial (or detrimental) suggestion.

UNBALANCED STATE Unbalanced Yang Type A's often offend others with their overly direct comments. They knowingly offend and look down on others without feeling remorse or guilt. They do not hesitate to express candid thoughts in any situation, even if it is inappropriate to do so.

BALANCED STATE Balanced Yang Type A's speak out for what they feel is right and just. They serve as a voice for others who are less fortunate or less confident about speaking up. They control their tendency to offend others by being humble and courteous to others.

Quick, Quick, Quick!

Yang Type A's tend to be the hastiest of all the body types. They simply like to get things done—now! In the process of finishing, they tend to forget minute details, but always seem to complete tasks quickly.

UNBALANCED STATE Yang Type A's may seem to forget that patience is a virtue. They may also fail to think twice about their actions, thus offending others around them. Yang Type A's have a tendency to jump to conclusions and make hasty judgments.

BALANCED STATE Balanced Yang Type A's challenge themselves to pay attention to detail while quickly moving through a task. In short they are both quick and efficient. Efficiency is something Yang Type A's need to cultivate, while quickness comes naturally to them.

Multitasking

Yang Type A's have the innate ability to multitask. Having three or more tasks at hand never seems to overwhelm Yang Type A's, and they benefit from obtaining high-paced, multifaceted work because it stops them from getting bored easily. Yang Type A's also make use of their time wisely and always seem to get the job done. To those who can only focus on one thing at a time, this may seem like a supernatural ability.

UNBALANCED STATE While Yang Type A's may be good at multitasking, they have trouble focusing efficiently on each task at hand. Since they are so focused on the finish line, Yang Type A's often forget to pay attention to detail. Skipping to conclusions and rushing through things are reflections of the Yang Type A's hasty nature.

BALANCED STATE Balanced Yang Type A's are aware of their own hasty nature. As a result they make a sincere effort to stay focused. When staying focused, balanced Yang Type A's improve their natural ability to multitask efficiently.

Anger and Sadness

Anger is the predominant temperament of Yang Type A's, and it's felt pretty much all the time. Even the littlest things can trigger anger in Yang Type A's, making them appear grumpy to other body types. If expressed in a subtle way, anger could actually benefit Yang Type A's, as it motivates them to take a stand against wrongdoing and injustice. They believe in doing what is right and simply cannot bear witness to atrocity. The Yang Type A's anger can easily explode into rage, however. My Sasang professor, who is also a Yang Type A, said that at a younger age he never once said a word when getting into an argument; instead he "spoke" with his fists. When their anger turns into rage, it is better for others to leave them alone or leave the scene as quickly as possible! Extreme anger affects no one as much as Yang Type A's themselves. After screaming, yelling, and/or attacking others, they plummet into the deep abyss of sadness. Extreme sadness, in this case, eats away at their strongest organ, the spleen.

UNBALANCED STATE Unbalanced Yang Type A's are always angry, even over the smallest things. This anger is based on selfishness and the inability to control their emotions. Occasionally, their anger may be directed at injustice and inhumanity, but they themselves fail to take action for the greater good. Instead, they simply bicker and complain and lose their faith in humanity. Unbalanced anger quickly gets out of control for Yang Type A's, eventually exploding into rage, which is then immediately followed by depression.

BALANCED STATE Balanced Yang Type A's are aware of their anger and make sure to keep it under control. Since anger is natural for them, it could eventually grow worse if simply suppressed and lead to injury of the spleen. Therefore, the spleen's anger needs to be expressed in a positive way. Balanced Yang Type A's direct their anger toward taking a stance against injustice and treating others with fairness. This is a valuable aspect of anger, which gives balanced Yang Type A's a sense of purpose and mission in life.

Yang Type B Emotional Balance

KEY TRAITS

Strongest Organ: Lungs
Strongest Sense: Hearing
Innate/Inborn Virtue: *In* (Compassion)
Inherent Abilities: *Chon Shi*—the ability to hear the "voice" of the heavens; inherent psychic ability

Sa Mu—the ability to engage and succeed in public affairs (an offshoot of the Yang Type B's strong lungs)

Predominant Temperament: Sorrow

COMPASSION—THE VIRTUE OF *IN*

Compassion, or *in* in Korean, is the strongest virtue of Yang Type B's, and is associated with the lungs. Born with strong lungs, Yang Type B's have a strong sense of compassion. This sense is the result of a distinctive ability to "hear" the voice of the heavens, a characteristic known as *chon shi*. Yang Type B's feel that it is their life's mission to lead and guide others through compassion. The virtue of compassion, however, does not manifest on its own, or by simply attempting to be compassionate while wondering, "Hey I'm showing compassion here. Why aren't you listening to me?!" It comes from a heartfelt attempt to accumulate knowledge and wisdom, which are the strongest inherent virtues of Yin

Type B's. The sincere effort to accumulate wisdom and the manifestation of *in* are the Yang Type B's keys to unlocking the door to the other two virtues: humility and righteousness.

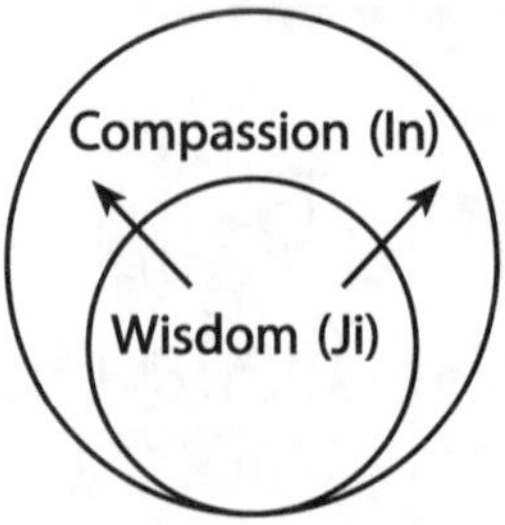

Figure 2.2. Yang Type B's compassion is derived from wisdom

UNBALANCED STATE Yang Type B's need to skillfully utilize their *chon shi* by helping and leading others. Unbalanced and unwise Yang Type B's may misinterpret the sound of their *chon shi*. Without learning how to put *chon shi* into action, Yang Type B's can lose their mind. They simply do not know what to do with those voices screaming inside their head. Through depression, anger, and frustration, they may lead others astray. Various tyrants of the past, such as Hitler or Stalin, were likely Yang Type B's. Without accessing the virtue of *ji,* Yang Type B's get easily disappointed in others and become excessively angry, constantly feeling that others are looking down on them. Unbalanced Yang Type B's may find themselves unable to lead, and thus unable to carry out their life's mission. Without guiding others Yang Type B's become ill, both mentally and physically.

BALANCED STATE Balanced Yang Type B's show compassion through wisdom. They make a constant attempt to slow down and listen to the needs of others, developing deep friendships. They know when to yield and do not become excessively distraught when others do not follow them. The balanced Yang Type B has the ability to express immense compassion and empower others through a gentle but firm embrace.

EMOTIONAL TENDENCIES

Natural-Born Leaders

The ability of Yang Type B's to lead and guide others surpasses that of other body types. Yang Type B's commonly assume the role of politician, CEO, or religious leader. They are gifted at convincing others of their capabilities. The leadership skills of Yang Type B's come from an inborn trait called *sa mu* in Korean, the ability to engage others and conduct public affairs. Their charisma makes it easy for them to motivate others. *Sa mu* derives from the strength of the lungs, the Yang Type B's strongest organ.

UNBALANCED STATE Unbalanced Yang Type B's use their leadership skills to lead people astray as a way to elevate their own standing. If Yang Type B's do not develop their leadership skills, they feel unworthy, sad, and eventually become ill.

BALANCED STATE Balanced Yang Type B's are leaders and mentors for those in need of direction and guidance. They use their innate virtue of compassion to help others find their way. Balanced Yang Type B's have extraordinary power in this regard, finding it their life's mission to guide and support others.

Keep in Mind

While Yang Type B's are natural-born leaders, not all leaders are benevolent or wise. Yang Type B's rush to the task of leading others, often without considering their responsibility. Others usually recognize their ability to lead and appoint them to high positions. Once in a high position, Yang Type B's often seek more authority and lose their connection with others in the process. Yang Type B's carry out public affairs, but they lack skill in private affairs. Oftentimes, those who are close to Yang Type B's shift their allegiance and turn away. Yang Type B's have trouble knowing and keeping track of who are their friends and who are their enemies. If they are not careful, Yang Type B's may be betrayed by seemingly close friends or comrades.

Sense of Hearing—Ingenious and Psychic Ability

Yang Type B's can "hear" the voice of the heavens through a trait referred to as *chon shi.* This gives them an extraordinary ability to decipher, comprehend, and discover the unknown and tap in to the metaphysical and the supernatural.

UNBALANCED STATE Unbalanced Yang Type B's use this ability to take advantage of others by tricking them. You can see this in the twisted politician, the cult leader, the cunning salesman, and the mad scientist. They may also have trouble translating the "messages" of *chon shi,* giving mixed messages to others and leading them astray. An ancient Buddhist adage states, "To know half the 'truth' is often more disadvantageous than knowing nothing at all."

BALANCED STATE Balanced Yang Type B's empower others by means of this "sixth sense." *Chon shi* may also give them the ability to further develop and contribute to the fields of medicine, politics, and the like. Sasang medicine itself was first established from the insight of a Korean Yang Type B doctor named Lee Je-ma. The seemingly supernatural discoveries of Yang Type B's greatly support and benefit society at large. For this reason they are often sought after for leadership and guidance.

Let's Climb Mt. Everest!

Yang Type B's push themselves to the limit. They put every ounce of energy into whatever cause they embrace. This tendency may result in unsurpassed strength or unnecessary anguish.

UNBALANCED STATE Unbalanced Yang Type B's push themselves and others beyond their limits, putting themselves and others in harm's way. It is common to see unbalanced Yang Type B's collapse from utter fatigue, forgetting their need for rest. They may also drive others past the point of no return.

BALANCED STATE Balanced Yang Type B's always do their absolute best to take care of themselves and others, being aware of their tendency to go overboard. They motivate others to move beyond their limitations but take the utmost care not to go too far too quickly. They recognize that taking charge does not need to take a toll on their health and well-being.

Sadness and Anger

Sadness, which originates from their strongest organ, the lungs, is the predominant emotion of Yang Type B's, which from time to time, may get out of control and cause them to sink into depression. The Yang Type B's depression can easily morph into extreme anger or rage. When this happens, it is better for others to leave them alone or flee the scene as quickly as possible. However, anger is most damaging to Yang Type B's themselves.

UNBALANCED STATE Unbalanced Yang Type B's are always sad, even about the smallest things. Occasionally, this sadness may help the Yang Type B empathize with the suffering of others. However, unbalanced Yang Type B's do not make an effort to alleviate the suffering of others around them. Instead, they simply fall deeper and deeper into their own despair. Unbalanced Yang Type B's may even find pleasure in leading others toward further suffering and sorrow, while elevating their own status. Sorrow quickly gets out of control for unbalanced Yang Type B's, eventually exploding into a rage that seriously compromises their health and further weakens the liver, their weakest organ, and injures their strongest organ, the lungs.

BALANCED STATE Balanced Yang Type B's are aware of their tendency to be overwhelmed by sadness and make sure to temper it. Since sorrow is natural for Yang Type B's, it could eventually grow worse if they simply suppress it. Suppressed sorrow could lead to injury of the lungs and explosive anger, causing injury to the liver. Therefore, the sorrow of the lungs needs to be expressed in a positive way. A balanced Yang Type B's sorrow is directed toward assisting and leading others toward a happier, more fulfilled direction in life. This valuable aspect of sorrow gives the Yang Type B a sense of purpose and mission.

I Am a Bull!

Yang Type B's have a tough, masculine nature. With their natural flair for leadership, this desire may lead to authoritarianism, haughtiness, and violence. Yang Type B's are often portrayed as powerful, charismatic, and almost super-human. At other times they may seem obsessive, domineering, and even dangerous.

UNBALANCED STATE The masculine nature of Yang Type B's can easily go to extremes. Without understanding their feminine side, they are unable to identify with the needs of others. They simply push, push, and push some more until someone collapses from exhaustion. They focus on being outwardly strong, but forget the importance of developing inner strength.

BALANCED STATE Balanced Yang Type B's are able to get in touch with their feminine side. They take the time to understand the needs of others, rather than forcing others to follow them. They are soft when softness is needed and strong when strength is needed. As leaders this quality helps Yang Type B's get in touch with the common people and gain their respect.

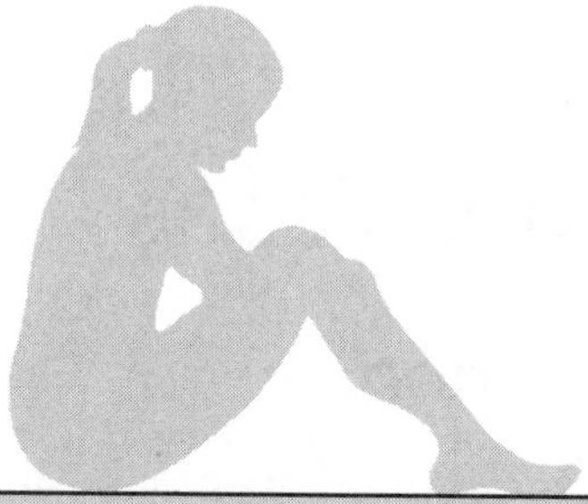

PART THREE

Eating and Exercising Right for Your Yin Yang Body Type

Body Type Foods

An Introduction

Since ancient times Asians have believed that food is medicine. Each has its own ability to harmonize the energies in our body and keep us healthy. In the Sasang medical clinic, diet modification is often prescribed as the first step in treating illness. Eating right for your body type may, in itself, be the answer to overcoming chronic or acute conditions. Herbs are generally prescribed for people who need a stronger boost to get things rolling. No matter how strong an herbal remedy is, however, it cannot take effect without a supportive diet.

The consumption of foods that correspond to our body type is an essential part of staying healthy and free of disease. Certain foods may be considered healthy for some, but not beneficial for our own system, while other foods that are considered unhealthy for others may actually be beneficial to us. Body type–specific foods can help us as follows:

- Avoid getting sick by strengthening the immune system.
- Lose or gain weight, depending on the metabolic needs of our system.
- Overcome chronic or acute illness alone or in conjunction with other medicines.
- Feel more energetic, sleep better, and feel healthier overall.

No matter how powerful and effective a treatment approach may be, it is essentially the body that heals itself from disease and illness. The best medicine in the world cannot cure even minor illness without the help of the body, which is constantly trying its best to keep us healthy and balanced. We overcome illness only when our body's energy is flowing smoothly and is in harmony. Eating body type–specific foods can help promote the smooth flow of energy from our stronger to our weaker organs, enhancing overall health.

FOOD ENERGY

According to Sasang medicine, each food has its own temperature, which is not based only on a hot or cold sensation in the mouth. Temperature is a way to classify the energetic nature of food. Foods that are classified as hot have a "hot" energetic nature and cold foods have a "cold" energetic nature. The energetic nature of a particular food gives us several hints about its effect on the body.

Foods can be classified into one of four energetic natures: warm, hot, cool, or cold. The energetic nature of a food determines which area of the body it travels to (see table 3.1 on page 112). After ingestion warm-natured foods travel to the lungs and support and stimulate their function; these warm-natured foods are therefore beneficial for Yin Type A's, born with weaker lungs. Hot-natured foods travel to the spleen and support and stimulate its function; thus hot-natured foods are beneficial for Yin Type B's, born with a weaker spleen. Cool-natured foods travel to the liver and support and stimulate its function, so cool-natured foods are beneficial for Yang Type B's, who are born with a weaker liver. Lastly, cold-natured foods travel to the kidneys and support and stimulate their function. Therefore, cold-natured foods benefit Yang Type A's, born with weaker kidneys.

Yang types have a tendency to accumulate too much heat in the body; hence they benefit from cool or cold foods, which help to reduce heat. Yin types have a tendency to accumulate too much cold within the body and therefore benefit from warm or hot foods. The cold accumulation of Yin types leads to stagnation and sluggish circulation. Since heat expands, consuming warm or hot foods can assist energy flow outward to the extremities. Yang types have the opposite issue: their energy has difficulty slowing down and following its designated course. Since cold has a contracting nature, cool and cold foods slow down the excessive flow of Yang types and bring their energy back to the core.

TABLE 3.1. ENERGETIC NATURE OF FOODS AND BODY TYPE

Food Nature	Function after Ingestion	Most Beneficial for This Body Type
Warm	Stimulates the Lungs	Yin Type A
Hot	Stimulates the Spleen	Yin Type B
Cold	Stimulates the Kidneys	Yang Type A
Cool	Stimulates the Liver	Yang Type B

Beneficial Food Energy and the Yin Yang Body Types

When discussing the nature of a particular food, we are simply referring to the temperature that is most prominent in that food. Actually, each food contains all four energetic natures or temperatures. Yet, of all four energetic natures, each food has its own predominant temperature. Cold foods, for example, also have cool, warm, and hot energies that are less apparent. Does this ring a bell? Each of us also has all four of the major organ energies (lungs, spleen, liver, and kidneys). Yet our body type is determined by which of the four major organs and temperaments are strongest. The energetic nature of food works the same way.

Since the four energetic natures are present to a certain degree in each food, they can at least partially benefit all four body types. If Yang Type A's are starving and grab a nutritious hot-natured food, it will not harm them. If they are suffering from hunger or malnutrition, any type of available food will suffice. However, if the consumption of hot-natured foods became habitual, they would eventually experience heartburn, headaches, and the like from overstimulation of the spleen and stomach. While this holds true in most situations, Yin Type B's need to be the most careful when it comes to food. Because they are born with a weaker digestive system, consuming cold foods in the winter or when they're sick could quickly exacerbate things for them, resulting in acute indigestion. See table 3.2 for general guidelines on the temperature of food.

TABLE 3.2. GENERAL FOOD TEMPERATURE GUIDELINES

Cool/Cold-Natured Foods	Warm/Hot-Natured Foods
Raw Foods	Cooked Foods
Most Vegetables	Most Spices
Chilled Foods	Warmed-Up Foods
Iced Foods	Spiced Foods

Keep in mind that food does not single out and influence only one organ or area of the body. Warm foods primarily support liver function, but they travel to other organs as well. No matter which food we eat, it eventually works its way into the bloodstream and flows throughout the entire body, bathing each of our organs. Foods that are considered healthy and compatible with our body type support the health of all organs in the body. However, foods that are not considered healthy or compatible with our body type may undermine the health of our entire system.

Changing the Energy of Food

Cooking or chilling a particular food can change or enhance its energetic temperature. Oysters, for example, are considered to have a very cold nature and are therefore not recommended for the Yin types. With their weaker digestive system, Yin Type B's almost always suffer from digestive discomfort after eating raw oysters. When oysters are cooked, however, their cold energetic nature is transformed into warmth, and most healthy Yin Type B's can digest cooked oysters without a problem. I recommend that Yin types cook foods that are cold-natured before ingesting them. Yang types, on the other hand, benefit from chilling otherwise warm or hot-natured foods. Drinking iced tea in the summer is much more soothing than hot tea to the stomach of a Yang Type A.

Determining the Energy of Your Food

Determining the energetic temperature of a particular food is not always an easy process. Foods and herbs that have a hot nature may not necessarily taste spicy. One of the hottest-natured herbs in Sasang medicine, called *bu ja,* is not spicy at all! Yet once *bu ja* enters the body, its hot nature immediately warms up the weak and cold spleen of Yin Type B's. Most herbalists would agree that it's those innocent, gentle-looking herbs that you sometimes have to watch out for! Fortunately, with a history of more than five thousand years, Eastern medicine has provided us with ample information in this regard. But there are many foods that have not been energetically classified because, historically, they were not available in Asia. Table 3.2 on page 113 gives a general list of food energies. If you are still having difficulty identifying the energetic nature of a particular food, log onto sasangmedicine.com and click "Learn more about the Yin Yang Body Types," "Sasang Discussion Forum," or "Contact Us" for more information.

Determining the energy of your food is not an impossible task! Your body is the perfect laboratory for a food energy experiment. Try sampling a small amount of food by itself to determine how it feels in your stomach. Does a particular food taste spicy to you? Does it cause you to break out in a sweat? Does it warm you up? If you answered yes to any of these questions, then it is likely a warm- or hot-natured food. Does a particular food make you feel cold? Does it help refresh your system on a hot day? Does it help reduce swelling? If so, you are probably eating a cool or cold-property food. Moreover, Yin types may also experience a stomachache if they eat cool or cold foods, while Yang types may experience the same symptoms if they eat warm- or hot-natured foods. However, this method of determining food energy may not be successful if you don't have a sensitive stomach or digestive system.

Keep in Mind—Food Choices

Sasang medicine continues to evolve and adapt to our eating styles and food choices. Some foods are still in the experimental stage and have not yet been energetically classified. If you are curious about the nature of a particular food, try following the method specified above or speak to a Sasang specialist by logging onto sasangmedicine.com.

FOOD ENERGY AND DIET

In this part each food is designated as a green, yellow, or red light to reflect its compatibility with each body type. Green-light foods are easily metabolized, yellow-light foods are less easily metabolized but do not harm the body, and red-light foods could sooner or later negatively affect your health. Keep in mind that each body type has its own food-nature requirements. Thus a green-light food for one body type may be a red-light food for another.

Green-Light Foods: More Than 60 Percent of Total Food Intake

These foods are easily digested, transformed into energy, and eliminated from the body. They offer ample support for the weakest organ of each body type. Each body type has a different list of green-light foods, depending on their stronger and weaker organs. An ideal diet consists of no less than 60 percent green-light foods.

Yellow-Light Foods: Up to 40 Percent of Total Food Intake

Even though yellow-light foods don't focus on supporting your weakest organ, they can still supply your body with its nutritional needs. Yellow-light foods are not digested as well as green-light foods, but they do not cause indigestion when consumed in moderate amounts.

There are two subcategories of yellow-light foods for each body type. Do you recall that Yang corresponds to warmth or heat, while Yin corresponds to cool or cold? The first subcategory of yellow-light foods is called "similar energy" foods; these are very closely related in temperature to green-light foods because they have the same Yin or Yang nature. The yellow-light foods for Yin Type B's, for example, have a warm nature, while their green-light foods have a hot nature. Even though warm foods are not as beneficial as hot foods for Yin Type B's, they may still have significant nutritional value because they have the same Yang nature. The second subcategory is referred to as "opposite energy" yellow-light foods. These foods are not as compatible as similar energy yellow-light foods, but can still be eaten in moderation and may have some nutritional value.

In most cases up to 40 percent of your entire diet should consist of similar energy yellow-light foods, while opposite energy yellow-light foods amount to 30 percent of the total yellow-light food intake. The 40/30 rule doesn't necessarily apply to all yellow-light foods, so make sure to read the amount of intake noted next to each food list. Table 3.3 spells out which foods fall into each category, according to body type.

TABLE 3.3. FOOD ENERGY AND BODY TYPE COMPATABILITY*

Body Type	Green Light	Yellow Light: Similar Energy	Yellow Light: Opposite Energy	Red Light
Yin Type A	Warm	Hot	Cold	Cool
Yin Type B	Hot	Warm	Cool	Cold
Yang Type A	Cold	Cool	Warm	Hot
Yang Type B	Cool	Cold	Hot	Warm

*Note that the green-light energy is the exact opposite of the red-light energy for each body type.

If taken in excessive amounts, yellow-light foods could eventually lead to minor digestive issues, such as slight gas and bloating. If you are trying to lose weight, avoid eating excessive amounts of yellow-light foods.

Red-Light Foods: Less Than 5 Percent of Total Food Intake

Foods in this category should be kept to a minimum because they overstimulate our stronger organs and cause damage to our weaker ones. If you have recently eaten a red-light food, do not panic! Most of these foods cause no immediate damage to the system, yet, if eaten habitually, they can lead to serious health issues such as chronic fatigue, allergies, indigestion, intestinal, and cardiovascular issues, regardless of your body type. Yin Type B's with a weaker digestive system should be especially careful when eating red-light foods. As a sensitive Yin Type B, I recall being rushed to the hospital several times in my childhood after eating too many red-light foods. Some people may not exhibit any symptoms whatsoever after eating red-light foods while others may notice them right away. Red-light foods should make up less than 5 percent of your diet.

From the Clinic

Mark, a pleasant and otherwise healthy Yin Type A, asked me why he always felt short of breath in the evening. After thorough investigation, it turns out that his Yang Type A girlfriend habitually cooked him pork for dinner. As a red-light food for the Yin Type A, pork was overstimulating his strong liver and weakening his already deficient lungs. Other than his difficulty breathing, Mark had no signs of indigestion or other discomfort. His breathing quickly improved after modifying the dinner menu to accommodate his body type.

Could there be yet another food category? Well, not exactly. Category X is an imaginary category that refers to a combination of green- and yellow-light foods. In reality it is very challenging to eat only green-light foods, since this category is usually more restrictive than the yellow-light category. We may not have easy access to green-light foods, or we may simply get sick and tired of eating them over and over again. Category X stretches the limits of what we can and cannot eat.

Do you recall the 60 percent green- and 40 percent yellow-light rule that I introduced above? Some may feel comfortable thinking, shopping, and cooking in ratios, but others with less time or patience can get along better with the Category X method described below. This free-thinking category gives you the chance to eat any combination of green- and yellow-light foods, keeping the following in mind:

- Always try to mix at least some green-light foods in with yellow-light foods.
- Continue to avoid red-light foods whenever you can.
- Stick closer to green-light foods when you are feeling ill or if you start to notice any digestive discomfort (bloating, gas, excessive fullness after meals), and/or stool-related issues.

Keep in Mind—Food Categories

For the purposes of this book, I have included fish and shellfish under the category of "meat." I have also included dairy and dairy substitutes, such as almond milk and rice milk, alongside meats under the category "meat and dairy" because they are significant sources of protein.

Yin Type A Foods

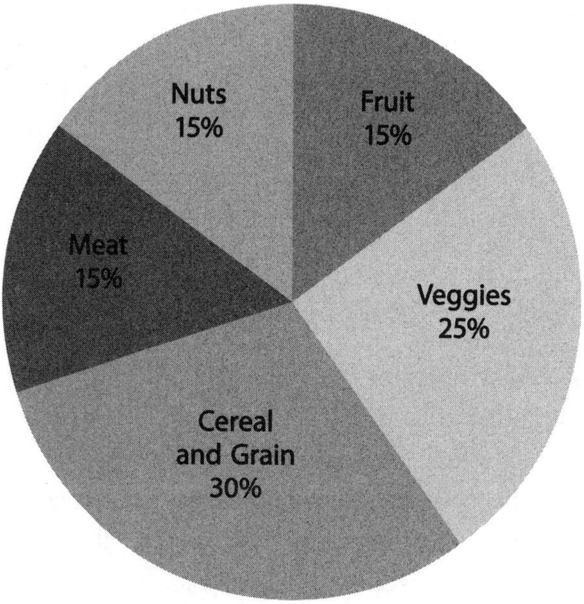

Figure 3.1. Breakdown of optimum food group percentages for the Yin Type A's diet (also see table 3.4 on pages 136–38 for details)

Yin Type A's often take great pleasure in eating. Not only does it give them an opportunity to socialize, but it also provides their stronger liver with comfort and gratification. With such a strong liver, however, Yin Type A's tend to absorb excessive toxins from their food, which can lead to weight gain and/or accumulation of toxins in the body.

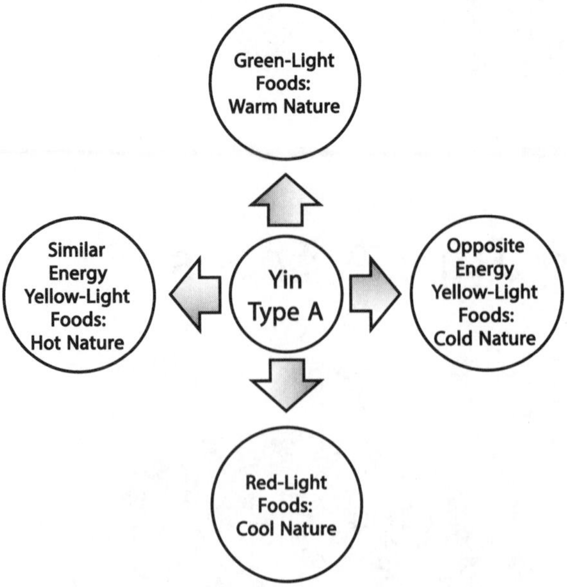

Figure 3.2. Yin Type A food energy summary

FOOD NAVIGATOR

The Yin Type A's weaker lungs are strengthened by the warm nature of green-light foods that offer immune support and energy. The hot-natured, similar energy yellow-light foods of Yin Type A's resemble the warm nature of their green-light foods but do not directly support their weaker lungs. The Yin Type A's cold-natured, opposite energy yellow-light foods are closer to red-light foods because cool and cold, which support the Yang Type organs, are opposite energies of warm and hot. Cool-natured foods are especially incompatible because they can overstimulate and congest the Yin Type A's naturally stronger liver. Refer to figure 3.2 for further illustration.

CEREALS, SEEDS, AND GRAINS FOR YIN TYPE A

The cereals and grains category is the Yin Type A's most important food group. These foods, which help supply the body with consistent energy throughout the day, are also usually high in fiber and therefore promote the passage of food through the intestines. Yin Type A's easily succumb to intestinal issues, such as constipation and diarrhea. I recommend that up to 30 percent of the entire Yin Type A diet be devoted to cereals and grains.

Green-Light Cereals, Seeds, and Grains for Yin Type A

> White or yellow sesame seeds, tahini (hummus), Job's tears, and whole grains such as brown rice, millet, quinoa, flaxseed, pumpkin seeds, sunflower seeds, and oats should constitute more than 60 percent of Yin Type A's cereal and grain intake.

Whole grains, such as brown rice, are not only rich in fiber but are also known to prevent cardiovascular disease and cancer. Even though millet is better known for its use as bird food, it is a nutritious food option for humans as well, since it is rich in minerals like magnesium, phosphorus, zinc, copper, and manganese. It also curbs the appetite because it expands within the stomach after ingestion. Hence, millet makes an excellent diet food for those who tend to overeat. Millet is also gluten-free, making it a safe alternative for those with gluten sensitivities. Rice and millet are staple foods in Asia, where they are greatly valued. At one point in Chinese history, rice was used as a form of money and as a status symbol. As a complex carbohydrate, rice is slowly but consistently broken down in the stomach and intestines to provide ongoing energy throughout the day. Flax seeds, with their high levels of omega-3 fatty acids, can help lower cholesterol. They also contain phytoestrogens, which help alleviate postmenopausal symptoms. Flax seeds are also gluten-free. Mahatma Gandhi once said that "wherever flax seeds become a regular food among the people, there will be better health."

Most Yin Type A's are sensitive and/or allergic to gluten products. Luckily, there are several great sources of gluten-free flour on the market. Quinoa flour, for example, is not only gluten-free but also filled with protein, iron, and fiber. This healthy gluten-free grain was considered sacred by the Incas, who referred to it as the "mother of all grains." Quinoa can also be prepared in its whole-grain form in cereals, salads, or your favorite pasta. Oats contain a type of gluten different from that of wheat and barley, making it easier for Yin Type A's to digest. However, it may still cause issues for those who are allergic or sensitive to gluten. Bob's Red Mill (bobsredmill.com) is a good source of gluten-free oats.

Yellow-Light Cereals, Seeds, and Grains for Yin Type A

Similar Energy: glutinous (sweet) rice should constitute less than 40 percent of Yin Type A's cereal and grain intake. (Keep in mind that even though sweet rice is also referred to as glutinous rice, it does not contain gluten.)
Opposite Energy: wild rice, black sesame seeds, and black rice should constitute less than 30 percent of Yin Type A's *yellow-light* cereals and grains.

These similar energy cereals and grains have a warm nature, while the opposite energy foods have a cold nature. Yellow-light foods are not harmful for Yin Type A's, but they may cause slight indigestion in the long run if consumed excessively.

Red-Light Cereals, Seeds, and Grains for Yin Type A

Buckwheat, barley, rye, corn, and wheat should constitute less than 5 percent of Yin Type A's cereal and grain intake.

Buckwheat is considered a cool-natured food. Since the Yin Type A has a strong liver, too much stimulation of this organ can lead to indigestion, headaches, and other toxicity-induced symptoms. Because Yin itself corresponds to cold, cool-natured foods are difficult for Yin types to digest. These foods "freeze" up their digestive system, causing indigestion, bloating, and possible weight gain. Although buckwheat has *wheat* in its name, it is not related to wheat at all and doesn't contain gluten.

Wheat and barley are Yin foods that should technically be in the yellow-light category for Yin Type A's because they have a cold nature. Yet about 50 percent of all Yin Type A's and 20 percent of Yin Type B's experience stomach and/or intestinal issues after ingesting wheat and barley, due to gluten-related food allergies. As a Yin food, wheat may also induce sinus-related allergies among the Yin types.

Breads, cakes, crackers, cookies, biscuits, croutons, pasta, pizza, muffins, and pastries are nearly always made with wheat (except for gluten-free versions now increasingly available). Surprisingly, gluten also shows up in other foods, such as hot dogs, soy sauce, and beer. Yin Type A's or Yin Type B's who have tried unsuccessfully to overcome chronic fatigue, indigestion, celiac disease, and/or allergies may benefit from either reducing or eliminating gluten altogether from their diet, while closely monitoring whether or not their symptoms improve. Meanwhile, try the many alternatives now to be found in gluten-free sections of grocery stores, natural food stores, and more and more restaurants and cafes, on Internet sites, and in cookbooks offering recipes that will satisfy cravings without hurting your system.

VEGETABLES AND SPICES FOR YIN TYPE A

Foods in the vegetables and spices category are usually easy to digest because they keep the energy flowing smoothly throughout the digestive system and the entire body. Most leafy-green vegetables nourish the blood with their iron and vitamin B content. Since vegetables generally have a cool or cold nature, it is advisable for Yin types to flash-steam or cook them lightly before eating. Be aware, however, that the vitamin content of vegetables is lost if they are cooked too long! I recommend that up to 25 percent of the entire Yin Type A diet consist of vegetables and spices.

Green-Light Veggies and Spices for Yin Type A

White beans (lima, navy, Great Northern), potatoes, sweet potatoes, radishes, carrots, lotus root, yams, cabbage, turmeric, bean sprouts, pumpkin, arrowroot, dandelion greens, bell peppers (green, red, and yellow), chickpeas (aka garbanzo beans), and asparagus should constitute more than 60 percent of Yin Type A's vegetable and spice intake.

Warm-natured vegetables and spices all strengthen and support the weaker lungs of Yin Type A's. In addition they have the following health benefits.

Lima beans are a rich source of unsaturated fat, which helps support smooth bowel function. They are also a significant low-fat source of protein. One cup of lima beans offers 29 percent of the recommended daily allowance (RDA) of protein. With a lower rating on the glycemic index, lima beans make a great source of energy for those with blood sugar issues. Potatoes offer a rich supply of vitamins B_6 and C, potassium, and fiber. While potatoes are nourishing in themselves, they are usually prepared in unhealthy ways. Try to avoid deep-frying potatoes or slathering excess butter on baked potatoes. One cup of chopped sweet potatoes offer 438 percent of the recommended daily allowance of vitamin A! Despite their significant starch content, researchers have discovered that sweet potatoes can actually control blood sugar levels when they're baked or boiled.* Dandelion greens are particularly beneficial to ingest during the spring and summer because they help gently cool the body and quench thirst. Dandelion greens and asparagus are both excellent sources of vitamins C, A, and K, plus calcium and iron. In Eastern medicine asparagus root is often used to support the function of the liver and kidneys, while turmeric and arrowroot are prescribed to prevent infection and treat inflammation. Chickpeas, also known as garbanzo beans, are a significant source of protein (9 grams of protein per 100 grams of chickpeas), phosphorus, and fiber. Recent studies suggest that ingesting this legume may help lower cholesterol in the bloodstream.†

---

*For example, see Ludvik, Bernhard H., Beatrice Neuffer, and Giovanni Pacini, "Efficacy of *Ipomoea batatas* (Caiapo) on Diabetes Control in Type 2 Diabetic Subjects Treated with Diet" *Diabetes Care* 27, no. 2 (February 2004): 436–40.

†For example, see Pittaway, J. K., K. D. Ahuja, M. Cehun, A. Chronopoulos, I. K. Robertson, P. J. Nestel, and M. J. Ball. "Dietary Supplementation with Chickpeas for at Least 5 Weeks Results in Small but Significant Reductions in Serum Total and Low-Density Lipoprotein Cholesterols in Adult Women and Men" *Annals of Nutrition and Metabolism* 50, no. 6 (2006): 512–18.

Caution about Beans

Make sure to thoroughly cook your beans! Most raw beans contain traces of toxic substances that are destroyed during the cooking process.

Yellow-Light Veggies and Spices for Yin Type A

Similar Energy: garlic, green onions (scallions), onions, shallots, sage, ginger, thyme, black pepper, jalapeños, chives, anise, cilantro, fennel, rosemary, wasabi, mustard seed, coriander, cardamom, and horseradish should constitute less than 40 percent of Yin Type A's vegetable and spice intake.

Opposite Energy: red beans, adzuki beans, kidney beans, black beans, mung beans, lettuce (romaine), kale, cucumber, burdock root, eggplant, celery, soybean paste (miso), tofu, and parsley should constitute less than 30 percent of Yin Type A's *yellow-light* vegetables and spices.

These similar energy vegetables and spices have a hot nature, while the opposite energy foods have a cold nature. Although yellow-light foods are not harmful for Yin Type A's, they may cause slight indigestion in the long run if ingested excessively (more than eight servings a week).

Yin Type A's should flash-steam or cook cold-natured vegetables during the colder months to avoid indigestion or other metabolic issues. In warmer climates or in the summer, raw vegetables can be consumed more often without this risk.

Spices, such as garlic, onions, and ginger, may add flavor to a meal but are rarely the main ingredient. Yin Type A's can enjoy these spices with just about every meal as long as they do not overdo it. Habitual consumption of excessively spicy foods can lead to heat accumulation and congestion in the Yin Type A's stronger liver.

Red-Light Veggies and Spices for Yin Type A

Lettuce (iceberg), alfalfa sprouts, artichoke, snow peas, tomato, Swiss chard, bitter gourd, bamboo shoots, and broccoli should constitute less than 5 percent of Yin Type A's vegetable and spice intake.

Cool-natured vegetables can easily overstimulate and cause congestion of the Yin Type A's stronger liver. But remember that cooking with or flash-steaming these vegetables changes their nature from cool to warm, making them easier to digest.

FRUITS FOR YIN TYPE A

Fruits are an excellent source of vitamins, fiber, and antioxidants for all body types, especially when they're in season. They are also easy for just about everyone to digest. Even though oranges, for example, are a Yin Type B fruit, the other body types can benefit from eating fresh oranges. Remember that humans are a product of nature and the seasons have a strong effect on our physical and emotional state of being. Mother Nature provides us with foods according to the seasonal requirements of our body. I recommend that up to 15 percent of the entire Yin Type A diet consist of fruits that are in season.

Keep in Mind—Sugar in Fruit

Individuals with sugar sensitivities, such as diabetes or hypo- or hyperglycemia, need to restrict their fruit intake. Additionally, fruit juice contains significantly less nutritional value and more sugar than whole fruit, especially if the pulp and skin have been removed in the manufacturing process.

Green-Light Fruits for Yin Type A

Pears, figs, apricots, plums (prunes), avocados, and longan should constitute the majority of Yin Type A's fruit intake.

Pears are one of the best foods for strengthening and supporting the Yin Type A's weaker lungs. Not only are they shaped like lungs, but they also benefit the lungs tremendously. Eating pears can help Yin Type A's avoid colds and coughing. There is a popular traditional fall dish in China prepared by steaming sliced pears sprinkled with a tablespoon of brown sugar to help prevent colds and soothe coughs and throat dryness. Brown sugar, when consumed in moderate amounts, can also be beneficial for the nondiabetic Yin Type A. Prunes are best known for their ability to promote bowel movements, helpful for Yin Type A's, who often have difficulty with elimination. Prunes, which are actually dried plums, also help to support lung function, reduce coughing, and even treat diarrhea! Longan, which translates as "dragon eye fruit" from Chinese, is sometimes squeezed into juice, consumed as a yummy dried fruit, or added to an herbal formula. It is commonly used in Sasang medicine to aid in digestion and to calm an unsettled spirit.

Yellow-Light Fruits for Yin Type A

Similar Energy: apples (all varieties), oranges (all varieties), tangerines, lemon, lime, mango, passion fruit, grapefruit, lychee, pomegranate, dates, cherry, peaches, and durian can constitute up to half of Yin Type A's fruit intake.
Opposite Energy: blackberries, strawberries, blueberries, grapes (raisins), pineapple, and bananas should constitute less than half of Yin Type A's *yellow-light* fruits.

It is safe and even beneficial for Yin Type A's to eat the similar energy and opposite energy yellow-light fruits when they are in season, but they may either be too cooling or too warming for Yin Type A's if eaten out of season or in excess. Keep in mind that locally grown fruits are fresher and easier to digest than imported ones.

Red-Light Fruits for Yin Type A

There are no red-light fruits for Yin Type A's! Yet, keep in mind that Yang Type B fruits (black currant, kiwi, grapes, persimmons, and star fruit) have a cool nature, which may cause liver congestion and constipation if consumed in excess by Yin Type A's.

NUTS FOR YIN TYPE A

While nuts are a healthy source of protein for all body types, they are especially beneficial for Yin Type A's. The flow of stool through the intestines of the Yin Type A tends to be sluggish, leading to bowel retention or constipation. While meat is the most efficient source of protein, it tends to cause constipation if consumed heavily. Yin Type A's cannot afford the risk of constipation, which can easily take a toll on their general health. Most nuts, if they have not been roasted, have substantial amounts of protein in the form of volatile oils, which help the passage of stool through the intestines, making them an excellent source of protein and intestinal health. I therefore decided to create a separate nut category specifically for the Yin Type A and recommend up to 15 percent of the entire Yin Type A diet be devoted to nut consumption.

Green-Light Nuts for Yin Type A

> Chestnuts, walnuts, pine nuts, ginkgo nuts, almonds, hazelnuts, acorns, macadamia nuts, and pecans should constitute more than 60 percent of Yin Type A's nut intake.

Nuts play an important role in the health of Yin Type A's. They are rich in palmitoleic acids and omega-3 essential fatty acids, which play a role in preventing cholesterol buildup. Studies have indicated that people who ingest nuts on a regular basis are less likely to experience coronary heart disease, high blood pressure, and stroke.* Nuts are also a great source of protein, minerals, and antioxidants, said to help prevent and fight against cancer. Almonds and walnuts have been known to reduce cholesterol concentration in the body. Almonds contain significant amounts of B vitamins, while walnuts are the only significant nonanimal source of omega-3 fatty acids. Chestnuts and walnuts, which are perhaps the best types of nut for Yin Type A's, strongly support the function of the lungs. Pine nuts promote kidney function. In Eastern medicine the kidneys are said to be responsible for hair growth, lower-back strength, and healthy teeth, so these areas of the body can benefit greatly from regular consumption of pine nuts.

Yellow-Light Nuts for Yin Type A

Peanuts and coconut should constitute less than 30 percent of Yin Type A's total nut intake.

This category only consists of opposite energy yellow-light foods because there are no hot-natured similar energy nuts in Sasang medicine. The nuts in this category have a cold nature and therefore benefit the Yang body types more than the Yin types. Eating more than five portions a week of these nuts could cause indigestion in Yin body types.

Red-Light Nuts for Yin Type A

There are no red-light nuts for Yin Type A's, but keep in mind that peanuts and coconuts, which are cold- and cool-natured, respectively, can interfere with digestion and bowel movement. Ingesting excessive amounts (more than five servings a week) of cold- and cool-natured nuts is not recommended.

---

*For example, see Richmond, Korina, Sheila Williams, Jim Mann, Rachel Brown, and Alexandra Chisholm, "Markers of Cardiovascular Risk in Postmenopausal Women with Type 2 Diabetes Are Improved by the Daily Consumption of Almonds or Sunflower Kernels: A Feeding Study" *ISRN Nutrition* 2013.

MEAT AND DAIRY FOR YIN TYPE A

Most meats offer an abundant supply of protein and are rich in one or more fat-soluble vitamins (A, D, E, and K). Most meats also contain ample amounts of iron, which is easier for the body to absorb than from plant sources. The Yin Type A's body cannot get along without these essential components of the diet, and there are no other foods that compare to meat protein when it comes to supporting the process of cell repair and cell reproduction, even though there are numerous nonmeat foods that are rich in fat-soluble vitamins.

The metabolism of the Yin body types is slower than that of the Yang types. Meat-derived protein can become toxic if it sticks around too long in the gut. The fat-soluble vitamins derived from meat also tend to linger in the body for a while, since they get absorbed into our fat tissue. Higher doses of these vitamins can lead to toxic accumulation. The body does not need a daily supply of fat-soluble vitamins, which are stored in the liver and fat tissue for days, if not weeks. Moreover, Yin Type A's, with their strong liver, tend to absorb more fat and energy from their food than the other body types. They should therefore consume meat in smaller portions. I recommend that no more than 10–15 percent of the entire Yin Type A diet consist of meat.

Green-Light Meat and Dairy for Yin Type A

Duck, beef, salmon, goat's milk, almond milk, yogurt, and cheese (made from sources other than cow's milk or soy milk) should constitute more than 60 percent of Yin Type A's meat and dairy intake.

Duck has more iron and less saturated fat than beef, making it a healthier choice for the blood and heart, while beef contains five times as much vitamin B_{12}, which plays a key role in supporting the brain and nervous system. Both of these meats are very rich in protein and selenium, both of which are important in metabolism. Salmon, also very rich in protein, has the added benefit of abundant omega-3 fatty acids, which help reduce inflammation and prevent heart disease and cancer. Unlike these other meats, salmon is also rich in vitamin A, essential to maintaining healthy vision. Like beef, it is a great source of vitamins B_6 and B_{12}.

Goat's milk is easier to digest than cow's milk because it has less lactose, an important factor for Yin Type A's, who tend to be lactose intolerant, especially in their adult years. It is also richer than cow's milk in vitamins B_3, B_6, and A and numerous essential fatty acids. The lactose-intolerant Yin Type A can also try almond milk or rice milk, which has absolutely no lactose or cholesterol. Since almonds are extremely healthy for Yin Type A's, almond milk can be a great substitute. Almond milk is low in fat and high in vitamin E, calcium, iron, and other essential nutrients.

Yellow-Light Meat and Dairy for Yin Type A

Similar Energy: chicken, lamb, quail, pheasant, Alaskan pollack, venison, and rice milk should constitute up to 40 percent of the Yin Type A's meat and dairy intake.
Opposite Energy: crab, clams, squid, shrimp, cod, trout, mackerel, herring, snapper, crawfish, flounder, tuna, halibut, and cheese (made from cow's milk) should constitute less than 30 percent of Yin Type A's *yellow-light* meats and dairy.

These similar energy meats are hot-natured; they support the function of the spleen, which controls the digestive system. Opposite energy meats, which have a cold nature, have an affinity for the kidneys. Since Yin Type A's have a comparatively slow metabolism, cold-natured meats tend to stick around longer in their bodies, possibly causing fat or toxic accumulation. Most cheeses derived from cow's milk contain traces of lactose, which may cause indigestion for Yin Type A's.

Red-Light Meat and Dairy for Yin Type A

Pork, cow's milk (raw or pasteurized), and soymilk should constitute less than 5 percent of Yin Type A's meat and dairy intake.

The nature of pork and soymilk are between cool and cold, making them great stimulants for the Yang types' weaker liver and kidneys, but a source of congestion and overstimulation for the stronger liver and kidneys of the Yin types. The cool nature of cow's milk also leads to congestion and overstimulation of the Yin type A's stronger liver.

In 2006 the American Centers for Disease Control reported that 77 percent of all mothers at least briefly breast-feed their infants.* Breast milk contains immunoglobulins that work to support and strengthen the immune system. The recent rise in breast-feeding may also contribute to healthier Yin Type A infants! Milk tends to produce phlegm, while interfering with the digestive system of Yin Type A's. Most infants can digest cow's milk, thanks to an enzyme in their gut called lactase. But Yin Type A's often become deficient in lactase as they get older. Yin Type A infants fed nothing but cow's milk may eventually develop indigestion or allergy-related symptoms. I recommend that the mother of a Yin Type A infant breast-feed whenever possible or use alternative sources of milk. Fermented milk products, such as yogurt and cheese, are often easier to digest, making them tolerable for most Yin Type A's. Yet these foods too may occasionally cause digestive issues. Yin Type A's are often sensitive to certain, rather than all, types of cheese.

TEAS FOR YIN TYPE A

Green-Light Teas for Yin Type A

Dandelion, chamomile, green, and/or white teas should be consumed daily by Yin Type A's after meals.

*From Mike Stobbe's "CDC: 3 Out of 4 New Moms in U.S. Now Breast-Feed their Infants," http://usatoday30.usatoday.com/news/health/2008-04-30-117201504_x.htm (accessed June 29, 2014).

There are over thirty different herbal remedies beneficial for Yin Type A's that are prescribed for specific health reasons. In this section I list several herbs that support the general health of Yin Type A's and are also easy to find. If you have a garden full of dandelions in the spring, don't fret; your weeds can be transformed into a healthy cup of tea. Dry the flowers and stems of your dandelions and boil 10 grams with one cup of water. Let the tea simmer for about five minutes and then strain. Drink up to three cups of warm tea a day. Consuming tea with meals can help with digestion and boost your metabolism. Green tea, in particular, contains abundant antioxidants that help prevent premature breakdown of tissues and cells within the body. Dandelion tea is often prescribed as a treatment for breast abscess or other abnormal tissue growth in the chest area. It makes a safe herbal tea for Yin Type A's to help detoxify the liver and promote blood flow. Chamomile tea assists with the Yin Type A's digestion and can prevent the feeling of fullness or fatigue after meals. Chamomile also calms the nervous system of Yin Type A's, alleviating stress and insomnia.

Yellow-Light Teas for Yin Type A

Similar Energy: ginger, cinnamon, clove, chai, licorice, and citrus (lemon, tangerine peel) teas should be consumed up to five times a week by Yin Type A's.

These hot-natured similar energy teas may serve as a helpful remedy for Yin Type A's suffering from nausea, motion sickness, phlegm, and/or indigestion. Yet in the long run the hot nature of these herbs may cause heartburn, acid reflux, or stomach irritation.

Red-Light Teas for Yin Type A

Pine needle, buckwheat, and quince fruit teas should be avoided by Yin Type A's.

Cool-natured teas can cause Yin Type A's excessive stimulation and congestion of the liver. Although consuming these teas would not cause any immediate problems, they should nevertheless be avoided whenever possible.

SUPPLEMENTS FOR YIN TYPE A

Coenzyme Q10, vinegar, turmeric, vitamin E, omega-3 and omega-5, ginkgo biloba, probiotics, baby aspirin

These warm-natured supplements support the Yin Type A's weaker lungs while promoting circulation. In Sasang medicine weaker lungs often contribute to poor circulation, since the heart relies on oxygen to carry out its job. Ginkgo increases memory by enhancing the circulation of blood to the brain from the Yin Type A's weaker lungs. Vinegar, turmeric, coenzyme Q10, and baby aspirin all help promote blood flow. Omega-3 and omega-5 fatty acids help reduce inflammation and cholesterol accumulation, while preventing heart disease and cancer. The daily intake of probiotics can greatly improve digestion and promote the immune function of Yin Type A's. Probiotics are actually microorganisms (beneficial bacteria or yeast) that help the body digest and fight against "bad" bacteria. Antibiotics tend to destroy both the good and the bad bacteria in the intestines, so Yin Type A's should take daily doses of probiotics when undergoing antibiotic treatment to replenish the good bacteria along the intestine wall. Herbs and supplements will be discussed further in part 4 on addressing health issues.

OTHER FOODS TO AVOID IN EXCESS

The following foods do not fit into any of the above categories but should be limited: refined (white) sugar, milk chocolate, and salt.

Refined sugar causes a sudden spike in blood sugar levels and leads to energetic imbalance within the body. The quick breakdown of refined sugar also leads to the release of free radicals into the bloodstream, where they scavenge the body, wreaking havoc along the way. Try using pure maple syrup or molasses instead of white sugar to sweeten food or drink. Milk chocolate should be avoided for the same reasons as cow's milk. If you love chocolate, I recommend that you consume dark chocolate instead of milk chocolate to avoid lactose issues. Excess salt in the diet overstimulates and causes damage to the kidneys and liver. The 2010 Dietary Guidelines for Americans, issued by the USDA, recommend limiting sodium intake to less that 2,300 mg a day. This is slightly less than a teaspoon. If you are fifty-one years old or older, of African American descent, or have high blood pressure, the recommended daily allowance is less than 1,500 mg.

See table 3.4 on pages 136–38 for a detailed summary of all Yin Type A food recommendations.

TABLE 3.4. QUICK REFERENCE OF YIN TYPE A FOODS

Food Group	Green-Light Foods (60% or more)	Yellow-Light Foods (40% or less)	Red-Light Foods (foods to avoid)
Cereals, Seeds, and Grains (30%)	Oats, white/yellow sesame seeds, millet, tahini (hummus), quinoa, Job's tears, brown rice, pumpkin seeds, sunflower seeds	Glutinous (sweet) rice, barley, black sesame, black rice, black sesame seeds	Buckwheat, rye, corn, wheat, and other forms of gluten. Many Yin Type A's are allergic to gluten.
Vegetables, Beans, and Spices (25%)	White beans (lima, navy, Great Northern), potatoes, sweet potatoes, radishes, carrots, lotus root, yams, cabbage, turmeric, bean sprouts, pumpkin, arrowroot, dandelion greens, bell peppers (green, red, yellow), chickpeas, asparagus	Garlic, green onions (scallions), onions, shallots, sage, ginger, thyme, black pepper, jalapeños, chives, anise, cilantro, fennel, rosemary, wasabi, horseradish, mustard seed, coriander seed, cardamom, red beans, adzuki beans, kidney beans, lettuce (romaine), celery, kale, cucumber, burdock root, green peas, black beans, eggplant, parsley	Lettuce (iceberg), alfalfa sprouts, artichoke, snow peas, tomato, bamboo shoots, Swiss chard, bitter gourd, broccoli. If these foods are cooked or flash-steamed, they transform into yellow-light foods for the Yin Type A, because their nature goes from cool to warm.

Food Group	Green-Light Foods (60% or more)	Yellow-Light Foods (40% or less)	Red-Light Foods (foods to avoid)
Fruits (15%)	Pears, figs, apricots, plums (prunes), avocados, longan	Apples (all varieties), oranges (all varieties), tangerines, lemon, lime, mango, passion fruit, peaches, grapefruit, lychee, durian, pomegranate, dates, blackberries, strawberries, blueberries, grapes (raisins), pineapple, raspberry	There are no red-light fruits for the Yin Type A. Yet, keep in mind that Yang Type B fruits (persimmon, black currant, kiwi, and star fruit) have a cool nature, which may cause liver congestion for Yin Type A's if consumed in excess.
Meat and Dairy (15%)	Duck meat, cow meat, salmon, goat's milk, almond milk, yogurt, cheese (made from sources other than cow's milk)	Chicken, lamb, quail, pheasant, Alaskan pollack, venison, rice milk, crab, squid, shrimp, calamari, mackerel, herring, crawfish, flounder, codfish, snapper, tuna, cheese (made from cow's milk)	Pork, cow's milk, soymilk
Nuts (15%)	Chestnuts, walnuts, pine nuts, ginkgo nuts, almonds, hazelnuts, acorns, macadamia nuts, pecans	Coconut, soybean, peanuts	Nuts are generally safe for Yin Type A's, but stay away from too much salt!

TABLE 3.4. QUICK REFERENCE OF YIN TYPE A FOODS (continued)

Food Group	**Green-Light Foods (60% or more)**	**Yellow-Light Foods (40% or less)**	**Red-Light Foods (foods to avoid)**
Teas	Dandelion, chamomile, green, white	Ginger, cinnamon, clove, chai, licorice, citrus (lemon, tangerine peel)	Pine needle, buckwheat, quince tea
Supplements	Coenzyme Q10, vinegar, aspirin, turmeric, vitamin E, omega-3 and omega-5, ginkgo biloba	No need to supplement with yellow lights!	Excessive use of any supplement can cause liver congestion in Yin Type A's, so try to stay away from quince fruit extract, graperoot extract, and devil's club extract, which have a cool nature.

Yin Type B Foods

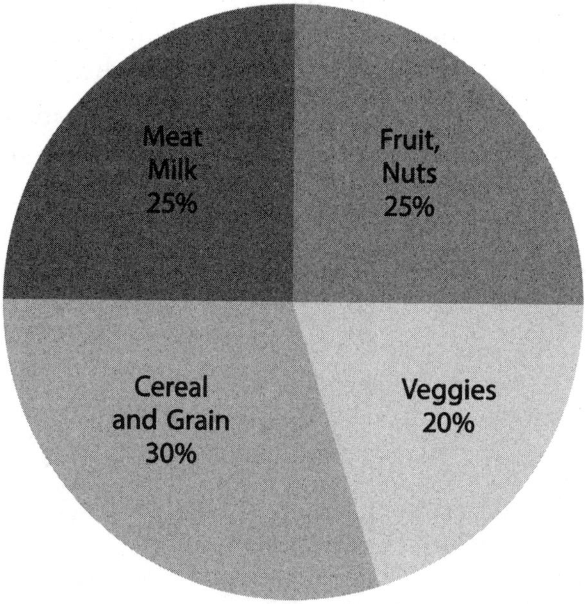

Figure 3.3. Breakdown of optimum food group percentages for the Yin Type B's diet (also see table 3.5 on pages 155–56 for details)

Born with a weaker digestive system, Yin Type B's have to be the most careful about their food intake. The ingestion of cold-natured foods may quickly lead to indigestion or illness. The Yin Type B's cold and weak spleen benefits from hot-natured foods, which help boost the digestive system. Cold-natured foods, on the other hand, "freeze up" and inhibit their spleen/digestive function.

Yin Type B's have an acute sense of taste to protect them from eating incompatible foods. This sensitivity gives them the ability to determine which foods have a hot or cold nature. The superprimed taste buds of Yin Type B's naturally cause them to avoid cold-natured foods and seek out warm- or hot-natured foods. An acute sense of taste may not always benefit them, however. It can cause extreme fear of food and inhibit them from eating things that are otherwise compatible for their body type. The oversensitive Yin Type B may become emaciated and weak, especially after mistakenly eating a red-light food. It is important for Yin Type B's not to let such sensitivity inhibit them from eating altogether.

Yin Type B's often lose their appetite right after ingesting red-light foods. When this happens they can try making themselves a cup of fresh ginger tea and slowly work green-light foods back into their diet. This is perhaps the best remedy for the Yin Type B's indigestion. See the Yin Type B section in "Maintaining a Healthy Digestive System" (pages 317–20) for more information.

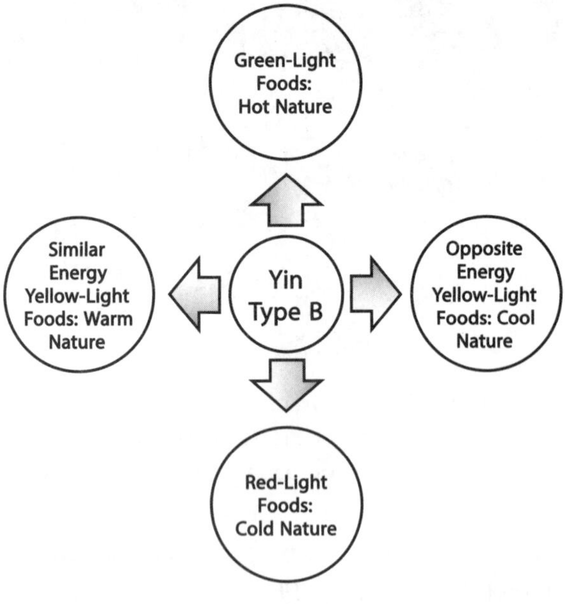

Figure 3.4. Yin Type B food energy summary

FOOD NAVIGATOR

The Yin Type B's weaker spleen is strengthened by the hot nature of this body type's green-light foods, which offer digestive support and energy.

The warm-natured, similar energy yellow-light foods for this body type resemble the hot nature of their green-light foods. The Yin Type B's cool-natured, opposite energy yellow-light foods are closer to red-light foods because cool and cold are opposite energies of warm and hot. A *cold* nature makes the Yin Type B's red-light foods the exact opposite of their *hot*-natured green-light foods and can overstimulate and congest their naturally stronger kidneys.

CEREALS, SEEDS, AND GRAINS FOR YIN TYPE B

Most cereals and grains have either a cool or a warm nature, making them most suitable for Yang Type B's and Yin Type A's. Warm-natured cereals and grains, however, can help support the Yin Type B's digestive system because they are easy to digest.

Cold-temperature cereals and grains tend to cause digestive stagnation in Yin Type B's. A bowl of cold cereal for breakfast every day can lead to symptoms such as fatigue, diarrhea, and chronic indigestion. I suggest cooking or warming up cereals and grains. Also, try adding hot-natured spices, such as cinnamon, ginger, or honey, to your cereals and grains to energetically warm them up. I recommend that up to 30 percent of the entire Yin Type B food intake consist of cereals and grains.

Green-Light Cereals, Seeds, and Grains for Yin Type B

Glutinous (sweet) rice should constitute more than 80 percent of Yin Type B's cereal and grain intake.

Glutinous rice is the only green-light grain for Yin Type B's. Does this mean that Yin Type B's should avoid most grains altogether? Have no fear, spices are here! Try choosing a few spices from the green-light spices on page 144 and mix them with your similar energy yellow-light grains. The warmer the food is, the more it benefits the weak spleen and digestion of the Yin Type B. Also, keep in mind that there are plenty of yellow-light grains that Yin Type B's can digest without difficulty.

Glutinous rice is a staple food in Asian culture, where it is greatly valued. It is the most warming of all grains and is therefore very gentle on the Yin Type B's sensitive digestive system. Rice, in general, is a complex carbohydrate that is broken down consistently and effectively in the stomach and intestines to provide long-lasting energy.

Yellow-Light Cereals, Seeds, and Grains for Yin Type B

Similar Energy: oats, white/yellow sesame seeds, pumpkin seeds, sunflower seeds, millet, tahini (hummus), quinoa, Job's tears, flaxseed, and brown rice should constitute up to 40 percent of Yin Type B's cereal and grain intake.
Opposite Energy: buckwheat, rye, and corn should constitute less than 30 percent of Yin Type B's *yellow-light* cereals and grains.

These similar energy yellow-light foods have a warm nature. Warm-natured foods are more beneficial for Yin Type A's than for Yin Type B's, but they need not be avoided. Preparing these grains with ginger, cinnamon, nutmeg, or other Yin Type B–friendly spices can transform them into green-light foods. Hummus can be made with roasted garlic and oats can be mixed with cinnamon to add flavor and make it easier for the Yin Type B's weak spleen to digest. Their soft texture also contributes in this regard. Even though Job's tears is especially helpful for the lungs, it can also strengthen the weak digestive system of the Yin Type B when cooked with sweet rice. In Eastern medicine Job's tears are often used to treat indigestion.

Buckwheat is a yellow-light food with a cool nature. The Yin Type B can digest it efficiently when warm or spiced up with green-light foods. A well-known dish in Korea called *mei-mil guksu* (buckwheat noodle soup) is made from buckwheat noodles that are dipped into a spicy radish sauce with grated ginger. The hot-natured sauce balances out the cool nature of buckwheat, making it easier for Yin Type B's to digest.

Red-Light Cereals, Seeds, and Grains for Yin Type B

Barley (especially from cold beer), wild rice, wheat, black sesame seeds, and black rice should constitute less than 5 percent of Yin Type B's cereal and grain intake.

Cold-natured grains have heavy and cloying qualities. If Yin Type B's eat these foods, they may experience indigestion or other discomfort. Gluten in barley and wheat often causes gas, bloating, headaches, and/or bowel issues for Yin types. For further information about Yin type gluten sensitivities, see pages 121–22.

Did you just eat a red-light food? Don't worry! Try making yourself a cup of fresh ginger tea and slowly work green-light foods back into your diet while temporarily omitting yellow- and red-light foods altogether. This is perhaps the best remedy for the Yin Type B's indigestion.

VEGETABLES AND SPICES FOR YIN TYPE B

Spices are an essential food for Yin Type B's. They are usually easy to digest and keep the energy flowing smoothly throughout the digestive system and the entire body. Spices are usually hot- or warm-natured. They can be mixed with the yellow-light foods to aid with digestion. I recommend using spices when preparing almost any food for Yin Type B's. Even though spicier foods are easier to digest and healthier for Yin Type B's, overconsumption can cause problems. Excessively spicy foods can be too harsh for the sensitive digestive system of the Yin Type B, leading to stomach and bowel issues. Generally speaking the colder Yin Type B's feel, the more spice they can tolerate.

Digestion Trick of the Trade

To promote the digestion of warm- or cool-natured foods, try preparing green-light with yellow-light foods. Spices such as ginger can be added to meats and vegetables for an extra digestive boost. The Yin Type B can drink ginger tea with meals to aid in digestion as well.

Most leafy-green vegetables nourish the blood, thanks to their iron and B-vitamin content. Since most vegetables have a cool or cold nature, it is advisable for Yin Type B's to flash-steam or fry them for five minutes or less. Steaming or sautéing vegetables is especially important during the colder months, when the Yin Type B's digestive system is most vulnerable. Keep in mind that overcooking vegetables should be avoided in order to retain their nutritional value. I recommend that up to 20 percent of the entire Yin Type B food intake come from vegetables and spices.

Green-Light Veggies and Spices for Yin Type B

Garlic, green onions (scallions), onions, shallots, sage, ginger, thyme, black pepper, jalapeños, chives, anise, cilantro, fennel, rosemary, wasabi, horseradish, mustard seed, cardamom, thyme, and coriander should constitute more than 80 percent of Yin Type B's vegetable and spice intake.

These vegetables and spices are all said to have a hot nature. Hot-natured foods strengthen and support the Yin Type B's weaker spleen and digestive function. Ginger, for example, is the most effective herb for bolstering the digestive system and can be considered a staple for Yin Type B's, to be mixed with just about any food. It can also be taken as a tea after meals to avoid indigestion and fatigue. Garlic and black pepper, with very strong antibacterial properties, can fight off colds and throat infections while strengthening the immune system. Even though wasabi may quickly burn a hole through the stomach of Yang types, it can unfreeze the "frozen" digestive system of Yin Type B's. It is also a great way to balance the cool/cold nature of sushi, making it edible for Yin Type B's. Chives are rich in B vitamins and vitamin C and promote the flow of blood through the body. Mustard seed and coriander are both commonly used in Eastern medicine to promote digestion and remedy gas, bloating, and stomach discomfort. Mustard seed is also used for clearing phlegm and coughing from a stubborn cold. Fennel is also used as an herb in the Sasang medical clinic to warm and support the function of the digestive system. It contains anethole, an organic substance with antimicrobial and antifungal properties.

Yellow-Light Veggies and Spices for Yin Type B

Similar Energy: turmeric, bean sprouts, pumpkin, chestnuts, arrowroot, dandelion greens, bell peppers (green, red, and yellow), potatoes, sweet potatoes, radishes, carrots, lotus root, yams, cabbage, white beans (lima, navy, Great Northern), chickpeas (garbanzo beans), and asparagus should constitute up to 40 percent of Yin Type B's vegetable and spice intake.
Opposite Energy: lettuce (iceberg), alfalfa sprouts, artichoke, broccoli, snow peas, Swiss chard, tomato, bitter gourd, and bamboo shoots should constitute less than 30 percent of Yin Type B's *yellow-light* vegetables and spices.

These similar energy foods have a warm nature. It is much easier to go from warm to hot than from cold to hot, making it is easy to transform warm-natured foods into hot-natured foods by adding spices or mixing them with hot-natured foods. Most beans, for example, can be prepared with aromatic vegetables like onions and garlic and seasoned with sage and thyme.

These opposite energy vegetables, with their cool nature, need to be flash-steamed or cooked for Yin Type B's. In warmer climates or in the summer, raw vegetables can often be consumed by Yin Type B's without the risk of indigestion. However, in the winter and in colder climates, the cooler nature of these foods may cause indigestion and intestinal issues down the road. While yellow-light foods are not harmful for Yin Type B's, they may cause slight indigestion in the long run if ingested excessively (more than eight servings a week).

Red-Light Veggies and Spices for Yin Type B

Lettuce (romaine), celery, kale, cucumber, taro root, burdock root, eggplant, parsley, mung beans, green peas, black beans, red beans (adzuki, kidney), and soybeans (miso, tofu) should constitute less than 5 percent of Yin Type B's vegetable and spice intake.

Because these red-light vegetables are cold-natured, if Yin Type B's eat these foods by themselves or uncooked, they will likely experience indigestion or other discomfort.

Can Yin Type B's eat lettuce? Even though lettuce is in the red-light category for Yin Type B's, they can still ingest lettuce during the warmer months of the year. A leaf or two can also be added to a sandwich without causing indigestion. During the cooler months, lettuce can be eaten if accompanied by such Yin Type B spices as ginger, garlic, pepper, and the like.

Are you frowning because there are foods in this red-light list that are yummy or nutritious? Don't worry! When these cold-natured foods are cooked or flash-steamed, they become warm-natured. Warm-natured foods are in the yellow-light category and can be consumed in moderation.

Did you just eat a red-light food without cooking or steaming it? Not to worry. The best remedies for red-light foods are green-light foods, which can help cleanse and strengthen the digestive system.

FRUITS AND NUTS FOR YIN TYPE B

Fruits are an excellent source of vitamins, fiber, and antioxidants for all body types. Especially when they are in season, fruits are also easy for just about anyone to digest. This is therefore the most lenient category, rarely causing digestive or other issues, even if consumed by other body types. Even though oranges, for example, are a Yin Type B fruit, the other body types can benefit from fresh oranges and orange juice when they're in season. Keep in mind that humans are products of nature. The seasons have a strong effect on our physical and emotion state of being. Mother Nature provides us with foods according to the seasonal requirements of our body.

The fruits in this section have enzymes that promote the digestion of meats and other heavy foods, making them a perfect addition to the Yin Type B's meal. Whether in whole or juice form, these fruits can also support the function of the spleen, preventing indigestion and other illness. I recommend that up to 25 percent of the entire Yin Type B diet come from fruits in season.

Most nuts fall into the similar energy yellow-light category for Yin Type B's because they have a warm nature. Since nuts are not as easily digested as green-light foods, I recommend ingesting them after a workout, after the body gets fired up, and only when hungry. If Yin Type B's eats nuts on a full stomach, they can easily feel bloated or gassy. Otherwise, nuts can be a rich source of protein and other nutrients for Yin Type B's.

Green-Light Fruits for Yin Type B

Apples (all varieties), oranges (all varieties), tangerines, mango, passion fruit, lemon, lime, grapefruit, lychee, pomegranate, dates, durian, cherries, and peaches should constitute more than 80 percent of Yin Type B's fruit intake.

Compared to other fruits, these fruits have a relatively high amount of citric acid, which is said to have a "hot" nature in Sasang medicine. These fruits also have relatively high amounts of enzymes, which help the stomach break down and convert food into energy. These fruits not only make for a delicious dessert, they also help improve the overall health of Yin Type B's. With a substantial amount of vitamin C, oranges (all varieties) are excellent at helping Yin Type B's fight off colds and also clear phlegm from the lungs and sinuses. Mangos, too, are a significant source of vitamin C and B vitamins, and contain several flavonoids, such as quercetin and astragalin, which help prevent certain forms of cancer. Dates are used in Sasang medicine to nourish and support the blood of Yin Type B's, alleviating vision issues and/or insomnia. Lychees make for a tasty dessert and aid in digestion. Durian is likely the hottest-natured fruit in this category. It strongly warms up the weaker spleen of Yin Type B's, offering them a healthy boost of energy. This fruit is often available at Asian markets when in season. Cherries are rich in fiber and vitamin C, and they are also the only known fruit source of melatonin. Melatonin deficiency has been associated with insomnia and lack of skin pigmentation. Cherries also contain lutein, which is believed to help with eye and cardiac health.

Yellow-Light Fruits and Nuts for Yin Type B

Similar Energy: apricot, avocados, pears, plums, figs, longan, chestnuts, walnuts, pine nuts, ginkgo nuts, almonds, hazelnuts, acorn, macadamia nuts, and pecans should constitute up to 40 percent of Yin Type B's fruit and nut intake.
Opposite Energy: black currants, kiwi, star fruit, raspberry, and persimmon should constitute less than 30 percent of Yin Type B's *yellow-light* fruits and nuts.

These similar energy yellow-light fruits are warm-natured, and therefore, in moderate amounts, they can supply plenty of fiber and water-soluble vitamins for the Yin Type B. Opposite energy yellow-light fruits are on the cool-natured side but do not pose a threat to the Yin Type B's spleen if they're eaten in season. Why does the season make such a big difference? During the warmer months when these fruits are available, the Yin Type B's body also tends to warm up. Warm external temperatures help to cultivate and build the warmth (or Yang) within the body of the Yin Type B. Yin Type B's often feel healthier during the summer and fall because of the accumulation of heat. If the weather is consistently warm or hot, it is okay for the Yin Type B to consume cooler-natured foods. Fruits are also the safest category of food for the Yin Type B because they are soft and usually easy to digest. I would still recommend that Yin Type B's not exceed eight portions a week of these yellow-light fruits.

Red-Light Fruits and Nuts for Yin Type B

Melon (watermelon, cantaloupe, honeydew), bananas, and peanuts should constitute less than 5 percent of Yin Type B's fruit intake.

Fruit is a gift of Mother Nature that crosses the boundaries of each body type. Yang types can enjoy Yin type fruits, while Yin types can enjoy Yang type fruits without having to worry about indigestion or other problems. The key is to consume red-light fruits in moderation and in season.

Most Yin Type B's can get away with eating melon (watermelon, cantaloupe, honeydew) in the warmer months without risking indigestion, even though melon is considered a very cold-natured fruit. It is best, though, for Yin Type B's to avoid eating melon on cooler days or during the cooler seasons.

Peanuts have a cold nature that could lead to bloating and gas if Yin Type B's overindulge themselves. Unlike other nuts they do not grow on trees, but on shrubs. Since trees are taller, they are considered to have more Yang than shrubs; hence peanuts have the most Yin nature of all nuts mentioned in this book. With so much Yin already hanging around in their system, Yin Type B's don't need to invite more inside.

MEAT AND DAIRY FOR YIN TYPE B

Meat is hardier and takes longer to digest than foods in other categories. Because of the Yin Type B's weaker digestive system, it could take more than an hour for meat to pass through the stomach of this body type. For this reason cold-natured meat, which is incompatible with their body type, could easily lead to a feeling of fatigue or grogginess after meals. Undercooked or rotten meat can also cause major health issues for Yin Type B's, who are better off avoiding meat if it has even the slightest unusual smell, taste, or color. Hot-natured meats, however, are not only easier to digest, but also help support the function of the digestive system. To be on the safe side, it is always a good idea for Yin Type B's to cook meat with green-light spices to ensure efficient digestion and reduce toxicity.

Despite being more difficult to digest than other foods, meat is an essential part of the diet for Yin Type B's because it supplies them with needed protein. I recommend that up to 25 percent of the entire Yin Type B diet come from meat intake.

Since ancient times it was common for the Chinese to drink rice milk after suffering from indigestion or recovering from illness. Glutinous rice is a green-light food for the Yin Type B, and therefore, when ingested as a milk, it can be an excellent way to reignite a weakened digestive system. Unlike glutinous rice soy has a cold-nature, making it very difficult for Yin Type B's to digest soy milk. Cow's milk has a cool nature and can be digested in smaller portions if ingested warm or lukewarm.

Green-Light Meat and Dairy for Yin Type B

Chicken, lamb, quail, pheasant, Alaskan pollack, anchovy, venison, and rice milk should constitute more than 80 percent of Yin Type B's meat and dairy intake.

These hot-natured meats and rice milk heat up and strengthen the weak digestive system of the Yin Type B. However, keep in mind that meats in general are more difficult to digest than other food groups. They contain long chains of polypeptide bonds that take a lot of effort to break down into energy. Even though these foods have a hot nature, it is still important to cook them with Yin Type B spices. The addition of spices will help Yin Type B's digest meats more effectively. Yin Type B's should also consume thinly sliced or ground, rather than chunky, pieces of meat. Consuming meat in stews or soups is another way to aid the digestive process. Larger, dryer, and shortly cooked portions of meat are harder to digest and can lead to bowel- and stomach-related issues for Yin Type B's.

Protein from meat is essential for cell repair and reproduction, preventing osteoporosis, and maintaining bone density. Among the foods listed above, chicken and lamb have the hottest nature of all meats. Their hot nature makes them easier to digest for Yin Type B's with their cold digestive system. Chicken and lamb also have high amounts of protein (chicken: 31 grams of protein per 100 grams; lamb: 28 grams of protein per 100 grams). Chicken is also a significant source of vitamin B_3, which helps prevent cardiovascular disease and high cholesterol.

Lamb, on the other hand, is a significant source of vitamin B_6, which is essential for supporting immunity, nourishing the blood, and aiding digestion. Quail has more protein than chicken and lamb, less sodium, and almost half the calories! It is also an even richer source of vitamin B_6 than chicken. Chicken and lamb can help the emaciated Yin Type B gain a few pounds, while quail is a good option for the heavyset Yin Type B who does not wish to gain weight.

Yellow-Light Meat and Dairy for Yin Type B

Similar Energy: duck, beef, croaker, salmon, sole, goat's milk, almond milk, and yogurt should constitute up to 40 percent of Yin Type B's meat and dairy intake.

Yin Type B's can consume up to eight servings a week of warm-natured meats and dairy products without any health risks. These foods should always be cooked with Yin Type B spices or prepared with green-light foods to make them hot-natured.

Red-Light Meat and Dairy for Yin Type B

Pork, shellfish (especially oyster, crab, and lobster), squid, mackerel, herring, octopus, flounder, codfish, snapper, halibut, tuna, and soymilk should constitute less than 5 percent of Yin Type B's meat and dairy intake.

These cold-natured meats are potentially harmful to Yin Type B's because they have a tendency to "freeze" up this body type's already cold-natured digestive system. Shellfish, shrimp, crabs, oysters, and halibut spend most of their time close to the ocean floor. According to Yin Yang theory, the deeper parts of the ocean correspond to Yin, making these fish more Yin than Yang. Since the Yin types already have abundant Yin, eating these foods can create stagnation and toxic buildup.

TEAS FOR YIN TYPE B

Green-Light Teas for Yin Type B

Ginger, cinnamon, clove, chai, licorice, and/or citrus (lemon, tangerine peel) teas should be consumed daily by Yin Type B's after meals.

There are over thirty-five different herbs that are beneficial for Yin Type B's, most of which are prescribed for specific health situations. This section lists a few herbs that can be ingested often as teas to support the general health of Yin Type B's. These teas are also easy to find. Ginger is by far the best herb for Yin Type B's, whose digestive system it helps to "unfreeze" and strengthen. Ginger also helps to prevent and treat common colds and boost energy. It can be consumed with meals to aid metabolism and to avoid stomachaches or bloating. The active ingredients in ginger—oleoresin and terpenes—help kill unwanted bacteria and regulate bowel movement. Cinnamon is used for the same reasons as ginger. The two spices are often mixed together to enhance each other's healing properties. Cinnamon is also rich in fiber, calcium, and iron. Clove tea makes an excellent after-dinner drink, as it also alleviates bloating and gas after a heavy meal. Tea made from organic lemon and/or tangerine peel can help rid the body of phlegm and ease coughing or wheezing.

Diary Entry: Ann, a 43-year-old Yin Type B

Ginger has so many uses! I drink it as a tea about three times a day after meals to enhance my digestion. When I feel a cold coming on, I make my ginger tea very strong, adding half of a fresh gingerroot to about 1½ cups of water. I let it boil and then simmer for about twenty minutes on a low flame and, voilà! I have the best cold remedy. After I ingest ginger, I feel its warmth fill my stomach. This is always a sign that it is starting to work its magic. I even use it during allergy season to reduce my allergy symptoms.

Yellow-Light Teas for Yin Type B

Similar Energy: dandelion, chamomile, white, green, genmai, and other similar warm-natured teas should be consumed up to five times a week by Yin Type B.

These warm-natured teas are somewhat beneficial for the Yang-deficient Yin Type B's. In moderation these teas can support the circulation and warm up their cold digestive system.

Red-Light Teas for Yin Type B

Peppermint, barley, mint, and black teas should be avoided by Yin Type B's.

These cold-natured teas have a tendency to freeze up the already cold digestive system of the Yin Type B. Consuming these teas regularly can lead to chronic stomachaches, bloating, and colds. Since teas are consumed warm, cold-natured teas, such as mint and peppermint, do not pose an immediate threat to Yin Type B's and can be ingested in moderation.

SUPPLEMENTS FOR YIN TYPE B

Vitamin C, ginger (extract), cinnamon (extract), enzymes (multienzymes), ginseng

Who hasn't heard of vitamin C?!? While this is arguably the most popular supplement on the market, few people realize that almost all major sources of vitamin C are from Yin Type B foods and herbs. Vitamin C can help prevent colds by giving the digestive and immune systems a boost. Since it is water-soluble, vitamin C is safer to ingest at higher doses. The famous author/professor Norman Cousins overcame his own bout of chronic illness by ingesting high doses of vitamin C and by using laughter as medicine to support the immune system.

Ginger has already been mentioned a few times for its essential role in supporting the Yin Type B's overall health. It is perhaps the strongest herb for enhancing the function of the spleen and digestive system. It also boosts the immune system and helps the system fight off colds. Cinnamon plays a similar role and is often consumed as a complement to ginger.

There are numerous brands of multienzyme ginger formulas on the market. While most of these are compatible with the Yin Type B diet, I suggest trying the Rainbow Light Advanced Enzyme System because it contains ginger, papaya, and fennel (which are all Yin Type B green-light foods). This formula offers an ample supply of enzymes to help in digesting foods. Many of my Yin Type B patients have used it to alleviate gas, bloating, and fatigue after meals.

Ginseng is often used in Sasang medicine to support and improve the function of the Yin Type B's weaker spleen. A weaker spleen can lead to chronic fatigue, indigestion, depression, and frequent colds. This herb has one of the strongest effects on the body, compared to other Sasang herbs. It should therefore be ingested as a supplement only after consulting with your Sasang counselor or another herbal specialist. Excessive use can cause high blood pressure if it is not administered properly. Ginseng is not to be used when you're suffering from a common cold because it helps the body absorb energy, rather than helping it push out bacteria and other unwanted visitors. Finally, since overdose or improper use of ginseng could have adverse health effects, closely follow the manufacturer's specified proper dosage range.

See table 3.5 on pages 155–56 provides a detailed summary of all Yin Type B food recommendations.

TABLE 3.5. QUICK REFERENCE OF YIN TYPE B FOODS

Food Group	Green-Light Foods (60% or more)	Yellow-Light Foods (40% or less)	Red-Light Foods (foods to avoid)
Cereals, Seeds, and Grains (30%)	Glutinous (sweet) rice	Millet, oats, white/yellow sesame seeds, tahini (hummus), quinoa, Job's tears, brown rice, buckwheat, rye, corn	Barley (especially from cold beer), wheat, wild rice, black sesame seeds, black rice
Vegetables, Beans, and Spices (20%)	Garlic, green onions (scallions), onions, shallots, sage, ginger, thyme, black pepper, jalapeños, chives, anise, cilantro, fennel, rosemary, wasabi, horseradish, mustard seed, coriander, thyme, cardamom	Turmeric, bean sprouts, pumpkin, chestnuts, arrowroot, dandelion greens, bell peppers (green, red, and yellow), potatoes, sweet potatoes, radishes, carrots, lotus root, yams, cabbage, white beans (lima, navy, Great Northern), chickpeas, lettuce (iceberg), alfalfa sprouts, artichoke, broccoli, snow peas, tomato, Swiss chard, bitter gourd, bamboo shoots	Lettuce (romaine), cucumber, taro root, burdock root, eggplant, kale, celery, green peas, black bean,s red beans (adzuki, kidney), soybean paste (miso), tofu
Fruits and Nuts (25%)	Apples (all varieties), oranges (all varieties), tangerines, mango, passion fruit, lemon, lime, cherries, grapefruit, lychee, pomegranate, dates, durian (fruits in season are the best choice)	Apricots, avocados, pears, peaches, plums, black currants, kiwi, star fruit, blackberries, raspberries, blueberries, strawberries, grapes (raisins), persimmon, walnuts, pine nuts, ginkgo nuts, almonds, hazelnuts, sunflower seeds, pumpkin seeds, acorn, macadamia nuts, pecans	Melon (watermelon, cantaloupe, honeydew). These fruits are considered to have a very cold nature. Moderate amounts of other cold-natured fruits can be ingested when in season.

TABLE 3.5. QUICK REFERENCE OF YIN TYPE B FOODS (continued)

Food Group	Green-Light Foods (60% or more)	Yellow-Light Foods (40% or less)	Red-Light Foods (foods to avoid)
Meat and Dairy (25%)	Chicken, lamb, quail, pheasant, Alaskan pollack, venison, rice milk	Duck, beef, croaker, salmon, sole, goat's milk, almond milk, yogurt	Pork, shellfish (especially oyster, lobster, and crab), shrimp, squid, mackerel, herring, crawfish, octopus, flounder, codfish, snapper, tuna, soymilk
Teas	Ginger, cinnamon, clove, chai, licorice, citrus (lemon, tangerine peel)	Most other warm-natured teas such as chamomile, white, green, genmai, dandelion	Peppermint, mint, barley, black
Supplements	Vitamin C, ginger (extract), cinnamon (extract), enzymes (multienzymes), ginseng	No need to supplement with yellow lights!	Excessive use of any supplement can quickly cause indigestion (gas, bloating) in the Yin Type B. Beware of these symptoms while supplementing!

Yang Type A Foods

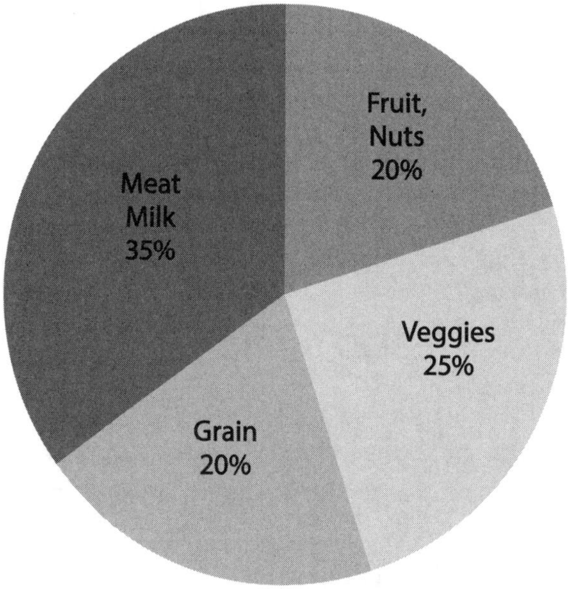

Figure 3.5. Breakdown of optimum food group percentages for the Yang Type A's diet (also see table 3.6 on pages 172–73 for details)

In Sasang medicine there is a saying that Yang Type A's can digest a rock. Of course I do not suggest that they try this! But this saying helps illustrate just how much stronger the Yang Type A's digestive system is than that of the other body types. Born with a strong spleen, the Yang Type A often needs to eat in order to quench an overactive and unsettled digestive system. If they do not satisfy their hunger quickly, Yang Type A's may become agitated, due to an accumulation of stomach and spleen heat.

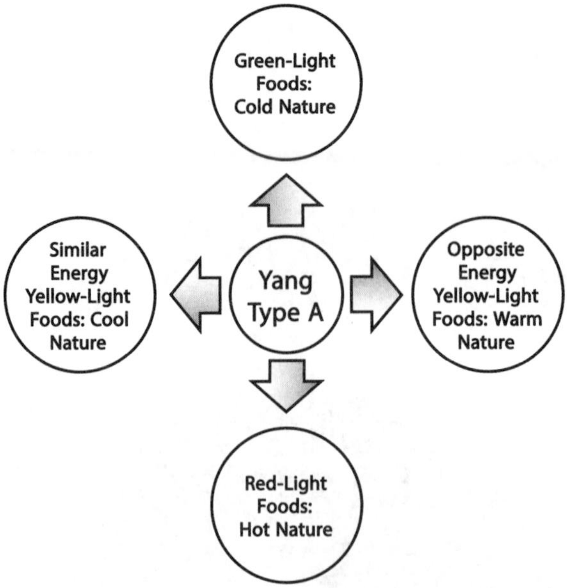

Figure 3.6. Yang Type A food energy summary

FOOD NAVIGATOR

The green-light foods in this section are devoted to nourishing and calming the stomach and spleen while supporting the Yang Type A's weaker kidneys. In Sasang medicine the kidney and spleen form a Yin Yang relationship, with the kidneys representing Yin and the spleen representing Yang. When Yin overreacts it takes away from Yang, and when Yang overreacts it steals energy away from Yin. The Yang Type A's green-light foods are cold-natured, supporting the kidney Yin and protecting it from abundant Yang. The Yang Type A's cool-natured, similar energy yellow-light foods resemble the cold nature of the green-light foods. The Yang Type A's warm-natured, opposite energy yellow-light foods are closer to red-light foods for them, because warm and hot, which support the Yin type organs, are opposite energies of cool and cold, which support Yang type organs.

CEREALS, SEEDS, AND GRAINS FOR YANG TYPE A

The cereals and grains category is an important food group for Yang Type A's. These foods help to cool and calm the excessive heat of their digestive system, while supporting kidney function. I recommend that up to 20 percent of the entire Yang Type A diet consist of cereals and grains.

Green-Light Cereals, Seeds, and Grains for Yang Type A

Wild rice, wheat, barley, black sesame seeds, and black rice should constitute more than 60 percent of Yang Type A's cereal and grain intake.

After ingestion these cold-natured foods travel to and calm the overactive stomach of Yang Type A's and support their weakest organ, the kidneys. Wheat especially enhances the Yang Type A's kidney and digestive function. The cold nature of wheat helps to cool stomach heat and, as a result, eases anxiety, insomnia, and nervousness. Anxiety, a common issue among Yang Type A's, is caused by stomach heat rising upward and bombarding the heart. Black sesame seeds support the function of the kidneys, assisting with reproductive health, and bolstering waist, hip, and lower-body strength. Most black foods are high in antioxidants and support kidney function. These foods include black rice, black sesame seeds, and black beans. One tablespoon of black sesame seeds provides nine percent of the daily recommendation of calcium intake! Rich in iron, fiber, and manganese, they also help reduce blood pressure by relaxing the vessel walls. Black rice, which is also rich in fiber and vitamin E, contains a flavonoid called anthocyanin, a compound said to help prevent heart disease and cancer. Wild rice is an excellent grain source of protein. It is also high in fiber, B vitamins, zinc, and manganese.

Yellow-Light Cereals, Seeds, and Grains for Yang Type A

Similar Energy: buckwheat, rye, and corn should constitute up to 40 percent of Yang Type A's cereal and grain intake.
Opposite Energy: oats, white/yellow sesame seeds, tahini (hummus), quinoa, Job's tears, brown rice, flaxseed, pumpkin seeds, sunflower seeds, and millet should constitute less than 30 percent of Yang Type A's *yellow-light* cereals and grains.

These similar energy cereals and grains, with their cool nature, have a greater amount of Yin, which helps balance the excessive Yang of the Yang types. Yin foods also support the lower body, which is generally weaker among the Yang types. These grains, if eaten in moderation, can therefore support the Yang Type A's weaker lower body. I suggest consuming up to twelve portions a week of these foods.

Even though Yang Type A's benefit from cold-natured foods, in moderation, opposite energy warm-natured cereals and grains can also be a valuable source of fiber for them. However, they may cause Yang Type A's slight indigestion in the long run if they're ingested excessively (more than eight servings a week).

Red-Light Cereals, Seeds, and Grains for Yang Type A

There are no red-light, hot-natured foods in this category for Yang Type A's. Grains and cereals have either a neutral, cool, or warm nature, with the exception of glutinous rice, an overall easy-to-digest food. The relatively gentle temperature of grains and cereals make them a safe source of nutrition.

VEGETABLES AND SPICES FOR YANG TYPE A

Yang Type A's have plenty of Yang, but are generally Yin-deficient. Yin, according to Eastern medicine, is the "mother" of blood. In other words it provides the moisture needed to form and replenish the blood. Thus, Yang Type A's have a tendency to develop anemia and other blood deficiencies. Most leafy-green vegetables are capable of nourishing the Yin and the blood with their higher proportions of iron and B vitamins. Vegetables mostly have a cool or cold nature, which is beneficial for the Yang Type A's stomach heat accumulation. Yang Type A's benefit more from eating raw vegetables because when they're cooked, vegetables lose their cold nature. I recommend that up to 25 percent of the entire Yang Type A food intake come from vegetables and spices.

Green-Light Veggies and Spices for Yang Type A

Lettuce (romaine), cucumber, taro root, burdock root, eggplant, kale, celery, green peas, red beans (adzuki beans, kidney beans), black beans, mung beans, and soybeans (miso, tofu) should constitute more than 60 percent of Yang Type A's vegetable and spice intake.

These vegetables and spices all strengthen and support the weakest organ of Yang Type A's, the kidneys, while calming their overactive digestive system. With such an active digestive system, foods are quickly broken down into sugar, potentially leading to an imbalance of blood sugar levels, a common issue among Yang Type A's. With a substantial amount of B vitamins and iron, these vegetables help nourish and balance the blood. As a rule of thumb, the darker green the vegetable, the higher the amount of iron and B vitamins it contains. Lettuce and kale contain significant amounts of vitamin A, which supports eye, immune, and bone health. In Eastern medicine cucumber is prized for its cooling and anti-inflammatory properties, and in the summer it is consumed regularly to quench thirst and prevent overheating. Mung and soy beans also have a cold nature and can calm the stomach and ease anxiety. Black beans contain high amounts of insoluble fiber, with one cup of black beans providing 60 percent of the recommended daily allowance. Black beans are also very rich in protein and iron: one cup provides 30 percent of the RDA of protein. Burdock root, which is often seen in Asian recipes, is also used to treat fever and sore throat. According to Eastern medicine, eggplant is said to nourish and strengthen the kidneys.

Eggplant skin is rich in antioxidants, which protect the body's cells from damage. As far as vegetables go, kale tops the charts in vitamins K, A, and C. Only 10 grams of kale supplies the recommended daily allowance of vitamin K, 25 grams for vitamin A, and 68 grams for vitamin C. It is also rich in glucosinolates, credited with lowering the risk of cancer of the bladder, prostate, and ovaries. Celery contains an active ingredient called phthalide, which helps to reduce blood pressure by dilating blood vessels and arteries. Keep in mind that your intake of celery may need to be restricted if you are taking medications for high blood pressure or circulatory disorders.

Yellow-Light Veggies and Spices for Yang Type A

Similar Energy: lettuce (iceberg), alfalfa sprouts, artichoke, broccoli, snow peas, Swiss chard, tomato, bitter gourd, and bamboo shoots should constitute up to 40 percent of Yang Type A's vegetable and spice intake.

Opposite Energy: potatoes, sweet potatoes, lotus root, carrots, cabbage, yams, bell peppers (green and red), radishes, pumpkin, white beans, turmeric, dandelion greens, chickpeas (garbanzo beans), asparagus, arrowroot, and bean sprouts should constitute less than 30 percent of Yang Type A's *yellow-light* vegetables and spices.

The above similar energy vegetables have a cool nature and could therefore support the weaker lower body of the Yang Type A, if ingested in moderation. I suggest ingesting up to eight servings of these foods each week.

The above opposite energy vegetables have a warm nature. Even though the Yang Type A benefits from cold-natured foods, in moderation these warm-natured foods can also be a valuable source of fiber, vitamins, iron, and beta-carotene. Keep in mind that a warm nature may cause slight indigestion in the long run if these foods are ingested excessively (more than eight servings a week).

Red-Light Veggies and Spices for Yang Type A

Garlic, green onions (scallions), onions, shallots, sage, ginger, thyme, black pepper, jalapeños, chives, anise, cilantro, fennel, rosemary, wasabi, horseradish, mustard seeds, cardamom, and coriander seeds should constitute less than 5 percent of Yang Type A's vegetable and spice intake.

If Yang Type A's eat a significant amount of the above hot-natured foods, heat will quickly accumulate inside the stomach, causing indigestion, acid reflux, frontal headaches, or stomachaches. Hot-natured foods can cause serious health issues in the long run for Yang Type A's because of their tendency to develop heat-related disorders. In small amounts these spices can occasionally be added to the Yang Type A's green-light foods to boost flavor. But be careful not to overdo it! While most cool-natured vegetables become warm-natured when cooked, some hot-natured vegetables actually mellow out too. Therefore, Yang Type A's do not have to worry about their health when cooking with moderate amounts of onions, green onions (scallions), chives, and garlic.

Did you just eat a red-light food? Don't worry! Chilled barley tea or natural mint iced tea can serve as a quick Yang Type A antidote for hot-natured foods.

FRUITS AND NUTS FOR YANG TYPE A

Being sensitive to heat, Yang Type A's often develop itchy and dry skin in the summer months. They also tend to be plagued with stomach heat–related conditions during this time often leading to acid reflux, bloating, a burning sensation in the solar plexus area, and/or frontal headaches. Fruits help to cool and moisten the Yang Type A's digestive system and skin. Eating seasonal fruits is an excellent way for Yang Type A's to keep cool and avoid heat-related issues. I recommend that up to 20 percent of the entire Yang Type A food intake come from fruit.

Green-Light Fruits and Nuts for Yang Type A

> Grapes, melons (watermelon), strawberries, bananas, pineapple, blackberries, and peanuts should constitute more than 60 percent of Yang Type A's fruit intake.

Grapes are a good source of vitamins C and K. They are used in Eastern medicine to strengthen the tendons and bones, promote urination in cases of edema (water retention), and nourish the blood. The cold nature of watermelon soothes the body when you're suffering from excess heat and calms the mind and body. It also helps to quench thirst. Strawberries and pineapple top all other fruits in this category when it comes to vitamin C content. They have 5½ times more vitamin C than grapes! Strawberries are used in Eastern medicine to promote digestion, calm a nasty cough, and soothe a sore throat. Like other fruits in this category, pineapple is good at clearing heat from the body, quenching thirst, and easing diarrhea due to excess exposure to heat. Bananas are a good source of vitamins C and B_6 and potassium, and are particularly beneficial for Yang Type A's in preventing illness of the kidneys, their weakest organ. Blackberries are one of the best foods for Yang Type A's because they help nourish and strengthen the kidneys. They are often used in combination with herbs in Eastern medicine to treat kidney and urinary disorders. Blackberries can be consumed regularly to support a sore or weak lower back and legs. Peanuts provide 47 percent of the recommended daily allowance of protein per 100 grams, and are a great source of iron (13 percent) and fiber (32 percent).

Yellow-Light Fruits and Nuts for Yang Type A

> **Similar Energy:** persimmon, black currants, kiwi, star fruit, and raspberries should constitute up to 40 percent of Yang Type A's fruit intake.

Opposite Energy: pears, figs, apricots, plums, dried plums (prunes), avocados, longan, chestnuts, walnut, pine nuts, ginkgo nuts, almonds, hazelnuts, acorns, macadamia nuts, and pecans should constitute less than 30 percent of Yang Type A's *yellow-light* fruits.

These similar energy cool-natured fruits, eaten in moderation, can support the Yang Type A's weaker lower body and counter the Yang Type A's tendency to overheat. I suggest ingesting up to twelve portions a week of these cool fruits.

Even though Yang Type A's benefit from cold-natured foods, in moderation these opposite energy warm-natured fruits and nuts can also be a valuable source of fiber and vitamin C. Keep in mind that their warm nature may cause Yang Type A's slight indigestion in the long run if opposite energy warm-natured fruits and nuts are ingested excessively (more than eight servings a week).

Red-Light Fruits and Nuts for Yang Type A

Apples (all varieties), oranges (all varieties), tangerines, lemon, lime, mango, passion fruit, grapefruit, lychee, durian, pomegranate, and dates should constitute less than 5 percent of Yang Type A's fruit intake.

Yang Types can enjoy most Yin type fruits, while Yin types can enjoy most Yang type fruits without having to worry about indigestion. The key, however, is to consume red-light fruits in moderation and in season.

Of all of the red-light fruits, durian has the hottest nature. This fruit can easily cause excessive stomach heat in Yang types. The Yang Type A is better off avoiding durian altogether.

MEAT AND DAIRY

I recommend that up to 40 percent of the entire Yang Type A food intake come from meat. That's a lot of meat, isn't it? Actually, without meat, the Yang Type A's stomach heat can burn out of control, leading to a number of symptoms, such as acid reflux, unsettled stomach, anxiety, high blood pressure, and tremors. Hunger is often a common cause of discomfort for Yang Type A's. Since meat takes a longer time to digest, it keeps the stomach occupied and out of trouble for longer periods. Protein from meat also helps to provide long-lasting energy that Yang Type A's cannot obtain any other way. It also provides them with plenty of energy for cell repair and cell reproduction.

Green-Light Meat and Dairy for Yang Type A

Pork, most fish (cod, mackerel, trout, flounder, herring), shellfish (clams, lobster, oysters, shrimp, prawns, scallops), crayfish, egg yolk (raw or boiled), cheese (made from cow's milk), cow's milk, and soymilk should constitute more than 60 percent of Yang Type A's meat and dairy intake.

This list consists of cold-natured meats and dairy products that are particularly beneficial for the Yang Type A's weaker kidneys and overactive digestive system, because they reduce excessive heat from the digestive system. Of all these meats, pork and shellfish have the most Yin, making them beneficial for the Yin-deficient Yang Type A. Pork is very rich in several B vitamins (thiamin, riboflavin, niacin, B_6, and B_{12}) and minerals (phosphorus, potassium, and zinc). Shrimp provides the most protein and crab provides the most zinc, compared to other shellfish.

Yang Type A's are prone to bone injury and osteoporosis because of their inherently weak kidneys. In Eastern medicine the kidneys are in charge of maintaining proper bone growth and strength. Yang Type A's therefore need to consider alternative ways to keep their bones strong. Regularly consuming cow's milk is a great way to strengthen the Yang Type A's bones. One cup of milk provides 28 percent of the recommended daily allowance of calcium. Cheese is another great source of calcium for Yang Type A's. Among all cheeses Romano, Swiss, and Ricotta have the most calcium. Romano cheese has 151 percent of the RDA of calcium per serving. The problem is, however, that it also has 122 percent of the

RDA of saturated fat! In smaller amounts Romano cheese can serve as a calcium-fortified, yummy addition to your favorite Italian recipe.

Caution about Cholesterol

Most of these meats and cheeses are high in cholesterol. The good news is that Yang Type A's can break down and eliminate food by-products better than the other body types. Even with more meat intake, they are less susceptible to cholesterol accumulation in the body. Still, it is important for Yang Type A's to guard against ingesting too much fat. Drinking mint or peppermint tea with meals can help counteract the accumulation of cholesterol in the body.

From the Clinic

At the age of three, Sarah often complained of pain in her solar plexus, which is directly above the fundus (the upper part of the stomach). Her mom realized that the onset of this pain always seemed to correspond to an empty stomach. The problem was that Sarah rarely mentioned that she was hungry. It was as if the pain stole her appetite away. Sarah's doctor diagnosed her condition as GERD (gastroesophageal reflux disease) and told her mom to give her antacid tablets. This seemed to work for her only during acute episodes, but it never stopped the problem from coming back. When Sarah turned four, she developed a taste for hard-boiled eggs. Like magic, her stomachaches disappeared!

Not only are eggs a substantial source of protein, but they also help to calm the Yang Type A's stomach heat, which can cause pain in the solar plexus. This is a common situation for Yang Type A's, due to a buildup of heat in the digestive system. Since the digestive system of the Yang Type A is so strong, it tends to overreact and get agitated easily. Protein takes longer to digest than other foods. Meat and dairy therefore keep the Yang Type A's stomach occupied without running the risk of overheating. All the Yang Type A's proteins (in the list above) help to cool stomach heat.

Yellow-Light Meat and Dairy for Yang Type A

> **Opposite Energy:** duck, beef, salmon, croaker, sole, goat's milk, almond milk, and yogurt should constitute less than 30 percent of Yang Type A's *yellow-light* meats and dairy products.

There are no similar energy yellow-light meats for the Yang Type A because meat either has a hot, warm, or cold nature according to Sasang medicine.

Opposite energy yellow-light meats and dairy products are a good source of protein and calcium for Yang Type A's. Calcium from the dairy products listed above also helps to calm their stomach heat. Yet since these foods have a warm nature, if taken in excess, they could cause further accumulation of heat in the stomach. Up to eight servings a week of these meats and dairy products are recommended. Also, keep in mind that if you are a Yang Type A who is suffering from signs of overheating such as fever, acid reflux, night sweats, or high blood pressure, you should avoid these meats and dairy products because they may exacerbate the problem.

Red-Light Meat and Dairy for Yang Type A

> Chicken, lamb, quail, pheasant, Alaskan pollack, anchovy, venison, and rice milk should constitute less than 5 percent of Yang Type A's meat and dairy intake.

Since Yang Type A's already have so much heat in the stomach and spleen area, these hot-natured foods are potentially harmful to them. After consuming chicken or lamb, Yang Type A's often experience excess gas, acid reflux, headaches, and/or belching. These symptoms may become acute if these meats are ingested during the warmer months or when the Yang Type A is ill. Rice milk is much more forgiving than the other hot-natured foods in this category due to its gentle effect on the digestive system. Even the Yang Type A can benefit from a limited amount of rice milk if no other milk is available.

TEAS FOR YANG TYPE A

Green-Light Teas for Yang Type A

Mint, peppermint, jasmine, and/or barley teas should be consumed daily by Yang Type A's after meals.

There are over thirty-six different herbs that are beneficial for Yang Type A's. Most of these herbs, made into teas, pills, or granules, are prescribed for specific health reasons. Listed here are four common herbs that can support the Yang Type A's general health. These teas are also easy to find. Try planting some mint or peppermint in your garden this fall. Come spring you'll have an abundant supply of herbs for fresh tea! Consuming tea with meals can help with digestion and boost your metabolism. Mint and peppermint are very cooling and soothing for the Yang Type A's overactive digestive system. These herbs can also help control allergies, colds, headaches, throat soreness, and indigestion. Researchers have recently discovered that jasmine tea may reduce cholesterol.* Jasmine tea has been the after-meal tea of choice for thousands of years in China. Cape jasmine (gardenia) has been historically used in Eastern medicine to treat inflammation, fever, infections, and headaches. Barley is an excellent source of fiber and iron. One hundred grams of barley contains 69 percent of the recommended daily allowance of fiber and 20 percent of the RDA of iron. Keep in mind that barley tea contains gluten, which may irritate the intestines of those with celiac disease or other gluten-related sensitivities.

Yellow-Light Teas for Yang Type A

Similar Energy: pine needle, buckwheat, and quince fruit teas should be consumed up to five times a week by Yin Type A's.

*For example, see Chan, Ping Ttim, Wing Ping Fong, Yuk Lin Cheung, Yu Huang, Walter Kwok Keung Ho, and Zhen-Yu Chen, "Jasmine Green Tea Epicatechins Are Hypolipidemic in Hamsters Fed a High Fat Diet" *Journal of Nutrition* 129, no. 6 (1999): 1094–101.

These cool-natured teas contain more Yin than Yang and are therefore somewhat beneficial for Yin-deficient Yang Type A's. In moderation these teas can support their circulation and cool down their easily over-heated digestive systems.

Red-Light Teas for Yang Type A

> Ginger, cinnamon, clove, chai, licorice, and citrus (lemon, tangerine peel) teas should be avoided by Yang Type A's.

Since Yang Type A's already have so much heat in the stomach and spleen area, these hot-natured teas are potentially harmful to them. After consuming these teas, Yang Type A's often experience excess gas, acid reflux, headaches, and/or excessive belching. Symptoms may become acute if these teas are ingested during the warmer months or when the Yang Type A is ill.

SUPPLEMENTS FOR YANG TYPE A

> Blackberry extract, goji (wolfberry) juice, calcium/vitamin D, fish oil, barley grass

Blackberry extract is very rich in nutrients, such as dietary fiber, vitamins C and K, folic acid, and manganese. The tiny black seeds in each blackberry are high in omega-3 and omega-5 fatty acids and protein. As if this weren't enough, blackberries also support the weaker kidneys of the Yang Type A.

Goji is another herb that supports the Yang Type A's kidney function. It is also used in Sasang medicine to support vision and calm the spirit. Several recent studies have reported positive effects of goji in the treatment of eyesight issues, such as macular degeneration and glaucoma, cancer, cardiovascular, and inflammatory diseases.* Since, in Sasang medicine, the kidneys are responsible for bone strength, the weaker kidneys of the Yang Type A often lead to weaker bones. Supplements with calcium can help prevent bone issues, such as osteopenia and osteoporosis, from developing. Vitamin D is usually taken with calcium to help the body absorb it better. Finally, I recommend that Yang Type A's ingest fish oil on a regular basis because its cold nature helps to nourish their weaker kidneys. Fish oil contains omega-3 fatty acids, which have an anti-inflammatory effect in the body. It has also been found to benefit those who are suffering from cardiovascular disease and arthritis.

See table 3.6 on pages 172–73 for a detailed summary of all Yang Type A food recommendations.

*For examples, see Bucheli, Peter, Karine Vidal, Lisong Shen, Zhencheng Gu, Charlie Zhang, Larry E. Miller, and Junkuan Wang, "Goji Berry Effects on Macular Characteristics and Plasma Antioxidant Levels" *Optometry and Vision Science* 88, no. 2 (2011): 257–62.; Luo, Qiong, Zhuoneng Li, Jun Yan, Fan Zhu, Ruo-Jun Xu, and Yi-Zhong Cai, "*Lycium barbarum* (Goji) Polysaccharides Induce Apoptosis in Human Prostate Cancer Cells and Inhibits Prostate Cancer Growth in Xenograft Mouse Model of Human Prostate Cancer" *Journal of Medicinal Food* 12, no. 4 (2009): 695–703; and "Side Effects and Benefits of Wolfberry (Juice)" www.zhion.com/herb/Wolfberry_goji_berry.html (accessed June 22, 2014).

TABLE 3.6. QUICK REFERENCE OF YANG TYPE A FOODS

Food Group	Green-Light Foods (60% or more)	Yellow-Light Foods (40% or less)	Red-Light Foods (foods to avoid)
Cereals, Seeds, and Grains (20%)	Wild rice, black rice, black sesame seeds, wheat, barley	Buckwheat, rye, corn, glutinous (sweet) rice, oats, white/yellow sesame seeds, tahini (hummus), quinoa, Job's tears, flaxseed, pumpkin seeds, sunflower seeds, white beans, brown rice	There are no red-light cereals and grains for Yang Type A's, but those with this body type shouldn't eat too many hot-natured grains, such as glutinous rice.
Vegetables, Beans, and Spices (25%)	Lettuce (romaine), cucumber, taro root, burdock root, eggplant, kale, celery, seaweed, mung beans, green, soy or red beans (adzuki beans, kidney beans), black beans	Lettuce (iceberg), alfalfa sprouts, artichoke, snow peas, tomato, Swiss chard, bitter gourd, bamboo shoots, potatoes, sweet potatoes, carrots, yams, lotus root, turmeric, bell peppers (green, red, yellow), radishes, pumpkin, chickpeas, asparagus	Garlic, green onions (scallions), onion, shallots, sage, ginger, thyme, black pepper, jalapeños, chives, anise, cilantro, fennel, rosemary, wasabi, horseradish, mustard seeds, coriander seeds, cardamom
Fruits and Nuts (20%)	Grapes, melon (watermelon), strawberries, bananas, pineapple, blackberries, peanuts	Black currant, kiwi, star fruit, persimmon, pears, figs, apricots, plums, dried plums (prunes), avocados, longan, chestnuts, walnuts, pine nuts, ginkgo nuts, almonds, hazelnuts, sunflower seeds, pumpkin seeds, acorns, macadamia nuts, pecans	Apples (all varieties), orange (all varieties), tangerines, lemon, lime, mango, passion fruit, grapefruit, lychee, durian, peach, cherries, pomegranate. Moderate intake of these fruits when in season will not cause health issues for the Yang Type A.

Food Group	Green-Light Foods (60% or more)	Yellow-Light Foods (40% or less)	Red-Light Foods (foods to avoid)
Meat and Dairy (35%)	Pork, most fish (cod, mackerel, trout, flounder, herring), shellfish (clams, lobster, oysters, shrimp, prawns, scallops, mussels), crayfish, egg yolk (raw or boiled), cheese (made from cow's milk), soymilk	Duck meat, cow meat, salmon, goat's milk, almond milk, yogurt	Chicken, lamb, quail, pheasant, Alaskan pollack, anchovies, venison, rice milk
Teas	Mint, peppermint, jasmine, barley	Pine needle, buckwheat, quince fruit	Ginger, cinnamon, clove, chai, licorice, citrus (lemon, tangerine peel)
Supplements	Blackberry extract, goji (wolfberry) juice, barley grass, calcium/vitamin D, fish oil	No need to supplement with yellow lights!	Hot-natured supplements such as ginger (extract), cinnamon (extract), ginseng

Yang Type B Foods

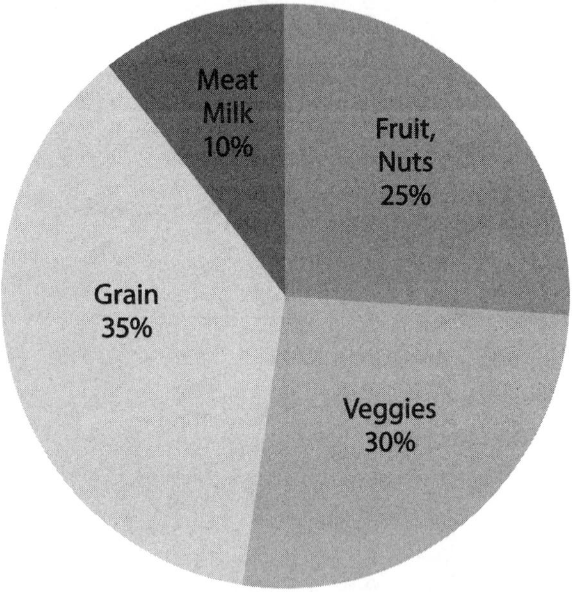

Figure 3.7. Breakdown of optimum food group percentages for the Yang Type B's diet (also see table 3.8 on pages 188–89 for details)

With so much Yang circulating through their upper body, Yang Type B's often appear to have the most energy of the four body types. They are always on the go and have the most trouble slowing down. It takes a lot of food to fuel their energy. Born with a weaker liver, however, Yang Type B's have difficulty digesting high-protein or fatty foods.

Just like a bull grazing in the pasture all day long, the Yang Type B benefits from a continuous supply of smaller, low-protein grain and vegetable-based meals. If Yang Type B's ingest too much protein in one sitting, they will likely vomit it up again, with no accompanying signs of discomfort, such as distention, gas, bowel issues, and the like. Their weakened liver will simply say no and send the food right back where it came from.

The cool-natured green-light foods in this section support and cleanse the weaker liver of the Yang Type B. In both Sasang and Western medicine, the liver is responsible for breaking down and eliminating fats and toxins from the body. A weaker liver cannot carry out this function effectively, hence the tendency to develop toxic buildup in the system. Luckily, Yang Type B's are also born with stronger lungs. In Sasang medicine the lungs can help the liver by sending it ample amounts of energy in the form of oxygen. As long as those macho lungs display compassion for the poor liver and don't hoard all the body's energy, the liver will be able to carry out its function efficiently.

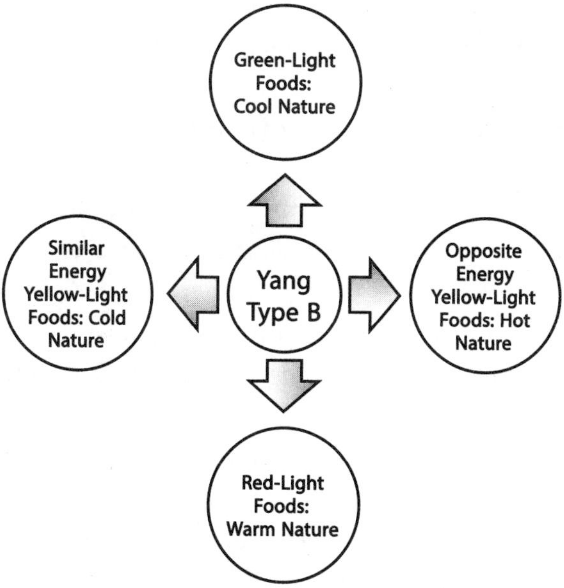

Figure 3.8. Yang Type B food energy summary

FOOD NAVIGATOR

The Yang Type B's weaker liver is strengthened by the cool nature of this body type's green-light foods, which offer digestive support and energy. The Yang Type B's cold-natured, similar energy yellow-light foods resemble the cool nature of this body type's green-light foods. The Yang Type B's hot-natured, opposite energy yellow-light foods are closer to red-light foods because warm and hot, which support the Yin type organs, are opposite energies of cool and cold. A warm nature makes the Yang Type B's red-light foods the exact opposite of their cool-natured green-light foods and can overstimulate and congest the Yang Type A's naturally stronger lungs.

CEREALS, SEEDS, AND GRAINS FOR YANG TYPE B

The cereals and grains category is an important food group for Yang Type B's because they help to cool and calm their excessive Yang, while supporting the weaker liver. I recommend that up to 35 percent of the entire Yang Type B food intake come from cereals and grains.

Green-Light Cereals, Seeds, and Grains for Yang Type B

Buckwheat, rye, and corn should constitute more than 60 percent of Yang Type B's cereal and grain intake.

Bukwheat has a cool energetic nature. After ingestion cool-natured foods travel to and support the Yang Type B's weakest organ, the liver. Buckwheat is one of the healthiest foods for the Yang Type B. One cup provides 68 percent of the recommended daily allowance of insoluble fiber. Buckwheat is also very rich in iron, niacin, and riboflavin. One cup of buckwheat also contains 98 percent of the recommended daily allowance of magnesium. Buckwheat is a nongluten alternative to rice or porridge. It contains a flavonoid called rutin, which acts as an antioxidant. Buckwheat has also been known to help in the reduction of cholesterol, likely due to its support of the liver function.

Yellow-Light Cereals, Seeds, and Grains for Yang Type B

Similar Energy: wild rice, black rice, black sesame seeds, and wheat should constitute up to 40 percent of Yang Type B's cereal and grain intake.
Opposite Energy: glutinous (sweet) rice should constitute less than 30 percent of Yang Type B's *yellow-light* cereals and grains.

Similar energy cold-natured grains, if eaten in moderation, can support the Yang Type B's weaker lower body. I suggest ingesting up to seven portions a week of these foods.

Glutinous rice can be a valuable source of fiber for Yang Type B's. Do bear in mind that its warm and slightly hot nature may cause Yang Type B's slight indigestion in the long run if they consume it excessively (more than seven servings a week).

Red-Light Cereals, Seeds, and Grains for Yang Type B

Oats, white/yellow sesame seeds, tahini (hummus), quinoa, Job's tears, brown rice, flaxseed, pumpkin seeds, sunflower seeds, and millet should constitute less than 5 percent of Yang Type B's cereal and grain intake.

These warm-natured foods can reverse the natural flow of energy from the stronger lungs to the weaker liver of the Yang Type B and therefore, should be avoided, if possible.

VEGETABLES AND SPICES FOR YANG TYPE B

Vegetables and spices make up another essential food group of the Yang Type B. These foods are usually easy to digest and keep the energy flowing smoothly throughout the digestive system. Unlike the other body types, Yang Type B's rely heavily on this group because of their difficulty in digesting meats. Vegetables are the main source of energy for Yang Type

B's, who need to consume a large quantity of vegetables to keep going, since they are the most active of the four body types. Keep in mind that they benefit more from eating raw vegetables, since cooking causes food nature to go from cool to warm or hot. I recommend that 30 percent of the entire Yang Type B food intake come from vegetables and spices.

Green-Light Veggies and Spices for Yang Type B

> Lettuce (iceberg), alfalfa sprouts, artichoke, broccoli, snow peas, Swiss chard, tomato, bamboo shoots, and bitter gourd should constitute more than 60 percent of Yang Type B's vegetable and spice intake.

These vegetables and spices all strengthen and support the Yang Type B's weakest organ, the liver. Raw vegetables also have a cold or cool nature, which helps calm and soothe the overactive Yang energy of Yang Type B's. These vegetables help nourish and balance Yang with their high B vitamin and iron content. Lettuce is very rich in vitamins A and K. Forty grams of lettuce provide the full recommended daily allowance of vitamin A. Lettuce also contains substantial amounts of vitamins C and B, folic acid, calcium, magnesium, and potassium. Artichokes have the most iron in the above group, claiming 26 percent of the recommended daily allowance in just 120 grams (one artichoke), and they make a good source of vegetable protein and calcium. Each artichoke contains 17 percent of the RDA of folic acid, which is essential in the process of gene formation in newborns. An added benefit of artichokes is their high vitamin C content, which is 20 percent of the RDA per serving! Tomatoes, too, are very high in vitamin C: one cup of tomato juice has 32 percent of the RDA. Also high in vitamins A and K, tomatoes contain a flavonoid called lycopene, known for protecting the skin against the sun's harmful UV rays. However, I wouldn't eat them in place of using sunscreen when frolicking about in summer sunlight! Broccoli tops all others in the above group when it comes to vitamins C and K. One cup of fresh broccoli contains 135 percent of the RDA of vitamin C and 116 percent of vitamin K and is also rich in fiber, plant-source protein, and vitamin A. Broccoli contains flavonoids that are believed to have antibacterial and antiviral properties, while helping to prevent prostate cancer and heart disease.

Yellow-Light Veggies and Spices for Yang Type B

Similar Energy: lettuce (romaine), most dark green vegetables, cucumber, taro root, burdock root, green peas, red beans (adzuki, kidney), black beans, mung beans, soybeans (miso, tofu), eggplant, kale, and celery should constitute up to 40 percent of Yang Type B's vegetable and spice intake.
Opposite Energy: garlic, green onions (scallions), onions, shallots, sage, ginger, thyme, black pepper, jalapeños, chives, anise, cilantro, fennel, rosemary, wasabi, cardamom, and horseradish should constitute less than 30 percent of Yang Type B's *yellow-light* vegetables and spices.

If eaten in moderation, these similar energy cold-natured vegetables can support the Yang Type B's weaker lower body. I suggest consuming up to twelve portions a week of these foods.

Even though the Yang Type B benefits from cool-natured foods, these hot-natured foods in moderation can be a valuable source of fiber, vitamins, iron, and beta-carotene. Keep in mind that a hot nature may cause slight indigestion in the long run if they're consumed in excess (more than eight servings a week). Since Yang Type B's have an abundant amount of Yang, they should avoid intensely spicy foods, which can aggravate their Yang energy.

Red-Light Veggies and Spices for Yang Type B

White beans (lima, navy, Great Northern), potatoes, sweet potatoes, radishes, carrots, lotus root, yams, cabbage, turmeric, bean sprouts, pumpkin, arrowroot, dandelion greens, bell peppers (green, red, yellow), chickpeas (garbanzo beans), and asparagus should constitute less than 5 percent of Yang Type B's vegetable and spice intake.

These warm-natured vegetables stimulate the excessive lung energy of the Yang Type B's. If Yang Type B's eat these foods, they will often experience shortness of breath, fullness in the chest, chest discomfort, or heat-related symptoms such as hot flashes, heatstroke, or excessive sweating. Warm-natured foods can cause serious health issues for Yang Type B's because they direct energy away from the liver and toward the lungs, causing further depletion of their already weak liver.

Did you just eat a red-light food? Don't worry! Large amounts of cool water or juicing with green-light vegetables can serve as a quick Yang Type B antidote to the effects of warm-natured foods.

FRUITS AND NUTS FOR YANG TYPE B

With the Yang types' tendency to overheat, they are prone to headaches and heat-induced exhaustion, especially in the summer months, a response to an excessive amount of Yang energy bursting upward toward the lungs and spleen. Fruits help to cool, settle, and ground the Yang Type B's excessive Yang energy, allowing it to flow more smoothly and more consistently throughout the body. Eating fruits in season is an excellent way for Yang Type B's to cool down and prevents the onset of heat-related issues. I recommend that up to 25 percent of the entire Yang Type B food intake come from fruits.

Green-Light Fruits and Nuts for Yang Type B

Persimmons, black currants, kiwi, star fruit, and raspberry should constitute more than 60 percent of Yang Type B's fruit intake.

All these cool-natured foods travel to the Yang Type B's weakest organ, the liver, to support its function. Persimmons are rich in vitamins A and C and they contain significant amounts of essential minerals, such as manganese and copper, that are important for blood cell growth and protection. Persimmons contain a compound called betulinic acid, known to have antitumor properties. In Eastern medicine they are used to calm and clear heat from the stomach and intestines, improving digestion and bowel movement. No other fruit in this category can compare with black currants when it comes to vitamin C. Every 100 grams of black currants supply 302 percent of the recommended daily allowance! Black currants are also a good source of calcium, vitamin A, and iron. Kiwi is next in line when it comes to vitamin C; each kiwi contains 155 percent of the RDA. They are also very rich in vitamin K (50 percent of RDA) and potassium (9 percent of RDA), and contain phytonutrients known to protect DNA from oxygen damage. This action can help prevent cell mutation leading to cancer cell formation.

Yellow-Light Fruits and Nuts for Yang Type B

Similar Energy: grapes, melon (watermelon), strawberries, bananas, pineapple, blackberries, blueberries, and peanuts should constitute up to 40 percent of Yang Type B's fruit and nut intake.

Opposite Energy: apples (all varieties), oranges (all varieties), tangerines, mango, peaches, passion fruit, lemon, lime, grapefruit, lychee, pomegranate, dates, durian, and cherries should constitute less than 30 percent of Yang Type B's *yellow-light* fruits and nuts.

The cold-natured, similar energy fruits listed above effectively nourish and cool the body during the warmer months of the year. These fruits, if eaten in moderation, can help support the weaker lower body of Yang Type B's and counter their tendency to overheat. I suggest ingesting up to twelve portions a week of these fruits.

Even though the Yang Type B benefits primarily from cool-natured foods, the above hot-natured opposite energy fruits, if eaten in moderation, are a valuable source of fiber and vitamin C. Keep in mind, however, that hot-natured fruits may cause slight indigestion for Yang Type B's in the long run if ingested excessively (more than eight servings a week). This is especially true of durian, which is the hottest-nature fruit in the above list.

Red-Light Fruits and Nuts for Yang Type B

Pears, figs, apricots, plums, dried plums (prunes), avocados, and longan should constitute less than 5 percent of Yang Type B's fruit and nut intake.

Although fruits have cooler and warmer natures, they are not limited to this or that body type. As long as you consume red-light fruits in moderation and in season, indigestion should not be a problem no matter which body type you are.

Did you notice that I did not include warm-natured nuts in the red-light food category? While some Yang Type B's have difficulty digesting warm-natured nuts such as walnuts, almonds, chestnuts, hazelnuts, and pecans, others may not be faced with this challenge. Nuts in general may serve as an easier to digest nonmeat protein source even for Yang Type B's. If you are a Yang Type B who feels bloated, experiences shortness of breath, or chest area discomfort after eating warm-natured nuts, then you may want to try cool and cold-natured nuts like coconut or peanuts instead. If you do not experience any of these symptoms, then ingesting moderate amounts of warm-natured nuts may help provide consistent energy throughout the day.

MEAT AND DAIRY FOR YANG TYPE B

The liver and its sister organ, the gallbladder, play a major role in the digestion of protein and fat in meat. A weaker liver makes it challenging for most Yang Type B's to digest meats. For this reason, Yang Type B's do not have their own green-light meats to indulge in. To preserve the health of their liver, it is advisable for Yang Type B's to consume no more than 10 percent meat in their diet. The rest of their dietary intake should come from vegetables, fruits, and grains. If Yang Type B's do eat meat, they should ingest only cold-natured meats, which are listed in "Yellow-Light Meat and Dairy for Yang Type B" (page 183).

Yang Type B's will often experience nausea after excessive ingestion of warm- or hot-natured meat. Even cold-natured meats may be difficult for them to keep down at times. While the other body types usually show signs of digestive distress, such as stomach pain, nausea, or body aches, Yang Type B's do not display any sign of discomfort, other than vomiting. Their energy level or appetite is also rarely affected. They simply go about their business as if nothing happened. If you are a Yang Type B who has trouble digesting meat, I suggest ingesting smaller portions in an easier-to-digest form, such as in soups or stews or plant-based protein drinks. Reducing meat portions may work for some but not others, who cannot ingest meat no matter how much they try. It's not necessary to force yourself to eat meat if you are a Yang Type B. There are numerous nonmeat, high-protein sources that could do the trick without causing issues (see table 3.7).

TABLE 3.7. ALTERNATE SOURCES OF YANG TYPE B PROTEIN

Compatibility for Yang Type B	Nonmeat Sources of High Protein (percent of RDA per 100 grams)
Green-Light Foods	**Grains:** Buckwheat (26%) **Vegetables:** Artichokes (6%), broccoli (6%)
Yellow-Light Foods	**Grains:** Black rice (17%), wild rice (8%), mung beans (6%), soybeans (33%), wheat (whole grain, 27%), barley (hulled, 25%), black sesame seeds (28%) **Vegetables:** Kale (6%), black beans (18%) **Nuts:** Peanuts (47%), coconut (uncooked, 7%)

Yellow-Light Meat and Dairy for Yang Type B

Similar Energy: pork, most fish (cod, mackerel, trout, flounder, herring), shellfish (clams, lobster, oysters, shrimp, prawns, scallops, crayfish, mussels), egg yolk (raw or boiled), cow's milk, and soymilk should constitute up to 40 percent of Yang Type B's meat and dairy intake.

Only if Yang Type B's can tolerate it should they ingest any of the above meats. These meats are generally cool- or cold-natured and are therefore potentially consumable for the Yang types. If Yang Type B's cannot tolerate meat, then even the above foods should be avoided. There is no need to force Yang Type B's to eat meat because they can absorb enough protein, vitamins, and minerals from the green-light grains, fruits, and vegetables.

From the Clinic

Brian's mom made numerous attempts to introduce meat into his diet. At eight years of age, he still could not eat meat. At first he would spit it out without swallowing. Later, he would try to swallow it, only to vomit shortly afterward. She has tried just about every type of meat in every form possible, from soup stock to small chunks of chicken, pork, turkey, and the like. Strangely, however, Brian never complained of indigestion. Nor did he show any other signs of nutritional distress. His skin has always been lustrous and his energy level was greater than that of most other healthy eight-year-olds. In consulting with me, she learned that Brian was a Yang Type B and that his inability to digest meat was a reflection of his body type. I reassured her that there was no need to worry and that Brian could get enough protein from Yang Type B green-light vegetables. I also suggested reintroducing small amounts of cold-property meats a few years later, when Brian's digestive system was more developed. Brian's mom was relieved to discover his body type and to further understand her child's needs.

Most Yang Type B infants can drink cow's milk and soymilk, as will many Yang Type B adults. If Yang Type B's don't have difficulty ingesting milk or eating the above meats, they should keep them as part of their diet but practice moderation. If they find milk products indigestible, I recommend supplementing with calcium and vitamin D to avoid deficiency.

Red-Light Meat and Dairy for Yang Type B

Duck, beef, salmon, croaker, chicken, lamb, quail, pheasant, venison, Alaskan pollack, goat's milk, almond milk, and yogurt should constitute less than 5 percent of Yang Type B's meat and dairy intake.

These warm- and hot-natured meats and dairy products are considered harmful to Yang Type B's. If Yang Type B's eat these foods, they will often experience indigestion or heat-related issues. Warm-natured foods can cause serious health issues for Yang Type B's because they direct energy away from the liver and toward the lungs, causing further depletion of their already weaker liver, which needs as much energy as it can get.

Did you just eat a red-light food? Don't worry! Large amounts of cool water or juicing with green-light vegetables can counteract warm-natured foods' effects on Yang Type B's.

TEAS FOR YANG TYPE B

Green-Light Teas for Yang Type B

Pine needle, buckwheat, and/or quince fruit teas should be consumed daily by Yang Type B's after meals.

There are over twenty herbs that are beneficial for Yang Type B's. Most of these herbs are prescribed for specific health-related situations. In this section I decided to list a few that support the general health of the Yang Type B. Buckwheat tea is a popular drink in East Asia (see pages 305–6 for more on this). It is usually boiled with water and then cooled in the refrigerator as a refreshing alternative to plain water. Pine needle tea has been used for thousands of years for its zesty taste and medicinal properties in both the Eastern and Western Hemispheres. It is very rich in vitamin C, works as a decongestant, and helps to boost the immune system. It has four to five times more vitamin C than fresh-squeezed orange juice! In Sasang medicine quince fruit (including the peel) is often used to treat indigestion, lower-body weakness, and lower-back and knee-joint pain. Quince is a good source of vitamin A, fiber, and iron.

Give It a Try!

Try collecting and preparing your own homemade pine needle tea! Follow the directions on this website for more details: http://www.ehow.com/how_2102192_pine-needle-tea.html.

Yellow-Light Teas for Yang Type B

Similar Energy: mint, peppermint, jasmine, and/or barley teas should be consumed up to five times a week by Yang Type B's.

These cold-natured, similar energy teas cool down the excessive Yang of the Yang Type B. The cold nature of these teas makes them suitable for ingestion especially during the warmer months or after a good workout. Keep in mind that barley contains gluten and could cause intestinal irritation for those with gluten sensitivities.

Red-Light Teas for Yang Type B

Dandelion, chamomile, green, and white teas should be avoided by Yang Type B's.

These warm-natured teas can overstimulate the already strong lungs of the Yang Type B and divert energy away from their weaker liver.

SUPPLEMENTS FOR YANG TYPE B

Quince fruit extract, graperoot extract, devil's club extract, cod liver oil

As mentioned above quince fruit helps support the weaker lower body of the Yang Type B and can be used for chronic lower-back, hip, knee, or ankle pain. An extract form can be purchased from theherbdoc.com. Graperoot extract also supports the lower body and contains an alkaloid called berberine, which is known for its anti-inflammatory and antibiotic properties. Graperoot extract is also used in cases of indigestion because it stimulates the flow of bile and compacted stool, preventing inflammation and bacteria accumulation along the digestive tract. Oregon graperoot extract is the most widely distributed and researched form of graperoot. Devil's club plays a major role in Sasang medicine as an important herb for grounding the excessive Yang of the Yang Type B. Like its cousin ginseng (a Yin Type B herb), it supports and strengthens the immune system. It has been traditionally used to fight against pneumonia, tuberculosis, tumor growth, and diabetes. Cod liver oil supports the function of the Yang Type B's weaker liver in accordance with the Eastern medical theory of "Like treats like."

See table 3.8 on pages 188–89 for a detailed summary of all Yang Type B food recommendations.

TABLE 3.8. QUICK REFERENCE OF YANG TYPE B FOODS

Food Group	Green-Light Foods (60% or more)	Yellow-Light Foods (40% or less)	Red-Light Foods (foods to avoid)
Cereals, Seeds, and Grains (25%)	Buckwheat, rye, corn	Wild rice, wheat, barley, black sesame seeds, black rice, glutinous (sweet) rice	Oats, white/yellow sesame seeds, tahini (hummus), quinoa, Job's tears, brown rice, pumpkin seeds, sunflower seeds, millet, flaxseed
Vegetables, Beans, and Spices (40%)	Lettuce (iceberg), alfalfa sprouts, artichoke, broccoli, snow peas, tomato, Swiss chard, bitter gourd, bamboo shoots	Lettuce (romaine), most dark green vegetables, cucumber, taro root, green peas, burdock root, eggplant, kale, celery, black beans, red beans (adzuki beans, kidney beans), mung beans, soybeans (miso, tofu), garlic, green onions (scallions), onions, shallots, sage, ginger, thyme, black pepper, jalapeños, chives, anise, cilantro, fennel, rosemary, wasabi, horseradish, coriander seeds, mustard seeds, cardamom	White beans (lima, navy, Great Northern), potatoes, sweet potatoes, radishes, carrots, lotus root, yams, cabbage, turmeric, bean sprouts, pumpkin, arrowroot, dandelion greens, bell peppers (green, red, yellow), chickpeas, asparagus

Food Group	Green-Light Foods (60% or more)	Yellow-Light Foods (40% or less)	Red-Light Foods (foods to avoid)
Fruits and Nuts (25%)	Black currants, kiwi, star fruit, coconut, persimmon, raspberries	Grapes, melon (watermelon), strawberry, banana, pineapple, blackberries, apples (all varieties), oranges (all varieties), tangerines, mango, passion fruit, lemon, lime, grapefruit, peach, lychee, pomegranate, dates, cherry, durian, peanuts	Pears figs, apricots, plums, dried plums (prunes), avocados, longan
Meat and Dairy (10%)	There are no green-light meats for the Yang Type B.	Pork, most fish (cod, mackerel, trout, flounder, herring), shellfish (clams, lobster, oysters, shrimp, prawns, scallops, mussels, crayfish), egg yolk (raw or boiled), cow's milk, cheese (made from cow's milk), soymilk	Duck meat, cow meat, salmon, chicken, lamb, quail, pheasant, venison, goat's milk, almond milk, yogurt
Teas	Pine needle, buckwheat, quince fruit	Mint, peppermint, jasmine, barley	Dandelion, chamomile, green, white
Supplements	Quince fruit extract, graperoot extract, devil's club extract, cod liver oil	No need to supplement with yellow lights!	Warm-natured supplements such as coenzyme Q10, vinegar, turmeric, vitamin E, omega-3 and omega-5, and ginko biloba

Balancing Your Diet

Previously, we discussed the function and actions of numerous types of herbs and foods for each body type. In this chapter we offer further guidance on what to eat, how much to eat, and when to eat to best serve your body type. The suggestions here refer to the healthy way to eat, rather than conforming to what is customarily accepted. For instance, when going out to lunch with your Korean boss, it is customary to choose what he or she orders from the menu. Choosing otherwise may offend your boss, but it may save your body from incompatible foods. Leaving room for dessert may be common practice in America, but filling up that room with sugary foods could make you feel heavy and groggy. Making the right choice for your health may at times leave you feeling like the oddball!

All this may seem like common sense, but that doesn't stop most of us from going off the deep end at times. It is human nature to see how much we can get away with, but it is also in our DNA to make positive changes for our health.

The end of the chapter provides a general outline of what a typical daily diet looks like for Yin and Yang body types and how to use these foods to balance your everyday life. These guidelines are not meant to be applied rigidly, but should be adapted to your individual needs. Modify them according to your lifestyle and you will reap the best of rewards. May this section provide you with a recharged desire for health and harmony!

THE FOOD PYRAMID AND YOUR BODY TYPE

Each of the body types has its own regimen for optimal food intake and categorization. In general Yang types need to eat more than the Yin types to satisfy their faster metabolism. Yin types often need to eat a bit less to compensate for a slower digestive system. Yang types benefit from eating more Yin energy foods, such as protein and raw veggies. Yin types, on the other hand, benefit from eating more Yang energy foods, such as cooked veggies, spices, and teas.

The USDA (United States Department of Agriculture) food pyramid offers basic guidelines for food intake, according to six major food groups: grains, fruits, vegetables, dairy, protein foods, and fruits, and provides us with a picture of how a balanced diet should look. While these suggestions offer considerable direction for those who are just getting started, they don't take into consideration the nutritional needs of each of us and our body type. A one-size-fits-all approach to diet can lead to imbalance, affecting the relationship between your stronger and weaker organs. With this in mind, in the previous chapter I have altered the suggestions provided in the USDA food pyramid to accommodate the needs of each body type. (By now, you have probably discovered your body type and have already graduated from using a generalized standard approach to nutrition and health.)

One area in which *Your Yin Yang Body Type* particularly deviates from the USDA is in the meat, cheese, and nuts category. The USDA lumps these foods into one single group, which contradicts Sasang medical principles. While meat, cheese, and nuts all contain significant amounts of protein, they have very different energies and characteristics. Meat, which closely resembles the protein structure of our cells, is a significantly different form of protein from that of plants or nuts. While this form of protein may be the most nourishing for the body's tissues, it tends to cause constipation in excessive amounts. Even though nuts do not provide us with as much protein per serving, they contain oils that actually promote smooth bowel movement, rather than hindering it, and unlike meat they do not contain cholesterol. Nuts are therefore an excellent source of protein for Yin Type A's, who have a tendency to get constipated and accumulate cholesterol in their system. I included a special Yin Type A Nuts category for this reason. So, if you're a Yin Type A, up to 15 percent of your diet can be devoted to going nuts! The excess stomach energy of the Yang Type A, on the contrary, needs something hardy like meat protein to keep occupied and avoid overheating. Meat, therefore, accounts for up to 40 percent of the entire Yang Type A diet. Keep in mind, however, that no matter which body type you are, each food group has a significant role to play in your diet.

Not only do each of the body types have their own food group emphasis, but they also differ when it comes to the foods themselves. Green-light foods help support our body type's weakest organ, thus enhancing our overall health. Yellow-light foods may help supply us with essential nutritional needs, but do not directly support our weakest organs. Red-light foods interfere with our health because they impede our energetic flow. Refer back to the earlier sections of this part to refresh your memory about these food categories.

WHAT TO EAT

Earlier on I introduced foods that were specifically compatible for your body type. This section offers general guidelines that apply to everyone, regardless of your body type.

How Do I Know Where to Get Good-Quality Foods?

Even though it would seem that living in the country offers us an advantage in acquiring good-quality food, this may not be the case. Higher demand often contributes to variety and enhanced quality when it comes to acquiring good-quality produce. Areas with larger populations almost always have a greater selection of organic and otherwise fresh foods. If you are living in a populated area, I recommend taking advantage of the slightly more expensive but healthier local whole food store produce. Fresh produce may also be available at a local farmer's market. Lastly, shopping at your nearby co-op is a great way to support local farmers, as well as stay healthy.

Driven by international consumer demand, organic products have become widely available within the last few years. In America most major supermarkets offer at least a few or have a section completely devoted to organic foods. Certified organic foods are free of pesticides and other artificial preservatives. Paying a few extra bucks for organic food may contribute substantially to greater health. The body can digest and assimilate organic foods more easily than processed or artificially preserved foods. Organic meats are a little more challenging to find than organically grown vegetables, nuts, and grains. Some companies will advertise hormone/antibiotic-free and/or grass-fed poultry or beef. If organic beef is not available in your area, choosing these alternatives may be the only option. However, before buying meat, it is advisable to do some research to confirm that you are getting a good-quality product. Look for the USDA label when purchasing organic foods.

Should I Supplement with Vitamins and Minerals?

Even though vitamins and minerals are natural components of most widely eaten body type foods, the market today is saturated with vitamin and mineral supplements of every kind. Many of us feel that we could simply supplement our diet with multivitamins and not worry about getting vital nutrients from vitamin- and mineral-rich foods. As tempting as it may sound to swallow a pill that meets all our nutritional needs, nothing can completely substitute for food in its natural form. However, some of us may not be able to absorb vitamins from food as efficiently as others, so we might need to supplement with certain vitamins or minerals.

Every vitamin and mineral listed in table 3.11 plays a significant role in keeping each body type healthy. Most are acquired from foods but some are produced by the body itself. Certain vitamins are especially beneficial for Yin types, while others work better for Yang types. Yang Type A's, for example, are prone to osteoporosis and weaker bones due to their inherently weaker kidneys. Vitamin D promotes the absorption of calcium from food into the bones, making it especially beneficial for Yang Type A's. The "Especially Good for . . ." column in table 3.11 offers further information about body type compatibility. Lastly, check out individual labels for the recommended daily allowance of each particular vitamin, based on your age and sex. If a particular vitamin/mineral is beneficial for your body type, I would recommend taking it in higher doses (slightly above the maximum RDA). Bear in mind, however, that excessive intake of certain vitamins can lead to toxicity. Even if a vitamin is deemed beneficial for your body type, keep it within the tolerable upper intake level (UL), which can be found by searching under, "UL, vitamins and minerals" on the Internet.

TABLE 3.11. VITAMINS AND THE BODY TYPES

Vitamins and Minerals	Function	Especially Good For . . .	Higher Amounts Found in
Vitamin A	Supports eyesight and immune function, maintains healthy skin	Yin types	Beef/chicken liver, milk, cheese, eggs, carrots, leafy vegetables, apricots, mango, papaya, peaches, peas, red peppers
Vitamin D	Facilitates the absorption of calcium for bone health	Yang types	Cod liver oil, salmon, mackerel, tuna, milk, sardines, beef, liver, eggs
Vitamin E	Antioxidant, improves circulation	Yin types	Almonds, pine nuts, peanuts, sunflower seeds, leafy-green vegetables, kiwi, mango, tomatoes, apricots, olives, spinach
Vitamin K	Helps heal wounds and prevents excess bleeding	All types	Leafy-green vegetables, soybean oil, cottonseed oil, olive oil, canola oil
Vitamin C	Antioxidant, helps absorb iron, supports immune activity	Yin types	Kiwi and citrus fruits, guava, mango, broccoli
Vitamin B	Supports the immune system, nervous system, overall energy, production of red blood cells, the absorption of iron	All types	Meat, liver, milk, yeast and its products, nuts, whole-grain cereals

TABLE 3.11. VITAMINS AND THE BODY TYPES (continued)

Vitamins and Minerals	Function	Especially Good For . . .	Higher Amounts Found in
Iron	Transports oxygen to the body's cells for proper function	Yang types	Eggs, meat (especially fish, liver)
Zinc	Supports the immune system, facilitates cell growth and wound healing	All types	Meat, leafy-green vegetables, whole grains, milk, eggs
Calcium	Essential for bone growth and strength	Yang types	Milk, probiotic yogurt, cheese
Potassium	Helps maintain electrolyte balance, prevents muscle cramps	All types	White beans, spinach, baked potatoes (with skin), apricots, yogurt, salmon, avocados, white mushrooms, bananas

The recommended dosage of each supplement depends on several factors, including body weight and the state of your health. Consult a physician if you believe that you are deficient in one or more of the above nutrients. Depending on your lifestyle and location, it may be challenging to consume sufficient amounts of these nutrients via food, and it may be necessary to take oral or injectable supplements. Only certain vitamin deficiencies can be determined through a blood test. Water-soluble vitamins, for example, quickly pass through the body and may not stick around long enough to be tested efficiently. Vitamin deficiency may also be due to health issues, such as malabsorption or disease. These issues should always be addressed by a professional.

Vitamins A, D, E, and K are referred to as fat-soluble vitamins. These vitamins are stored in the liver and fat tissue of the body after ingestion. It is not necessary, and is potentially dangerous to overload the body daily with fat-soluble vitamin supplements. Water-soluble vitamins, such as B vitamins and C, are easily eliminated from the body and therefore are less likely to causing toxicity. Nevertheless, excess intake of any supplement may cause side effects. Consult a medical professional if you experience an adverse reaction, such as indigestion, constipation, or lack of appetite, after ingesting supplements for any of the above nutrients.

The Carbohydrate Controversy

Carbohydrates, or "carbs," are one of the most misunderstood types of food out there. Most diets boast a low-carb profile, giving carbohydrates a bad reputation and making us believe that avoiding them altogether is the key to remaining healthy. Before dismissing carbohydrates as a "bad" food, it is important to consider these factors:

- Complex carbohydrates are an essential part of keeping your brain and red blood cells happy because they are slowly broken down into glucose, which is a main source of energy for brain and red blood cell function.
- Carbohydrates provide the body with much quicker sources of energy, compared to protein or fats, which take the body a longer time to digest. Longer processing times make proteins and fats essential for longer-term survival; they are also essential for cell and tissue repair. Carbohydrates, by contrast, provide the body with quicker, on-demand energy to get through the day.
- Carbohydrates are easier to digest than proteins and fats. Many high-protein/low carbohydrate diet plans claim that intense protein and fat intake leads to quicker weight loss. These statements are only half true. Under this kind of regimen, the body is forced to break down and digest fat tissue without carbohydrate sources of energy, thus contributing to weight loss. Yet, starving the body of otherwise readily available energy is not necessarily a healthy way to lose weight. Moreover, excess consumption of protein and fat causes an increased accumulation of toxins in the liver, kidneys, and gallbladder, leading to significant health issues down the road.

What Exactly Are Carbohydrates?

Carbohydrates are similar to proteins in the sense that they consist of polypeptide bonds. Once these polypeptide bonds are broken down, they are transformed into glycogen, which provides the body with energy in the form of sugar (glucose). It takes the body much longer to break down plant and animal fat and protein than it does to break down carbohydrates.

What Is the Difference between Simple and Complex Carbohydrates?

Simple carbohydrates are what give carbohydrates a bad reputation. They are broken down rapidly into sugar, sending off a cascade of free radicals swimming throughout the bloodstream; these damage the body's tissues. Most sweet-tasting, high-sugar foods are simple carbohydrates. These foods often give us a rush of intense energy (a so-called "sugar high") but cause us to crash soon afterward.

Now, if you think that simple carbohydrates are not necessarily bad for everyone, you are right! Even simple carbohydrates have their place in the diet and are necessary, in smaller amounts, to keep us healthy. While refined sugar in cake, cookies, processed snack foods, and candy is hardly healthy, simple carbohydrates from fruit and other naturally sweetened foods, often contain vital minerals, fiber, and vitamins, which enhance our health.

Complex carbohydrates, also known as starches, are complex chains of sugar that are broken down much more slowly than simple carbohydrates, but more quickly than fats and protein. The slower but steady breakdown of complex carbohydrates gives us a sustained level of energy throughout the day. Actually, complex carbohydrates are the body's primary source of fuel! These foods often contain the essential nutrients of vitamins, minerals, and fiber. Plants store energy in the form of starch and transform complex carbohydrates into cellulose to construct cell walls. Vegetables are therefore a rich and essential source of complex carbohydrates. See table 3.12 for examples of simple and complex carbohydrates.

Choosing to eat more complex carbs and reduce simple carb intake may be one of the best health choices you'll ever make! When it comes to blood sugar issues, such decisions are crucial. Simple carbs can quickly cause blood sugar levels to spike. Because complex carbs are broken down much more slowly, they can help balance blood sugar levels

TABLE 3.12. SIMPLE AND COMPLEX CARBOHYDRATES

Type of Carbohydrate	Food Examples
Complex	Whole grains (millet, oats, wheat germ, barley, wild rice, brown rice, buckwheat, oat bran, (whole-grain) breads and pasta, fresh (whole) fruit (prunes, apricots, oranges, plums, pears, grapefruit, apples), legumes, spinach, green beans, broccoli, potatoes, carrots, radishes, asparagus
Simple	**Helpful in moderation:** 100 percent pure fruit juice (without added sugar or high-fructose corn syrup), milk (better to limit for Yin Type A's), unrefined (natural) sugar, honey
	Better to limit: Candy, soda, corn syrup (aka high-fructose corn syrup), milk chocolate, refined sugar, cake, and other sweets

while providing the body with enough fuel to get through the day. If you suffer from blood sugar issues, I suggest that you consult with a professional to further discuss how to balance your carb intake.

How Much of My Diet Should Come from Carbohydrates?

As with all other types of foods, carbohydrates need to be consumed in balance. The Centers for Disease Control and Prevention recommends that 45–65 percent of the total intake of foods should be from carbohydrates. This amounts to 225–325 grams a day, based on a 2,000-calorie intake. Each body type also has different requirements when it comes to carb intake. The diet of Yin Type A's, for example, consists of only up to 15 percent meat, requiring them to consume a considerable amount of carbohydrates for energy. The Yang Type A's diet, on the other hand, consists of up to 40 percent meat; therefore, they have less carb consumption than the other body types. Yang Type B's often have difficulty digesting meat; as a result, substantial carb intake is the only way for their body to get the energy it needs. Finally, the diet of Yin Type B's consists of about 25 percent meat, which gives them energy from protein, while approximately 60 percent comes from carbohydrate intake.

In the previous section, every food group is given a percentage, according to the nutritional requirements of each body type. Following these percentage guidelines will help ensure that you are getting enough and not overdoing your carb intake.

Meat versus Vegetable Sources of Protein

There is no right or wrong when it comes to deciding whether or not to be a vegetarian. Accordingly, the Sasang approach does not attempt to take sides on this issue. Yet each body type has its own requirements regarding the amount of meat intake. Let's take Yang Type B's, for example, whose weaker liver causes most of them to vomit after ingesting even small amounts of meat. An individual of this body type may actually become a vegetarian out of pure necessity, rather than choice. Without an abundant supply of meat, Yang Type A's may easily become irritable, as their overactive stomach scavenges for something hardy to tear up and break down. The decision of whether or not to become a vegetarian comes a bit more easily for the Yin types, who do not react as strongly either way.

Eating according to the Season

Striking a balance between human and nature has long been a focus in Asian philosophy and medicine. Throughout Chinese and Korean history, countless monks and scholars have renounced their societal duties and retired to natural surroundings, either to meditate or to write. Many profound books have been written by these monks and scholars, such as the *Tao Te Ching* by the famous monk Lao Tzu, and *The Collected Songs of Cold Mountain* written by a hermit-poet named Han Shan (Cold Mountain). Born from this desire to connect with nature came the idea of eating according to the season. Warm- or hot-natured foods were traditionally consumed during the colder months, and cool- or cold-natured foods during the warmer months. Also, with a lack of refrigeration, foods were often eaten soon after they were produced or available. Fruits were most often consumed soon after they fell or were plucked from the tree. Meat was often dried in the fall for consumption during the winter, when other sources of food were less readily available. Eating according to the season, in conjunction with increased physical activity, likely contributed to quicker metabolism and less obesity in ancient China and Korea.

With the advent of refrigeration, the need to eat according to the season diminished. We could store just about anything in the refrigerator for weeks before it began to spoil. And oh that precious freezer—food can last forever in there (as long as you don't mind the taste of freezer burn)! Yet this could not compare to the taste of fresh fruit or garden-fresh vegetables. Foods that have been sitting in our refrigerator or packed with preservatives to prevent spoilage do not provide the quality of nutrition that our body needs. Interestingly enough, foods that are in season often have time-appropriate characteristics that help support our health. Local fruits that ripen in late summer and fall support the function of the lungs. Thus, consumption of these fruits in the fall can help prevent the onset of colds and flus, which often occur around this time. Domestic animals often fatten themselves up in the early winter to protect themselves from the cold. Eating meat with more fat in the winter can provide the body with more energy and warmth to get through it.

The seasons also have a direct influence on the Yin and Yang of each body type. The colder seasons cultivate Yin and the warmer seasons cultivate more Yang within the body. If the Yin types eat too many Yin (cool or cold) foods in the winter, they will likely experience bloating, indigestion, and bowel issues. The Yang types may experience the same issues if they have too many Yang (warm or hot) foods during the cooler seasons. Yet, the Yin types can get away with moderate consumption of cool or cold foods during the Yang cultivating warmer months, just as the Yang types can get away with moderate consumption of warm or hot foods in the Yin cultivating cooler months. Keep in mind that both environmental (seasonal) and internal (body type) factors play a central role in our health and well-being.

Spices and the Yang Types

The Sasang diet categorizes spices as a yellow- or red-light food for Yang types. Does this mean that Yang types should cut down on or refrain from eating spices? Many of us would argue that spices give life to our meals! If you are a Yang type, rather than omitting spices altogether, try spicing for flavor, rather than for heat. Despite the fact that garlic, for example, is in the Yang Type A's red-light category, it can still be added in moderation to any meal for added taste. Remember: It is time for the Yang types to cut down if eating spicy foods becomes an everyday desire.

HOW MUCH TO EAT

The Sasang approach is not another weight-loss regimen, but a way to enhance your overall well-being. The body type–specific diet plans in this chapter can help you regulate your weight by keeping your energies in balance without promising a quick and easy solution. You can lose excess weight only through a balance between eating, exercising, and emotion, in accordance with the needs of your body type. For those of you who would like to lose weight, following the guidelines in this section is an indispensable part of the process. I would also recommend that you check out "Shedding Those Extra Pounds" (pages 325–45).

It is difficult to gauge how much food to eat simply based on our appetite, which can fluctuate with our moods. Stress tends to trigger an increase in appetite in some while decreasing it in others.

According to the Centers for Disease Control and Prevention and the Estimated Energy Requirements (EER) of the Institute of Medicine, caloric intake depends on three major factors—age, activity level, and gender. While Sasang medicine focuses on body type–compatible foods, it does not provide specific guidelines on caloric intake. Keeping an eye on your total caloric intake is also an important factor involved in harmonizing and balancing your health. Table 3.9 on page 202 offers general guidelines for caloric intake, based on these three factors.

Total food intake also varies according to body type. Yin types generally benefit from consuming fewer calories than the general guidelines in table 3.9 suggest to avoid overwhelming their digestive system, while Yang types need to consume more calories to satisfy an overactive digestive system. Factors such as obesity, diabetes, and congestive heart failure also play a significant role in regulating your total caloric intake. Deviating from these recommendations may be advisable, based on your individual needs.

Do you find that reducing your meal size is a challenging, if not impossible, task? If so, cardiovascular exercise may be the answer to burning off those extra calories. Monitor your caloric reduction by using a treadmill, an elliptical machine, and/or a stationary bicycle. These machines often have calorie monitors that allow you to keep track of how many calories you're burning. Whether it is from increasing exercise or eating less, try to stay within the caloric intake guidelines.

TABLE 3.9. SUGGESTED CALORIC INTAKE BASED ON AGE AND GENDER*

Gender	Age (years)	Sedentary	Moderately Active	Active
Toddler	2–3	1,000	1,000–1,400	1,000–1,400
Female	4–8	1,200	1,400–1,600	1,400–1,800
	9–13	1,600	1,600–2,000	1,800–2,200
	14–18	1,800	2,000	2,400
	19–30	2,000	2,000–2,200	2,400
	31–50	1,800	2,000	2,200
	51+	1,600	1,800	2,000–2,200
Male	4–8	1,400	1,400–1,600	1,600–2,000
	9–13	1,800	1,800–2,200	2,000–2,600
	14–18	2,200	2,400–2,800	2,800–3,200
	19–30	2,400	2,600–2,800	3,000
	31–50	2,200	2,400–2,600	2,800–3,000
	51+	2,000	2,200–2,400	2,400–2,800

*From WebMD.com

How Many Calories Did I Ingest?

To determine the amount of calories in a particular food, take a look at the label. The Nutritional Facts section of the label often lists the number of calories in a single serving. If this information is not available, the following website is an excellent source, offering detailed information on the caloric content of each type of food, as well as other nutritional information: www.webmd.com/diet/healthtool-food-calorie-counter.

Without a food scale, how do you know exactly how many grams of each food you are consuming? The following website offers a visual comparison of different food portions: www.webmd.com/diet/healthtool-portion-size-plate.

How Many Calories Do I Burn Off When I'm Exercising?

Table 3.10 offers an estimate of approximately how many calories you burn per hour during each exercise. The amount of caloric reduction depends on your body weight. The heavier you are, the more calories your body burns. In other words it takes more energy for you to burn off the same number of calories if you are heavier.

TABLE 3.10. CALORIES BURNED DURING EXERCISE*

One Hour of Exercise	130–lb. Person	155–lb. Person	205–lb. Person
Aerobics	384	531	605
Backpacking/hiking	413	572	651
Ballet, twist, jazz, tap	266	368	419
Bowling	177	245	279
Cross-country skiing	413	572	651
Cycling (moderate)	472	654	745
Fishing	177	245	279
Golf (walking and pulling clubs)	254	351	400
Running	472	654	745
Swimming (breaststroke laps)	590	817	931

*From NutriStrategy.com

Do I Always Have to Monitor My Caloric Intake?

Keeping track of your daily caloric intake and your serving sizes can be a drag. While it is not something that I recommend you do continuously, a week or two could provide you with valuable feedback if you are attempting to lose or gain weight. After a few weeks of diligently keeping track of your food intake, you will likely develop a sense of how to regulate your serving sizes. Even if you are not concerned about losing or gaining weight, keeping track of caloric intake and serving sizes can help determine if you are eating enough or too much of one food or another.

WHEN TO EAT

It is customary for the average American to eat three meals a day. While most of us would accept this as the norm, inquisitive historians would likely differ. The three-meals-a-day custom can be traced back to the European upper class of ages ago. Other peoples, such as the ancient Greeks, often ate only one meal a day, even after hours of intense labor! Grazing on frequent healthy snacks, instead of eating three larger meals, provides the body with a consistent supply of energy throughout the day without overwhelming the digestive system. While it is possible to get hungry for your next meal within hours, the transit from mouth to anus takes up to eighty hours! Consuming frequent smaller meals, however, takes considerably less time to digest.

Did You Know?

Most of us tend to eat until we feel full, keeping our hunger satisfied from one meal to the next. Have you ever tried eating until you are satisfied but *not* full? Doing so could keep the digestive system operating efficiently without getting overwhelmed. Snacking throughout the day or in between meals on moderate amounts of healthy foods can help stop us from eating too much in one serving.

Healthy Snacking throughout the Day

The dietary advice provided in this section is based on the typical three-meals-a-day routine, but even though this approach may be challenging, you might try eating smaller, more frequent meals throughout the day. You may still get hungry for larger meals, even with added snacks in between. Keeping a close eye on your total daily food intake is one way to stay on top of things: keep track of the amount you are snacking and subtract that from your overall daily calorie intake.

Keep in Mind—Healthy Snacks

The term snack in this book should not be confused with snack foods. Simple carbs, such as oily, salty, and sweet-tasting finger foods, do not qualify as healthy snacks. Healthy snacking is simply a miniature version of a full meal, divided into smaller portions throughout the day.

Try the "two zipper bag principle" when preparing your snacks, devoting one bag to fruits and veggies and the other to nuts and grains. Pick away at both bags throughout the day, making sure you do not eat too much in one serving. When preparing your zipper bags, keep in mind your total caloric intake and provide yourself with enough, and not too much, nutrition throughout your day.

Timing Your Meals

Another way to keep your digestive system operating smoothly is to eat an early dinner. There are several reasons why this can keep you thin and healthy. For starters, as noted above, it takes a long time to completely digest a meal. Secondly, when you sleep, your heartbeat and metabolism both slow down considerably. Allowing ample time to digest dinner before bedtime can help you avoid waking up with an upset stomach from lingering undigested foods.

Body Type Energy Cycles

Up until now we have seen how each body type corresponds to different organ strengths, personality traits, foods, and herbs. Each body type also corresponds to different times of the day (see figure 3.9). Morning, for example, corresponding to Yang, is also associated with the Yang types, who have more energy during this time of day. The evening corresponds to Yin and is associated with Yin types, who have more energy in the evening. Thus the Yang types benefit from consuming larger meals earlier in the morning, while the Yin types can promote their digestive health by eating larger meals in the afternoon or early evening.

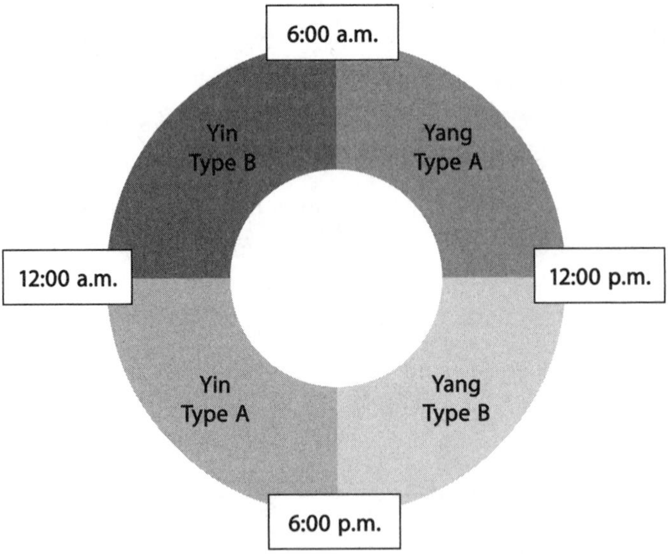

Figure 3.9. Most energetic time of day for each body type

BODY TYPE GUIDELINES FOR DAILY FOOD INTAKE

We all have our own preferences when it comes to making daily food choices. The Sasang approach is not meant to radically change your diet or restrict your way of life. Instead, it provides you with the tools necessary to make informed decisions based on the health requirements of your body type. This, in turn, helps you avoid getting sick and improves your health by introducing foods that nourish your weaker organs. Adding plenty of green- and yellow-light foods for your body type into your diet is one way to get the ball rolling. Yet with just a shopping list of foods in hand, it is difficult to know where to start on the path to health and harmony.

Tips for Becoming a Healthy Eater

Try slowing down. Eating on the run may help you get to work more quickly, but your digestive system will eventually have to pay the price. The more slowly you eat, the more time your body has to digest food efficiently.

Spend a little more on food. Sure, we all want to save as much money as we can, yet splurging on good-quality food is probably the best way to spend your money. Think of your body as an investment opportunity that always yields abundant dividends in the form of good health.

Remember to eat. Sometimes we get so busy that food is the last thing on our minds! If you do this often, try setting your phone alarm to remind you to eat. The "two zipper bag principle" comes in handy for this type of schedule, too.

Maintain a routine. We are creatures of habit. Eating at set times throughout the day helps to train our body to anticipate when food is on the way. By the time we take that first bite, our body will already be prepared and ready to get to work. Shocking the system with larger meals at random times throughout the day may contribute to weight gain and indigestion.

The sections that follow will set you in the right direction by offering helpful tips for each meal of the day, according to your body type. Before we jump into the specifics, let's review a few basic principles:

- Keeping track of your caloric intake will keep you in the driver's seat.
- Eating smaller meals more frequently is easier on the digestive system than three larger meals a day.
- Each meal size is slightly different, depending on whether you are a Yin or a Yang body type, so refer to the percentages listed under each meal below.
- The Sasang approach is meant to serve as a guide, rather than dictating your food intake.

YIN TYPES—WHAT TO EAT AND WHEN

The size and nature of each meal of the day varies considerably, depending on whether you are a Yin or a Yang body type. Yin types have a harder time getting their Yang flowing in the morning, the Yang time of day. This section will offer tips on how to cultivate Yang in the morning while kick-starting the circulatory system to provide energy throughout the day.

Breakfast for Yin Types

Eating a healthy body type–compatible breakfast is a great way to start your day. Since it takes a bit longer for Yin types to get their digestive system going in the morning, if you're a Yin Type A or a Yin Type B, try making this a lighter but well-planned meal. Devote most of your breakfast to green-light foods and throw a few yellow-light foods in there as well, if you wish. Avoid overwhelming your digestive system by consuming a heavier, difficult-to-digest breakfast. Breakfast for Yin types should be approximately 20 percent of total daily food intake.

Tip #1: Eat Soft and Warm Foods

Yin corresponds to cold, while Yang is associated with heat. Lacking in Yang, Yin types need to consume warmer foods and fluids in the morning to boost the digestive system. Yin types are therefore better off avoiding cold smoothies or other chilled foods for breakfast, which

Yin Type B Trick of the Trade

Nobody benefits more from warm- or hot-natured foods than Yin Type B's. If you are a Yin Type B, try consuming ginger every morning, ingested as tea or sprinkled over your breakfast for an extra kick! Ginger's warm nature promotes digestion while supporting the flow of Yang energy, giving Yin Type B's more overall spunk that could last throughout the day.

tend to freeze things up, slowing down their metabolism. Softer and warmer foods, such as porridge, warm cereals (i.e., oatmeal), or soups, are digested more quickly and easily, helping to increase metabolism and promote efficient breakdown of foods. Consuming tea with breakfast could also help kick-start metabolism and digestive function, like warming up the engine of a car before pulling out of the driveway. Refer to the food chapter for your specific body type for tea suggestions.

Tip #2: Promote Flow with Whole Grain and Nuts

A good night's sleep not only gives us a chance to let go of daily stress, it also replenishes energy and damaged cell tissue. Yet while we are asleep, our body is much less active than during the day. Lack of movement can lead to stagnation of the body's energy and blood flow, causing morning stiffness and soreness of the joints and/or muscles. Whole grains and nuts contain volatile oils that help promote the flow of energy and food through the digestive system, picking up and eliminating unwanted by-products along the way. So it's a good idea for Yin types to incorporate whole-grain foods and nuts into their breakfast as a way to unblock energy that accumulated while we were asleep.

Tip #3: Boost Your Circulation

On page 134 I discussed several supplements that help promote blood and energy flow for Yin Type A's. For a smooth ride throughout the day, these supplements are best consumed in the morning. Vinegar, perhaps the most accessible and effective supplement for Yin Type A's, strongly promotes circulation, reduces inflammation, and counteracts toxic buildup within the body. Try mixing up to two tablespoons of apple cider vinegar with one cup of water and drink up. If it is taken after meals, vinegar can aid in digestion. Taken on an empty stomach, it is absorbed faster, making it slightly more potent.

Tip #4: Tread Lightly

Eating a heavy or greasy breakfast in the morning can fatigue and slow down the Yin types' digestive system. In order to cultivate rather than smother their Yang, Yin types are better off consuming a lighter breakfast. This is even truer for those who enjoy working out in the morning. A heavy meal directly before a workout puts an extra load on the system, ultimately causing exhaustion and indigestion. Try eating enough breakfast until you're satisfied, rather than getting too full.

Lunch for Yin Types

The afternoon is often the busiest part of the day, demanding more from our mind and body. Rushing back to work directly after eating lunch may confuse the digestive system, as it tries to focus on breaking down food, rather than doing anything else! Activity directly after eating lunch can lead to fatigue and sluggishness throughout the rest of the day, especially for Yin types, who have a slower metabolism compared to Yang types. An ideal lunch for Yin types has more calories than breakfast but fewer calories than dinner and should be approximately 30 percent of total daily food intake.

Tip #1: Drink Tea after Lunch

There are several theories that explain why obesity is less prevalent in China than it is in the United States. Some may think that it has a lot to do with Americans consuming greasy or oily foods. Actually, while in China, I was surprised to discover how greasy and oily Chinese food could be! The Chinese, however, drink plenty of green tea after meals. Could green tea be the secret to staying slim? While this may be only one of several reasons the Chinese tend not to be obese, there is no doubt that tea assists with Yin types' digestion because warmth (Yang energy) helps to break down food. Drinking tea after lunch may also help prevent midday energy loss.

Tip #2: Save Dessert for Dinner

Even if you score 100 percent on eating a great lunch, all your effort may go to waste by following it with a heavy dessert. Save cakes and other goodies for after dinner, when your body is less in need of energy. But even then, tread lightly on these foods so that your system doesn't have to work the graveyard shift. The golden rule is to give your body enough time to digest everything before going to bed.

Tip #3: Nap after Lunch

In Spain it is customary to take a one- to two-hour hour siesta after lunch. Similar customs in Italy and China involve taking a long break for lunch to relax and socialize with friends. Studies have shown that napping in the afternoon can improve the health of our cardiovascular system.* Since most workers in the United States do not have time to rest after lunch, I recommend simply closing your eyes and taking deep breaths, even if it is for only a few minutes. Ideally, resting up to half an hour replenishes the body's energies and gives you enough time to digest the bulk of your lunch. The trick is not to fall into a deep sleep, which takes away from quality sleep at night and may leave you feeling drowsy for the rest of the day!

Dinner for the Yin Types

As noted above nighttime corresponds to Yin, while daytime corresponds to Yang, which means Yin types have more energy in the evening while Yang types are more energetic in the morning. Yin types thus digest dinner more easily than Yang types. So Yin types consume approximately 50 percent of their total daily food intake for dinner.

---

*For example, see Naska, Androniki, Eleni Oikonomou, Anotnia Trichopoulou, Theodora Psaltopoulou, and Dimitrios Trichopoulos, "Siesta in Healthy Adults and Coronary Mortality in the General Population *Archives in Internal Medicine* 167, no. 3 (2007): 296–301.

Tip #1: Drink Tea after Dinner

Remember our lunch tea tip? Well, here it is again for dinner. Keep in mind, however, that most teas on the market have at least some trace of caffeine. Green tea has one quarter to one-half the amount of caffeine as a cup of coffee. Many of us find getting to sleep difficult after consuming caffeine from the afternoon onward. I suggest choosing a noncaffeinated tea to follow your dinner, such as ginger, chamomile, dandelion root, licorice root, or cinnamon.

Tip #2: Eat Warm/Hot Energy Foods

Since Yin corresponds to the evening, Yin types often enjoy more energy at night than during the day. If Yin types ingest Yin cool or cold-natured foods in the evening, they may feel heavy and groggy, rather than energetic and perky. Avoiding these foods late in the day will keep your Yang energy intact.

YANG TYPES—WHAT TO EAT AND WHEN

With a stronger metabolism than that of Yin types, Yang types have less difficulty digesting larger and heavier meals. This is not an invitation, however, to indulge in greasy and fatty foods, which may aggravate even the most active Yang type digestive systems. In order to soothe a frequently overactive digestive system, Yang types benefit from consuming Yin-natured foods. This section will offer tips on how Yang types can cultivate Yin and sustain energy throughout the day.

Breakfast for Yang Types

As mentioned earlier Yang types feel more energetic in the morning, the time of the day when Yang is abundant. To take advantage of this window of opportunity, Yang types benefit from filling up in the morning with Yin-natured (cool/cold) foods, which help them build up enough energetic momentum to carry them through the rest of their day. Breakfast should be the largest meal of the day for Yang types and should be approximately 50 percent of their total daily food intake.

Tip #1: Consume Protein-Rich Foods

Yang types easily burn up their food, transforming it quickly into energy. Protein is a great source of sustained energy, with its long amino-acid (polypeptide) chains, taking longer to digest than most other foods. While a lot of protein in the morning could cause indigestion for Yin types, it is an essential part of the Yang type breakfast. High-protein foods, such as sausages, eggs, bacon, and/or ham, can help kick-start the Yang Type A's energy. As we learned earlier, protein can easily overwhelm the weak liver of Yang Type B's. Yet without an ample supply of protein, they are easily fatigued. Don't fret! Plant and nut sources of protein are an excellent alternative, since they are much easier on the liver. Liquid forms, such as beef or chicken broth and protein drinks, are another alternative to meat intake for the Yang Type B.

Tip #2: Ingesting Calcium

An overactive digestive system can easily cause heartburn, acid reflux, and/or anxiety for Yang types. Since we go the longest time without food when we sleep at night, the morning is especially challenging for Yang types. Yang types often experience these symptoms if they have gone without eating throughout the night or skipped a meal. Ingesting calcium (i.e., milk and yogurt) can both calm an overactive stomach and reduce these symptoms.

Tip #3: Go Easy on the Spices

While Yin types benefit from slightly spicy or aromatic foods in the morning to cultivate their Yang, Yang types are better off avoiding these foods early in the day. With their Yang nature, spicy foods promote circulation, while hardy and heavier foods have a Yin nature, which nourishes and fortifies the tissues and organs. Yang types could certainly enjoy spices in their food, but are better off avoiding intensely hot foods especially in the morning to tame their wild Yang energy.

Tip #4: Drink Plenty of Water

The kidneys and liver absorb by-products from food and other metabolic processes every second of the day. Like other organs they rely on the heart to keep things flowing to and through them. When we sleep everything in our body slows down, including circulation, causing a by-product buildup in the liver and kidneys. The weaker kidneys and liver of Yang types therefore need to be flushed with plenty of water in the morning. I suggest making a habit of drinking two to three cups of water first in the morning.

Tip #5: Balance Food Intake with Exercise

Morning exercise makes an already overactive digestive system metabolize foods even faster. While exercise is a great way for Yang types to stay in shape, it also may stimulate their appetite even further. So, when exercising, keep track of your caloric intake to avoid binge-eating. Consuming protein after your workout, however, is an excellent way to refuel your cells and tissues and calm an overactive digestive system.

Lunch for the Yang Types

With the afternoon as the busiest part of the day, more action equals more heat buildup in the body. Activity-generated heat easily overwhelms Yang types, who should make lunch a substantial 30 percent of their total daily food intake to give their heat-filled active stomach something to occupy itself.

Tip #1: Make the Time to Eat

Always on the go, Yang types rarely make time for life's basic necessities, and with afternoon as the busiest time of the day, Yang types often skip lunch or eat on the run. If you're a Yang type, be sure to set aside adequate time for lunch.

Tip #2: Eat Cool/Cold-Natured Foods

Since Yang corresponds to heat, the digestive system of Yang types can easily get overheated. The more active we are, the more heat accumulates in our digestive tract. Fresh fruits and vegetables are an excellent source of fluid and could also help calm an overactive/overheated digestive system. Eating ample amounts of vegetables or salad for lunch and fruit for dessert could do the trick (don't forget to choose vegetables and fruits based on your specific body type).

Tip #3: Hydrate with Cold-Natured Fluids

Drinking cool or cold water after lunch can help soothe the digestive system of Yang types, as well as balancing their metabolism. You may also want to prepare chilled shikye to drink throughout the day instead of water (see pages 321–22 for more information about this healthy beverage for Yang types).

Tip #4: Leave Stress at Work

While this tip may apply to all the body types, it is especially important for Yang types to calm their mind while eating lunch. Since Yang corresponds to activity, Yang types tend to overcharge themselves during the day. Excessive anger or agitation during lunchtime causes us to eat faster, losing control of our food intake and increasing the possibilily of gaining weight.

Dinner for Yang Types

As mentioned earlier it is easier for Yin types to digest dinner than it is for Yang types. Yet, dinner is still an essential source of fuel for Yang types and should amount to approximately 20 percent of their total daily food intake.

Tip #1: Drink Mint Tea with Dinner

Mint, as an herb, has a cold nature that makes it easy to digest and soothing for the stomach for the Yang types. As a warm tea, it promotes the Yang type's digestion.

Tip #2: Consume Calcium after Dinner to Alleviate Insomnia

Ingesting calcium before breakfast and after dinner is another way to calm the overactive digestive system of Yang types, who are prone to heartburn, acid reflux, anxiety, irritability, and/or insomnia due to heat buildup in the stomach. Going to bed on an empty stomach can often bring on such distress. Since calcium, as a mineral, has a heavy nature, it can ground and settle the energy of the stomach. A cup of milk or chewable calcium before bed helps alleviate these symptoms.

Tip #3: Eat Yin Foods at Night

For the most part, raw foods tend to be Yin-natured. The energy of food often changes to Yang when it is cooked. Some extremely cold-natured foods, such as pork or shrimp, still retain some of their cool Yin nature when they're cooked. Since nighttime also corresponds to Yin, eating raw or cold-natured foods for dinner is an efficient way to replenish Yin and strengthen the liver and kidneys, our Yin organs. Yang types should try adding raw vegetables or salads, sushi or sashimi, fresh fruits, and/or berries to their dinner.

Tip #4: Take It Easy after Dinner

Yang types could use some rest after dinner. With their Yang energy so active during the day, most Yang types tend to experience a loss of energy in the evening. Resting and/or meditation after dinner helps to soothe their overactive digestive system and replenish deficient Yin energy. Taking the time to breathe deeply and relax consistently throughout the day is an even better option.

Exercise according to Your Yin Yang Body Type

In Sasang medicine health depends on the smooth flow of energy from each body type's strongest to weakest organ. Performing consistent exercise is one of the most efficient ways to promote this energy flow. Yet stress, lack of exercise, eating on the run, and life itself can easily get in the way. In this section, we attempt to fine-tune what type and how much exercise you need, according to your age, weight, and body type.

Modern researchers continue to discover just how important exercise is. Table 3.13 on page 218 lists just a few conditions that benefit tremendously from exercise.

EXERCISE TIPS

Walking from one room to another may be considered exercise for some, while for others it may consist of a rigorous seven-day-a-week cardio and weight-lifting routine. Exercise requirements differ greatly from one person to another and from one body type to another. Even though each body type has its own specific exercise needs, there are general guidelines that apply to everyone. Keep these suggestions in mind when exercising to enhance your general health and well-being. Each of the following eight general tips can be applied to all four body types.

TABLE 3.13. CONDITIONS IMPROVED BY EXCERCISE

Condition	How Exercise Helps
Heart Disease	Strengthens the heart muscle and improves circulation
Stroke	Improves circulation, reducing blood-clot formation
High blood pressure	Has a direct effect on lowering blood pressure
Type 2 diabetes	Improves the body's utilization of insulin
Stress	Promotes release of endorphins, which trigger positive feelings
Osteoporosis	Helps the bones better absorb calcium
Smoking/drinking addictions	Stimulates neurotransmitters that enhance feelings of well-being
Constipation	Helps stimulate movement within the intestines, known as peristalsis
Insomnia	Relaxes the mind and reduces stress
Memory	Increases the flow of oxygen to the brain
Headaches	Enhances circulation and oxygen flow to the neck and shoulder muscles to help release tension

General Tip #1: Set Time Aside to Exercise

Several of my patients have lamented to me how disappointed they are that they've gained weight, even though they are on their feet all day long at work. Unless you are a full-time athlete, exercise at work does not count as *true* exercise. When we are at work, our mind is usually focused on work. When we exercise our mind is focused on exercising. The mind is the driving force for optimum health. Setting time aside to exercise helps the mind focus on health rather than work. It reduces stress and promotes joy by releasing endorphins into the bloodstream.

If this is your first time getting an exercise routine going, start by setting aside fifteen minutes devoted strictly to working out. As the weeks go by, slowly expand your workout time, dividing it into small sections throughout the day, if needed. A short walk during your lunch break, for example, may energize you during a long day at the office. As time goes on, try gradually increasing the frequency and intensity of your workout. Never push yourself to the point of exhaustion or pain. A little muscle soreness that lasts no more than a day after a workout, however, is to be expected when stretching your limits.

General Tip #2: Stretch before and after Your Workout

The hustle and bustle of modern society make it difficult for many of us to slow down. Even our exercise routines often allow little time for warming up and cooling down as we rush off to work. This puts an extra load on the body, which is already under stress from numerous other demands we place on it every day. Light stretching before your workout makes it easier for your muscles to stay loose without getting overwhelmed. In addition warming yourself up with a gentle workout or shower before strenuous exercise prevents muscles and tendons from becoming overly sore. Stretching after your workout helps the muscles rid themselves of excess tension. Ideally, stretching is most beneficial if done periodically throughout the day. Stretch as often as you can to loosen up those ever-tightening muscles. Keep in mind, though, that stretching a muscle past the point of pain does more harm than good for the body. A gentle pulling sensation of the muscle you are stretching is a sign that you are doing the stretch correctly.

A healthy stretching routine does not simply focus on a single area of discomfort. The body has complementary muscles and tendons that constantly push and pull one another. Stretching the lower back, for example, indirectly loosens a tight neck and shoulders. Hence, if the upper back aches, try adding lower-back stretches to your routine. If your lower back aches, stretch out your upper back, too.

Here are a few common techniques that can be incorporated easily into a daily stretching routine.

Keep in Mind—Why Stretch Out

The body has two major muscle groups, referred to as extensors and flexors, also called antagonist muscles because they oppose one another. Without antagonist muscles we would not be able to move our limbs back and forth. Practically everything we do requires greater use of our flexor muscles than our extensor muscles; thus, our flexor muscles can get much stronger than our extensor muscles, causing us to hunch over as we age. Stretching engages our extensor muscles, helping us to maintain good posture, alleviate muscle and tendon pain, and keep us flexible as we age.

In addition, stretching should always be done slowly and steadily without sudden movement. Prevent muscle spasms by breathing slowly while easing in and out of a stretch. Breathing also enhances the effects of stretching by oxygenating the muscles and tendons. Inhalation itself also helps to stretch the muscles of the chest and upper back by expanding the lungs.

NECK ROTATION

* Before getting out of bed in the morning, lie on your back while gently and slowly rotating your neck as far as you can to each side, looking over one shoulder and then the other without strain.
* Repeat the rotation back and forth five times while breathing deeply. If you don't feel a stretch, try rotating your head a bit further. If you feel any discomfort, reduce the extent of the rotation.

LOWER-BACK STRETCH

* Lie on your left side with a pillow beneath your head in a comfortable position on a flat surface.
* Bend both of your knees to about a 90-degree angle and rest them on the floor comfortably beside you.
* Gently rest your left hand on your right rib cage or on your bent right knee to add a little pressure to the stretch.

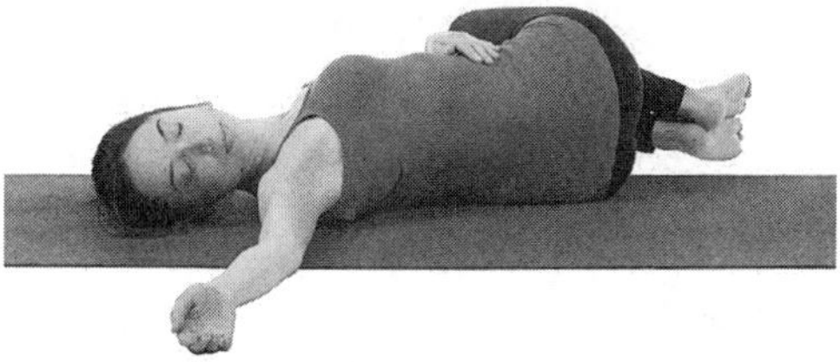

Figure 3.10. Lower-back stretch

* Draw your right shoulder toward the floor or bed, reaching the right arm straight out to your right side.
* Gaze up toward the ceiling or off over your right shoulder.
* Take about three deep breaths in this position, then repeat the stretch in the opposite direction. You should feel a gentle stretch in your lower back and hips. (See figure 3.10.)

CHILD'S POSE

* Kneel on a mat or the floor. Reach your arms straight out in front of you on the floor or mat.
* Bend your knees and reach your hips back toward your heels as far back as you can without putting too much strain on your arms, back, or legs.
* Take about five deep breaths in this position while gently swaying left and right. (See figure 3.11.)

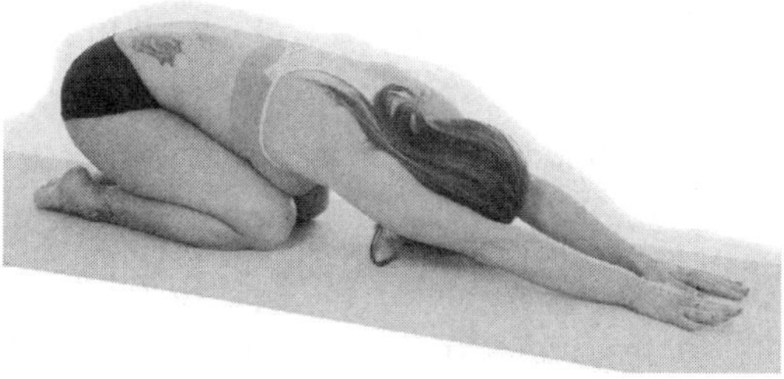

Figure 3.11. Child's pose

UPPER-BODY STRETCH

* Standing up tall, take a deep breath while rolling your shoulders up and back, drawing your shoulder blades together and extending your chest forward. Hold your breath for a few seconds or until you feel the urge to breathe out.
* Release your shoulders and relax your chest as you exhale.
* Repeat this movement five times in the morning, afternoon, and evening.

* This exercise stretches the pectoralis muscles, which go from the sternum to the shoulder, and encourages the flow of blood and energy through the chest and upper body.

General Tip #3: Balance Your Workout Intensity

No matter how short on time you are, never rush into an intense workout or you will place excess stress on your bones and muscles and wind up fatigued. Moreover, alternating the intensity of your workout is an ideal way to enhance circulation and avoid excess wear and tear on your joints by continuously straining the same muscle group.

The intense part of a workout is also referred to as the anaerobic phase. During anaerobic exercise, the body breaks down its own tissues (fat, muscle, etc.) as a source of energy, rather than using oxygen as a source of energy. The aerobic phase of a workout relies on oxygen to obtain energy through rapid or deep breathing. For those who are interested in losing weight, anaerobic exercise may sound appealing, since the body breaks down its own fat tissue in this phase! True, anaerobic exercise is an excellent way to break down fat tissue, but spending too much time in the anaerobic phase of exercise causes inflammation and trauma to the muscles and other tissues of the body. It also causes the body to fatigue more quickly, since it is literally "feeding" on itself. A healthy workout consists of a balance between anaerobic and aerobic phases (see table 3.14). Spending most of your workout in the aerobic phase will give the body a chance to replenish itself consistently without fatiguing, as this puts less stress on the organs, muscles, and tendons while strengthening the heart and promoting circulation. This is especially true for those suffering from arthritis, heart disease, or high blood pressure. Yet, in a balanced workout, you can also kick it up a notch by adding short spurts of anaerobic exercise.

TABLE 3.14. AEROBIC VERSUS ANAEROBIC EXCERCISES

Aerobic Exercise Examples	Anaerobic Exercise Examples
Recreational swimming, walking, bicycling, light jogging, light weight lifting (over a prolonged period, doing multiple repetitions), and other cardiovascular activities	Sprinting, swim racing, weight lifting (with heavy weights in short spurts), boxing, and other intense workouts

General Tip #4: Pace Your Breath during a Workout

Deep breathing is an essential part of any workout. The more we move our body, the more oxygen it demands. We naturally breathe more heavily when we're working out, allowing our body to absorb more oxygen at a quicker pace. Take this opportunity during a workout to pace your breathing. If you are walking, jogging, or bicycle riding, start with three steps/cycles while inhaling and three steps/cycles while exhaling. Count each step or cycle while controlling your inhalation and exhalation throughout the workout. When you're lifting weights or doing push-ups, exhale on the exertion and inhale when you release your muscles. Exhale when you're pushing or pulling weights upward, and inhale when you're moving them downward. This method of breathing, which helps prevent excessive buildup of pressure and tension in the body, also optimizes muscle oxygen uptake. While exercise serves many functions, perhaps it is the stimulation of breathing that offers us the greatest benefit.

Exercise and Meditation

While some exercises require us to focus strictly on the movements involved, others give our mind a chance to wander. Rhythmic exercises, such as walking and swimming, require less thinking, allowing our mind to entertain random thoughts or engage in meditation. If you are a person who equates the word *meditation* with closing your eyes, sitting, or remaining as still as possible and can never picture yourself meditating or sitting in one place for more than a minute, try meditating during your cardio workout by letting your body do the exercise while you focus on breathing, relaxing, and clearing your mind. As long as you are capable of relaxing your mind, meditation is possible, no matter where you are or what you are doing. Meditation directly after your workout may be equally rewarding, since this is usually the time when the mind and body are most in sync. (Also see information about active and passive meditation on page 226.)

General Tip #5: Establish Timing and Consistency

The human body relishes routine. If you ate dinner at 6:00 p.m. yesterday, for instance, your body will gear itself up for taking in food at 6:00 p.m. today. At 5:50 p.m. your body will produce more saliva as your gastric juices begin to churn. When this happens you may start to feel hungry or feel your stomach growling. Exercise works in much the same way. If you exercised yesterday morning, your body will gear itself up for exercise around the same time today. If you continue to exercise and eat around the same time each day, your body will always perform at its highest capacity. Surprising your body with random eating and exercise can throw off its natural cycle. This does not mean you have to exercise every day. Giving your body a break between workouts is also important. However, exercising and eating on a consistent schedule can greatly promote mind-body balance, weight loss, and other exercise goals.

General Tip #6: Exercise in the Morning

Our heart slows down when we sleep, decreasing circulation throughout the body. Although we may toss from side to side, there is minimal body movement throughout the night. The body also uses this time to replenish its tissues, shedding the old and building anew. Therefore, by morning the body has accumulated a fair share of toxins and by-products. Our joints, like a bend in a river, are where fluids tend to accumulate. This is why arthritic pain is often worse when we wake up and diminishes when we get up and move around. Working out in the morning can help get our engine turning over and stimulate more energy and blood flow throughout the day. If your schedule does not allow for morning exercise, afternoon or evening workouts will suffice. Just keep in mind that working out directly before bedtime often affects our ability to enter a deep sleep.

General Tip #7: Make Exercise Itself a Joy

Exercise gives us a natural high through the release of endorphins. Do you work out simply to feel good? While many of us do, others tend to push themselves too far, saying, "I have to be stronger than my friends!" or "I have to lose more weight!" I invite you to take the time to enjoy your workout, giving it a chance to make you happier. Yes, losing weight or getting stronger is certainly a feasible goal, but a workout can provide a whole lot more. Exercising regularly is one of the most effective ways to deal with stress, anxiety, and/or depression. Setting time aside to exercise means giving your mind and body the attention and acknowledgment they deserve.

Pushing yourself too hard during a workout only leads to excess fatigue and tissue damage. I have treated just as many patients with aches and pains from an excessive workout schedule as I have those who do not exercise enough. A little soreness after a workout goes a long way. There is no need to push past this point.

General Tip #8: Work Out to Music

By now we've discussed how different herbs, foods, and exercises benefit each body type, but music also has a role to play. Music facilitates both the slowing down and the speeding up of our mind and our body's energy. The excessive Yang of Yang types can be calmed by the soothing sounds of soft or slow (Yin) music, while the deficient and sluggish Yang of Yin types can get an occasional boost from loud or vibrant (Yang) music. Slower and softer music helps slow the racing heartbeat of Yang types, reducing anxiety, and promoting the flow of energy downward to nourish the weaker liver and kidneys, while loud or vibrant music can increase circulation of Yin types, alleviating stress and pain. No matter which body type you are, there is always room for both Yin and Yang music, depending on your taste and mood. Yet if you are an overly stressed Yang type who listens only to vibrant music, how about a soft tune to balance things out a bit? Are you a Yin type who needs a little push in the morning? Try starting the day with a little rock 'n' roll! Listening to music during the day or during your workout can serve as a simple but effective way to keep in balance, get the rhythm going, or slow it down.

EXERCISE CATEGORIES

This book includes four major exercise categories: cardiovascular, stretching, meditation, and strength training (see table 3.15). Each of these methods in its own way is beneficial for all the body types. Cardiovascular exercise, for example, focuses mainly on strengthening the heart and lungs, and therefore improves overall circulation and regulates blood pressure. Stretching relieves tight or spasmodic muscles, helping our muscles breathe and absorb oxygen. Meditation helps to relax and enhance the connection between our mind and body. Strength training encourages the muscles to do what they do best—flex and extend.

An ideal exercise routine provides a balance between each of the four categories. Balancing an exercise routine is a difficult task because it requires us to know when to slow down and when to pick up the tempo. Excessive weight lifting, for example, results in excessive muscle fatigue and burden on the heart. Although meditation can help reduce stress, hours of daily meditation might keep us from getting other things done! Cardiovascular exercise late in the evening might interfere with our sleeping and waking patterns.

Active and Passive Meditation

Your Yin Yang Body Type divides meditation into two major categories:

Active meditation involves the process of clearing and calming your mind, focusing only on your breath, and/or listening to calming music while performing rhythmic exercises, such as running and bicycling. This technique, which is also referred to as Yang meditation, benefits Yin types because it promotes balance and harmony while cultivating their weaker Yang energy.

Passive meditation includes qi gong, tai chi, yoga, or other contemplative exercises performed in a standing, sitting, or kneeling position. This technique, also referred to as Yin meditation, benefits Yang types because it soothes their overactive Yang.

TABLE 3.15. BENEFITS OF CERTAIN EXERCISES

Exercise Category	Examples	Effects
Cardiovascular	Running, bicycling, dancing, zumba, aerobics, treadmill, elliptical, trampoline, jump roping	Increases general circulation, supports lung and heart health, increases elimination of toxins
Stretching	yoga, general stretching	Enhances flow of oxygen to the muscles, reduces muscle fatigue, increases range of motion, reduces tension and headaches
Meditation	Active: Can be done while participating in any form of exercise Passive: qi gong, tai chi, zen, chanting, deep breathing	Calms the mind, increases energy flow and circulation, reduces stress, enhances self-image
Strength training	Weight lifting, push-ups and sit-ups (core strengthening), Pilates	Increases muscle strength, supports joint function, enhances endurance

EXERCISE AND THE BODY TYPES

While each of the four exercise categories is beneficial for just about anyone, every body type has its own emphasis. Yang body types derive greater benefit from Yin exercises. Yin types, by contrast, benefit more from Yang exercises (see table 3.16). So, what is the difference between Yin and Yang exercise? Yin, by nature, is quiet and sedentary; Yin exercises involve less movement than Yang exercises. Yang is active and lively by nature, so Yang exercises involve quick, rhythmic movements. Yin exercises include stretching, breathing, and weight lifting. Yang exercises include running, jogging, brisk walking, bicycling, hiking, rock climbing, and modern dance.

All body types can benefit from both Yin and Yang exercises, but

TABLE 3.16. YIN AND YANG EXERCISES

Yin Exercises	Yang Exercises
Meditation (passive), qi gong, tai chi, stretching, yoga, weight lifting, golfing, walking, fishing, dancing (slow pace), bowling	Cardio (jogging, running, swimming, aerobics, biking), hiking, wrestling, dancing (fast pace), meditation (active)

too much of one or the other can lead to an imbalance of Yin and Yang in the body. Because Yin and Yang are in opposition, if one gets stronger, the other gets weaker. The stronger organs have the tendency to "steal" energy away from the weaker organs. Yin Type B's, for example, are born with stronger kidneys and a weaker spleen. As the kidneys get stronger, the spleen will get weaker because of their Yin Yang relationship. A weakened spleen may cause digestion-related issues, such as stomachaches, bloating, feeling tired after meals, and diarrhea. Exercise, which is excellent at conflict resolution, can encourage communication between the stronger kidneys and the weaker spleen, helping to resolve these issues. In Sasang medical theory, keeping healthy depends on the smooth flow of energy from our stronger to our weaker organs. Body type–specific exercise, food, herbs, and the like all promote the flow of energy from the stronger to the weaker organs.

The remainder of the chapter provides a detailed approach to body type–specific exercises.

EXERCISE AND YIN TYPE A

With their inherently weaker lungs, Yin Type A's often breathe shallowly, which makes it difficult for them to absorb enough oxygen. Since breathing is something we often take for granted, shallow breathing is an issue that often goes unnoticed. Cardiovascular exercise, which should comprise 50 percent of the Yin Type A's total workout, strengthens the lungs by promoting deeper respiration. Yin Type A's often feel lighter after cardio exercise because this deeper respiration feeds their body's oxygen-thirsty cells. Yin Type A's can strengthen their lungs

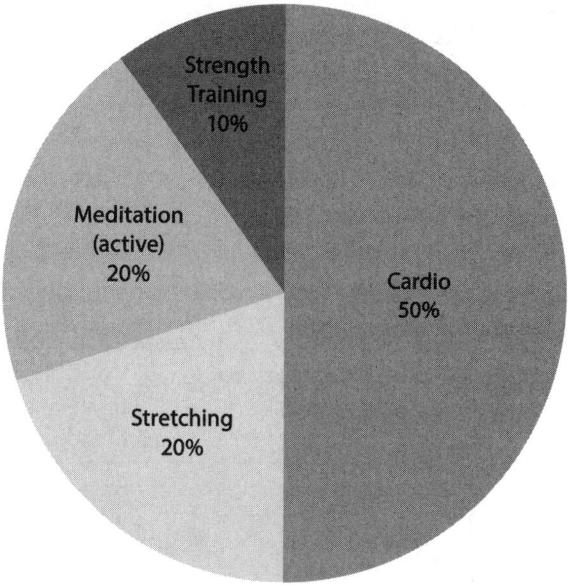

Figure 3.12. Breakdown of optimum exercise category percentages for Yin Type A

by breathing in and out as deeply as possible during exercise. It is also important for Yin Type A's to avoid holding their breath while exercising, even during the most difficult exercise routines. Although exercise is an excellent way to establish the habit of breathing deeply, making an attempt to breathe deeply all the time can greatly improve the Yin Type A's health.

The stronger liver of Yin Type A's can easily get itself in trouble, absorbing too many by-products from the digestive system. A balanced liver is proficient at breaking down and efficiently releasing toxins after absorbing them. Cardiovascular exercise not only promotes breathing, it also promotes blood flow, which in turn assists in the elimination of toxins.

In Sasang medicine the liver and kidneys are said to supply energy to the lower body while the lungs and spleen feed the upper body. The stronger liver of Yin Type A's promotes a sturdier and more developed lower body. Their weaker lungs result in a weaker upper body, hence the need for cardiovascular exercises to strengthen it.

TABLE 3.17. EFFECTS OF EXERCISE ON COMMON YIN TYPE A AILMENTS

Cause (Inherited)	Effect	Exercise Remedy
Strong liver	Toxic buildup	Exercise to promote circulation
Weaker lungs	Shallow breathing, respiratory issues	Maximize breathing during meditation and cardio
Stronger lower body (due to liver strength)	Weaker upper body (lungs, heart)	Upper-body strength training, cardio, deep breathing (yoga), hiking
Lack of circulation (due to excessively strong liver)	High blood pressure, vascular disorders	Refrain from excessive weight lifting, move your body, and, most of all, sweat!

Tip #1: Sweating Is Essential for Yin Type A

Are you a Yin Type A who has difficulty sweating? Sweating is an issue for most Yin Type A's because the skin pores are controlled by the lungs. Healthier lungs are able to control the opening and closing of the skin pores, allowing us to sweat regularly. The weaker lungs of the Yin Type A often result in either a lack of, or too much, sweating, as the skin pores get jammed shut or stuck in the open position. A lack of sweat means Yin Type A's have difficulty ridding themselves of toxins and other excesses. If you are a Yin Type A who sweats too much while feeling hot or under stress, it is likely that your liver is producing too much heat, which is released through the skin pores. This is certainly not a bad sign; it is simply a way that your body releases heat from its strong liver. If Yin Type A's don't sweat when they're hot, toxic heat may accumulate inside their liver, eventually leading to health issues.

If it is difficult for you to sweat even during cardiovascular exercise, try dressing in layers and covering your head with a hood during your workout. Certain Yin Type A's may also notice that they start to sweat twenty minutes or so into a workout. Try prolonging or intensifying your cardio workout if you aren't building up enough sweat. If all else fails, go into a sauna before or after your cardio workout and sweat it out! Since sweating may lead to dehydration, make sure you drink plenty of water before, during, and after your workout.

Tip #2: Cardiovascular Workout for Yin Type A

As we have seen, cardiovascular activity is the most important exercise for Yin Type A's. To understand why let's take a closer look at the concept of Yin and Yang. Yin is absorbing while Yang is dispersing. Yin types tend to absorb toxins and toxic by-products more than Yang types. Since Yin is associated with absorption, Yin Type A's tend to absorb too much of everything. Health is a balance between absorbing and excreting. While the body needs to absorb energy from food, it also needs to excrete unnecessary by-products and toxins. Strong absorption may interfere with circulation, causing a buildup of toxins and food by-products in the body.

Cardiovascular activity is a quick and efficient way to work up a sweat and increase circulation. The body releases toxins through the pores when we sweat, which is why perspiration can smell unpleasant. Increased circulation leads to more efficient elimination through defecation and urination. Hence the combination of both of these benefits can tremendously enhance the health of Yin types.

Tip #3: Kick-starting Your Engine as a Yin Type A

Yin Type A's have a tendency to be laid-back, and may be reluctant to get started on an exercise routine. Especially after a stressful day, the couch may be more inviting than the gym. Moreover, Yin Type A's usually have more energy in the evening, often making it difficult for them to wake up in the morning after they have been up late at night. An early work schedule may also interfere with the intention to work out in the morning. However, once Yin Type A's get started, they tend to keep going and can easily become "addicted" to exercising and find it difficult to slow down. Try establishing a balance between too much and too little exercise. This will help you stay consistent without lagging behind or overstressing your mind and body.

Tip #4: Heavy Lifting for Yin Type A

Weight lifting encourages the body to absorb more energy and blood in its tissues, producing increased muscle mass. If our muscles get too large or too tight, however, there is less room for everything else to flow by or through them. Yin Type A's have the ability to accumulate the greatest amount of muscle mass, due to their strongly absorbent liver. Excessive muscle tissue easily turns into fat when we stop working out consistently. Heavy weight lifting without sufficient cardio exercise greatly increases our chances of developing hypertension and other cardiopulmonary issues down the road. In short, less weight and more repetition can help strengthen your muscles without the threat of weight gain or compromised circulation.

Tip #5: Maximize Breathing to Strengthen Your Lungs as a Yin Type A

Breathing deeply during exercise will help strengthen the weaker lungs of Yin Type A's. Refer to General Tip #4 (page 223) for more details on how to breathe during exercise.

Tip #6: Vinegar before Exercise for Yin Type A

As noted earlier Vinegar is one of the most beneficial supplements for Yin Type A's because it helps promote circulation. Taken with water before you exercise, vinegar can loosen and prepare your muscles for action. Exercise also helps the body absorb and circulate vinegar throughout the vascular system, enhancing its capability to alleviate joint pain and arthritis, general body aches, and cardiovascular issues. Add two tablespoons of apple cider vinegar to one cup of water and drink up. Add or lessen the amount of vinegar, depending on your tolerance.

EXERCISE AND YIN TYPE B

The weaker spleen of Yin Type B's is easily affected by cold. Even on a warm summer day, the spleen of Yin Type B's often suffers from a heat deficiency. Do you recall that heat corresponds to Yang? Yin Type B's are the most deficient in Yang compared with the other three body types. Cardiovascular exercises, which comprise 40 percent of the Yin

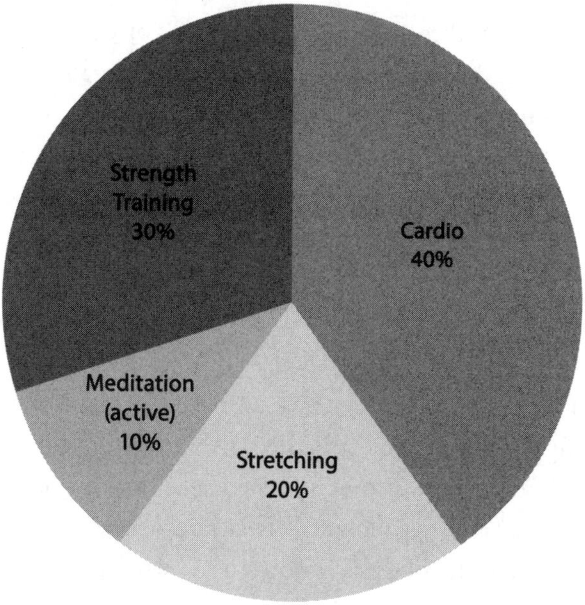

Figure 3.13. Breakdown of optimum exercise category percentages for Yin Type B

Type B's workout, help warm up their body from the inside out, sending Yang and heat to the spleen. You may wonder, "Where is all of this cold coming from?" As the primary internal source of cold energy, the Yin Type B's stronger kidneys behave like an air conditioner stuck on a high setting! In order to keep warm, they have to keep moving.

Keep in Mind

In Sasang medicine the kidneys are considered the "air-conditioner," while the spleen is the "heater" of the body. Born with a weaker spleen and stronger kidneys, Yin Type B's are prone to Yin cold-related issues, which in Eastern medicine are associated with common colds, sadness and grief, lack of appetite, and diarrhea.

The spleen is also energetically linked to the muscles of the upper body, whereas the kidneys correspond to the lower-body muscles. A stronger spleen reflects stronger and better-developed upper-body musculature. The weaker spleen of Yin Type B's often results in a lack of upper-body muscle development, making them look frail. Tired Yin Type B's are often hunched over, as if their neck is too weak to support their head. Weight lifting and other core-strengthening exercises that focus on strengthening the upper body constitute 30 percent of the total Yin Type B workout, and also serve another significant role, as we are about to see.

Besides cooling down the body, the kidneys are also responsible for eliminating fluid, excess minerals and protein, and by-products from the body via urine. Being the strongest of the Yin Type B organs, the kidneys often get into trouble, as they simply flush out too much protein, thinking that life would be easier without dealing with it at all! A lack of protein contributes to excessive weight loss and leaves the body feeling drained of energy. Weight lifting and other core-strengthening exercises encourage the body to absorb more protein by telling the kidneys to absorb rather than eliminate. Weight lifting can also encourage weight gain for the emaciated Yin Type B.

From the Clinic

As a junior high school student, Doug was a recluse. He disliked associating with others and lived in his own world. Sad and lonely, he developed some unhealthy habits, such as excessive consumption of alcohol. Yet, with the willpower of a horse (typical of Yin Type B's), he decided to start a weight-lifting regimen. As his muscles took shape, he also felt a deep sense of accomplishment, which led to making healthier decisions overall. Doug is now a doctor who treats young people with addiction-related issues.

Tip #1: Warm Up That Spleen!

The spleen needs warmth to digest food effectively. The weaker spleen of Yin Type B's has a tendency to lose heat and be afflicted by cold. Cardiovascular exercise is an excellent way to warm the Yin Type B's spleen, stimulate the appetite, and promote digestion. Take advantage of your increased appetite by eating slightly larger portions after your

TABLE 3.18. EFFECTS OF EXERCISE ON COMMON YIN TYPE B AILMENTS

Cause (Inherited)	Effect	Remedy
Strong kidneys (which produce cold)	Colder body	Warming exercises (cardio), sauna, hot tub
Weaker spleen (which promotes digestion and warmth)	Lack of digestion	Warming exercises (cardio), sauna, hot tub, spicy foods
Stronger lower body (due to kidney strength)	Weaker upper body (chest, shoulders)	Upper-body strength training, cardio, deep breathing (yoga), hiking
Overall lack of energy (due to weak digestion)	Easily fatigued, excessive sweating	Exercise in moderation, never pushing yourself too hard

workout. This is also a window of opportunity for protein ingestion, which otherwise may be too heavy for some Yin Type B's to digest.

The excessively cold nature of the Yin Type B's kidneys singe the heat of the spleen. An abundance of cold energy leads to indigestion, fatigue, and chilliness. The winter is an especially difficult time for Yin Type B's, when cold tends to sneak into the body, leading to indigestion, flu, chronic headaches, fatigue, and/or the inability to get warm. Regular cardiovascular exercise, saunas, and hot baths are a great way to warm up the spleen and tame the cooling energy of the kidneys, thus preventing these symptoms. The catch is to remember not to cool your body off directly after exercise. Try to preserve your body heat by covering your skin directly after exercise or taking a warm bath or shower.

Tip #2: Consume Ginger before Exercise

As we saw on page 144, ginger is one of the most beneficial foods for Yin Type B's. Consumed as tea before you exercise, ginger can loosen and prepare your muscles for action. Exercise helps the body absorb and circulate ginger throughout the vascular system, enhancing its ability to address indigestion, fatigue, and coldness. Thinly slice and peel one inch of fresh gingerroot and bring it to a boil in two cups of water. Let it simmer for twenty minutes and drink it warm, increasing or lessening the amount of ginger to your liking.

Tip #3: Now's Your Chance for Protein Intake!

Since the spleen governs appetite regulation, a cold spleen causes a reduction of appetite while a warm spleen stimulates it. Exercise is a great way to warm up the spleen and increase the appetite of Yin Type B's, whose cold spleen often reduces it. A healthy appetite is therefore a sign of sufficient Yang energy. Take advantage of this opportunity to ingest protein or other nutrient-rich food. If you do not have much of an appetite, try delaying the intake of protein-rich or hardy foods until after your workout or ingesting warm-property foods.

Tip #4: The Dangers of Excessive Sweating

Unlike Yin Type A's, who easily absorb energy, Yin Type B's easily dispose of it. When Yin Type B's overexercise, they can quickly lose what little Yang they originally had through profuse sweating. While sweating is a great way to release toxins, it can also signal exhaustion for Yin Type B's. It is common for Yin Type B's to sweat profusely when they are exhausted. This type of sweat usually flows from the face and upper body like a water fountain, forming a thin layer of moisture above the skin and feeling sticky, wet, and uncomfortable. Sweating a lot during an intense workout, however, is a natural occurrence for any of the body types. This type of sweat may also drip down from the face but slowly, drop by drop. The unhealthy, profuse sweat of the Yin Type B is accompanied by extreme fatigue and a constant desire to hit the sack. Called "Yang collapse," this is a result of complete exhaustion and/or depletion of Yang energy as it escapes from the body through the pores. Since Yin types are deficient in Yang energy to begin with, Yang collapse could cause serious health issues down the road. If you sweat in this way during an intense workout, you've taken things a bit too far. It's time to slow down and modify your exercise routine. Try to avoid getting to this point by regulating your workout, challenging yourself in short spurts rather than forcing yourself to perform a prolonged anaerobic workout.

EXERCISE AND YANG TYPE A

Yang Type A's owe their swift metabolism and efficient digestive system to an inherently stronger spleen. Yet, a stronger spleen often leads to an overactive digestive system, which produces excess accumulation of heat. This condition, referred to as "spleen fire," is marked by an upward rebellion of energy that bombards the heart, causing anxiety, anger, rage, and/or palpitations. Passive meditation, which accounts for 30 percent of the workout for Yang Type A's, can help curb their propensity for anger by promoting a harmonious flow of spleen energy.

Since the spleen is the body's internal source of heat, the strong spleen of Yang Type A's can make them feel as if they're standing next to an oven on a hot summer day. Accordingly, Yang Type A's often suffer from heat-related issues, such as fever, anger, excessive appetite, and heartburn. Passive meditation and stretching have a homeostatic effect on the body, which helps regulate body temperature and reduce excessive heat accumulation.

The kidneys also control water metabolism by regulating absorption

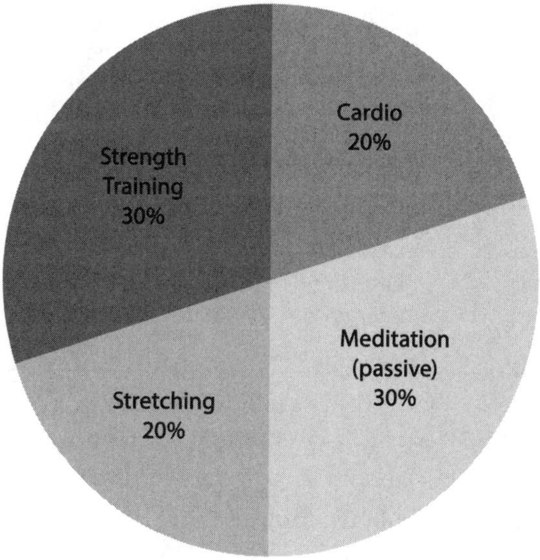

Figure 3.14. Breakdown of optimum exercise category percentages for Yang Type A

and excretion of fluids from the body. Born with weaker kidneys, Yang Type A's are prone to water retention in the abdomen and legs. Lower-body and abdominal strength training, which accounts for 30 percent of the Yang Type A's workout, helps to increase muscle tone of the lower extremities, and reduce the tendency of the abdomen, hips, ankles, thighs, and knees to retain water.

Because Yang Type A's are born with more Yang, their upper body is naturally stronger than the lower half. This is also because their stronger spleen, considered a Yang organ, is located in the upper half of the body. Lower-body strength training can help support and condition the weaker lower body of Yang Type A's and prevent lower-back, knee, ankle, and/or heel discomfort.

TABLE 3.19. EFFECTS OF EXERCISE ON COMMON YANG TYPE A AILMENTS

Cause (Inherited)	Effect	Remedy
Strong spleen (in charge of digestion)	Overactive digestive system and excessive upper body energy	Passive meditation, stretching, gentle walking/hiking
Weaker kidneys (in charge of water metabolism)	Water retention in lower body, dehydration	Lower-body and abdominal strength training with weights, squats, sit-ups, etc.
Stronger upper body (due to spleen strength)	Upper-extremity strength, leg weakness	Balance with lower-body strength training (see above)
Too much Yang!	Easy to burn out, lose energy	Ample rest, controlled exercise, (passive) meditation

Tip #1: The Dangers of Excessive Sweating

Sweating can be beneficial no matter what your body type, since it helps to release toxins from the body. However, in certain situations excessive sweating can be a sign of extreme fatigue. This type of sweat usually flows rather than drips from the upper body. Because it signals extreme fatigue, both the Yin Type B and the Yang Type A need to avoid excessive sweating. This condition is called Yang collapse in the Yin Type B, a dire situation in which Yang escapes from the body, leaving the Yin Type B feeling exhausted and weakened. For the Yang Type A, this condition is referred to as Yin collapse, meaning Yin escapes from the body. Although the mechanism of these situations is different, the results are equally detrimental, since the body relies on a balance of Yin and Yang to survive. These situations can be avoided by pacing your workout and refraining from pushing too hard.

Tip #2: Keep It Cool

As we have seen, exercise is an efficient way to warm up the body. On a cold winter day, this would appeal even to Yang types, who have more internal heat than Yin types. If Yang Type A's are not careful, though, they can easily become overheated and excessively fatigued. A continuous supply of cool water during a workout can keep their system cool and lubricated to prevent overheating. A cooler room, less clothing, and a handy water bottle during your workout will all ensure that you don't get overheated.

Tip #3: Alternate Your Rhythm

An intense workout is considered Yang, while a lighter one is considered Yin. Because of their Yang nature, most Yang Type A's like to jump right into a workout, getting it done quickly and out of the way. Although it may feel contrary to your nature, try slowing down periodically during a workout to protect your Yang energy, rather than expending it. Alternating aerobic (e.g., walking) and anaerobic (e.g., jogging) exercise every few minutes is one way to balance your workout.

Tip #4: Know Your Strengths and Weaknesses

Yang Type A's are born with a strong upper body. This strength gives them a natural advantage in sports and exercises that utilize the arms and upper torso, so Yang Type A's have a natural talent for wrestling, boxing, judo, upper-body weight lifting, and gymnastics. They can potentially outperform other body types in these sports with less effort. Yet, Yang Type A's have to work twice as hard as Yin types when it comes to sports that focus on lower-body strength, such as soccer, running, and bicycling. While it is great to cultivate your innate talents, it is equally important, for the sake of optimum health, to bolster your weaknesses.

Tip #5: Drink Plenty of Fluids

Weaker kidneys mean Yang Type A's lack the ability to feel thirsty—even if their body gets dehydrated! As a result Yang Type A's often suffer from dehydration after exercise or excessive body movement. Loss of fluid from dehydration causes the blood to thicken, making it extra hard for the already weaker kidneys of Yang Type A's to filter unwanted by-products. Drinking fluids before, during, and after a workout is an essential part of supporting the Yang Type A's kidneys' health.

Tip #6: Get into the Groove

Yang Type A's can easily get started with exercise, but once they get started, they find it challenging to maintain a consistent workout schedule. This is not because of laziness but rather from a lack of patience and an all-or-nothing attitude. This is why Yang Type A's earn the title of "jack of all trades but master of none." Challenge yourself to work out on a consistent basis and try to avoid giving up and trying something else. Make your exercise routine fun and enjoyable while refraining from pushing yourself too hard.

Tip #7: Direct Energy to the Kidneys

The overall well-being of Yang Type A's depends on the health of their kidneys. A two-step meditation technique, combined with guided imagery, can strengthen and keep your body healthy and your organs happy. First, focus the mind on a particular part of the body. Then, imagine the flow of positive energy, warmth, or blood to your area of focus. Eastern medicine holds that the mind drives the healing process. When the mind is filled with positive thoughts, the body becomes motivated to fight off the invasion of bacteria, viruses, or fungi. When the mind is consumed with negative thoughts, the body loses its motivation and succumbs to illness. There are hundreds of different guided imagery techniques out there. For the sake of brevity, I would like to offer a simplified version of guided imagery that I have implemented effectively in my own practice.

GUIDED IMAGERY FOR THE KIDNEYS

* Stand straight with both legs together. Place your hands (palms downward) above the kidneys, which are located slightly below the center of your back. Arch your back slightly while inhaling and exhaling slowly and deeply. Continue breathing slowly for up to two minutes while arching your back. On each inhale imagine that you are sending light, warmth, and energy to your kidneys. On each exhale imagine that you are releasing tension, turbidity, and toxins from your kidneys. After two minutes reverse the motion by bending your body forward and reaching toward your toes, relaxing everything in your body. Hold this position while breathing in and out for another two minutes. During this time continue with the above imagery on each inhale and exhale. This process can be repeated several times a day. Try this technique first thing in the morning and before going to bed at night. Because this meditation is designed to guide energy to the kidneys, rather than giving your muscles a workout, each movement should be gentle and comfortable.

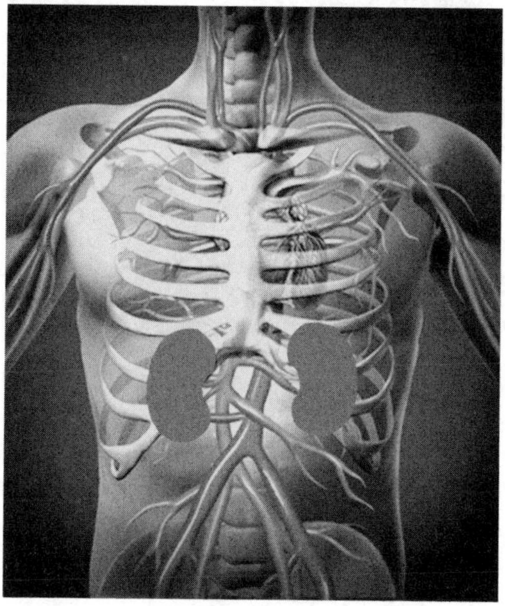

Figure 3.15. Location of the kidney

EXERCISE AND YANG TYPE B

Yang Type B's owe their enhanced upper-body strength and dignified appearance to an inherently stronger pair of lungs, which supply abundant energy to the face, chest, neck, and arms. Yet, stronger lungs may lead to hyperventilation, a condition that stems from abnormally rapid breathing. This results in excess oxygen and a lack of carbon dioxide in the body, an imbalance that often causes Yang Type B's to feel faint, dizzy, and/or experience anxiety attacks. In Eastern medicine overly rapid breathing is often due to jam-packed energy in the chest, neck, and head, with the resulting symptoms specified above. Passive meditation, which accounts for 50 percent of the workout for Yang Type B's, can help soothe their overactive lungs, encourage the downward movement of energy, and promote balance and harmony in the body.

In Sasang medicine the lungs correspond to the emotion of grief, making it common for Yang Type B's to feel sorrowful. Without an avenue leading away from their sad circumstances, they can fall more and

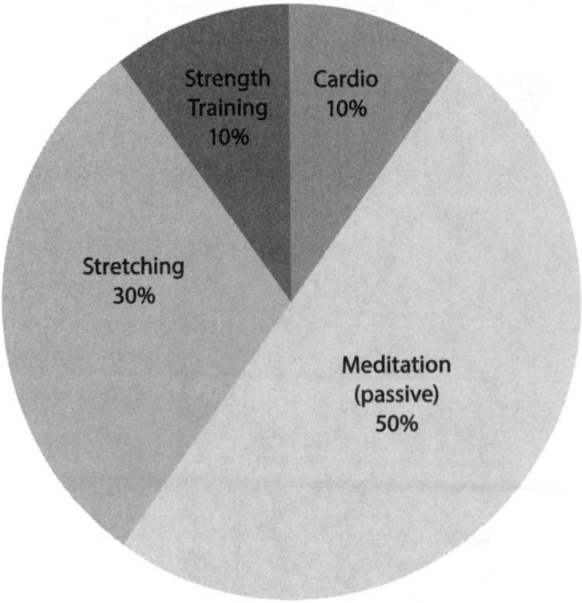

Figure 3.16. Breakdown of optimum exercise category percentages for Yang Type B

more deeply into the abyss of depression. The sadness of Yang Type B's easily morphs into sudden bursts of anger, which severely compromise their overall health. Exercises such as meditation, stretching, and light cardio are especially beneficial for Yang Type B's, as they offer refuge from excessive anger and sadness.

Since the lungs are situated in the upper half of the body, Yang Type B's naturally have stronger chest, arm, and neck muscles. Yet they tend to experience a lack of balance and coordination because of a surprisingly weak lower body. It is difficult for others to imagine how weak this area can be, given how exceedingly robust Yang Type B's appear above the waist!

Unlike the Yin Type A's stronger liver, which absorbs too many toxins, the Yang Type B's weaker liver has trouble absorbing anything at all. A weaker liver makes it difficult for Yang Type B's to absorb and hold on to energy from food. In Eastern medicine there are several ways to "exercise," to preserve energy and promote the health of your liver. One of these is qi gong, a type of meditation combined with stretching and breathing that enhances the flow of energy within your body. Refer to Tip #6 below for details.

TABLE 3.20. EFFECTS OF EXERCISE ON COMMON YANG TYPE B AILMENTS

Cause (Inherited)	Effect	Remedy
Strong lungs (fill the chest with oxygen)	Excess development and stagnation of upper-body energy	Meditation, yoga, stretching, gentle walking/hiking
Weaker liver (cannot absorb energy)	Lack of sustainable energy	Qi gong exercises and stretching
Stronger upper body (due to lung strength)	Upper extremity strength, waist and hip weakness	Lower-body light strength training, walking, stretching
Too much Yang!	Easy to burn out, lose energy	Meditation, ample rest, light exercise

Tip #1: Don't Push It!

Recommending that Yang Type B's take it easy is like training an eagle to walk instead of fly. It is the eagle's nature to fly, just as it is the Yang Type B's nature to move and take control. Excessive movement, however, results in fatigue and heightened stress levels. When engaging in exercise, it is necessary to keep yourself from pushing too hard. Meditative exercises, such as yoga, qi gong, and tai chi, provide an excellent way to balance your energies.

Tip #2: Balance Mind and Body

The mind of Yang Type B's is constantly active because their strong lungs provide the brain with an ample amount of oxygen. This gives Yang Type B's a keen sense of intuition and insight. Too much thinking, however, can cause Yang Type B's to become frustrated and lose their patience with others. With such an active mind, it is hard for them to live in their own skin, often thinking outside their body and losing track of its basic needs, such as eating and sleeping. Meditative exercise, which enhances the connection between mind and body, helps their mind relax and stay grounded.

Tip #3: Be Active in the Morning

Yang Type B's quickly lose their energy in the evening, so exercise at this time can cause even more fatigue and exhaustion. As with the other body types, exercise during Yang (morning) time provides energetic momentum for the rest of the day. Yet be vigilant about that all-or-nothing attitude and avoid using up every ounce of your energy in the morning!

Tip #4: Avoid Heavy Lifting

With so much Yang energy and pressure buildup in their upper body, it is common for Yang Type B's to be afflicted with high blood pressure. Lifting heavy loads can therefore be dangerous, as it increases systemic pressure and the potential for blood vessel injury. Their weaker lower body also tends to give out easily when lifting heavier items. Lighter and more repetitious lower-body, weight-bearing exercises can help strengthen the Yang Type B's weaker quads, gluteus, and calf muscles.

Tip #5: Stretch Your Upper Body

The Yang Type B's excessive upper-body strength often turns into neck, chest, and shoulder tightness, so releasing this area through stretching can bring a significant level of comfort (see pages 220–22 for more on specific neck, chest, and shoulder stretches).

Tip #6: Directing Energy toward the Liver

The overall well-being of Yang Type B's depends on the health of their inherently weaker liver. As discussed under Yang Type A exercise, the two-step meditation technique combined with guided imagery can strengthen and keep your body healthy and your organs happy. (See the Yang Type A's "Tip #7: Direct Energy to the Kidneys" on pages 240–41 for more information.) Here are a few simplified meditation techniques for the Yang Type B that I use in my own practice. They are most effective when practiced in sequence.

MEDITATION TECHNIQUE #1

* Lie down facing upward.
* Place both hands directly above the lower half of the rib cage (even though the physical location of the liver is under the lower half of the right side of the rib cage—see figure 3.17—Eastern medicine holds that liver energy flows bilaterally along both sides of the body, so the left hand plays just as significant a role in this exercise).

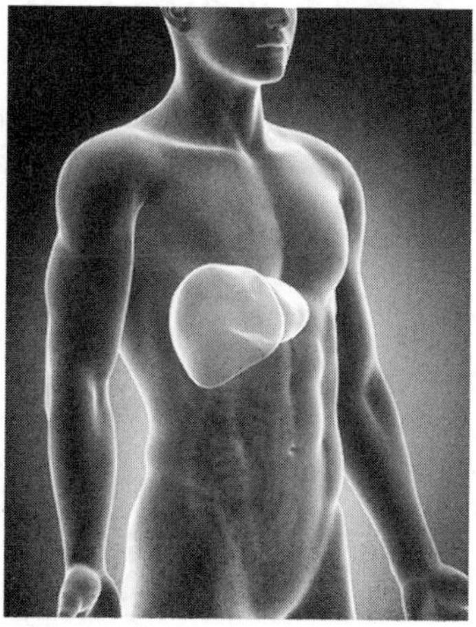

Figure 3.17. Location of liver.

* Take deep breaths and imagine with each inhale that you are sending light, warmth, and energy through your hands and into your body. On each exhale imagine that you are releasing tension, turbidity, and toxins from your liver.
* Continue breathing slowly for up to two minutes, with your hands resting on the lower rib cage.
* After two minutes place your hands on your chest and slowly rub in a downward motion toward the liver. Continue this movement for another two minutes, imagining a flow of energy, warmth, and light from the chest (lungs) to your liver, while inhaling and exhaling slowly.
* Try this technique first thing in the morning and before going to bed at night for several minutes at a time. The purpose of this movement is to guide energy to the liver, rather than to give your muscles a workout, so keep each movement gentle and comfortable.

MEDITATION TECHNIQUE #2

* Stand up with both feet about shoulder-width apart.
* Place your left hand over your liver (see figure 3.17).
* Reach upward with your right arm, take in a slow, deep breath, and lean toward your left side (keeping your right arm straight and your left hand over your liver).
* Exhale slowly as you return to an upright position. While performing this movement, imagine that you are sending energy, light, and warmth through your left hand into your liver.
* Continue this exercise on the opposite side, placing the right hand over the left lower rib cage, reaching upward with your left arm, and stretching toward your right side.
* Try repeating this exercise ten times on each side.

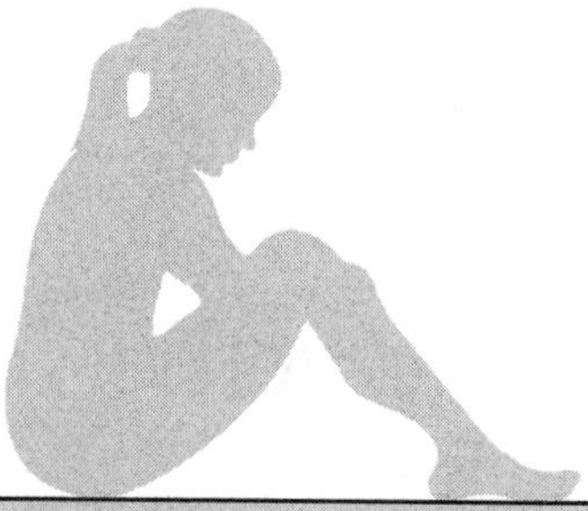

PART FOUR

Addressing Health Issues Based on Your Yin Yang Body Type

Healing with Sasang Medicine

An Introduction

Rather than simply eliminating illness, the Sasang approach focuses on supporting our vulnerable areas and helping the body heal itself. This method puts faith in our natural ability to fight off illness, pulling it out from the roots, rather than merely masking its symptoms.

This section includes a list of common syndromes and remedies that are categorized according to each of the four body types. While each body type has up to three different food and/or herbal remedy recommendations per health condition, the foods and herbs listed are not to be used in place of the advice of a doctor when you are ill. If you have a significant health issue, it is important to seek the help and knowledge of a health care professional. This section offers general advice to prevent and alleviate common, nonacute health issues in accordance with your body type.

According to Eastern medicine, food is the first line of defense in avoiding and/or fighting off illness. As we learned in part 3, eating according to our body type helps cultivate and strengthen the weaker aspects of our mind and body. The weaker lungs of Yin Type A's, for example, are nourished and supported by foods that bolster the lungs.

The deficient spleen of Yin Type B's is strengthened by foods that support the spleen. The Yang Type A's weaker kidneys benefit from foods that strengthen the kidneys. And, finally, the weaker liver of the Yang Type B's gains strength from foods that enhance the liver. Body type–specific foods keep us healthy by encouraging blood and energy flow to our constitutionally weaker organs.

Herbs and other supplements are the second line of defense in fighting off illness and are used when the illness has taken hold. The herbs in this part of the book are offered as stand-alone remedies for early stages of illness or in conjunction with other approaches. If your health issue lingers on, it may be necessary to obtain a thorough analysis from a medical doctor, naturopath, or trained professional in Sasang medicine. Though I offer one to three herbal remedies for each health condition, a Sasang herbal formula written by a Sasang medical professional often consists of ten to fifteen different herbs, prescribed in larger doses and offering more powerful ammunition in fighting off illness, based on the specific needs of the patient.

Sasang medicine is not the only solution for everyone or every health situation. Acute medical issues often require the use of Western medical remedies alone or in conjunction with Sasang medicine. When you are ill, it is crucial to use common sense in choosing the correct path toward wellness. If a particular method is not proving helpful despite giving it enough time to kick in or an illness is progressing rapidly, try a different approach. It is also recommended that you contact your doctor and a Sasang practitioner before ingesting herbs when on medications in order to avoid negative interactions.

TREATING ILLNESS ACCORDING TO YOUR BODY TYPE

There is no such thing in Sasang medicine as a universal cold remedy, arthritis formula, or the like. As mentioned above herbal treatment focuses on supporting the weaker organ of each body type. The common cold will affect each of the body types differently, depending on their weaker and stronger organs. Yang Type A's, for example, cannot share cold remedies with Yin Type A's. If they did, the Yin Type A's cold might easily get worse! This is because Yang Type A's have weaker kidneys while Yin Type A's have weaker lungs. When Yang Type A's catch a cold, their kidneys need to be supported. When Yin Type A's get a cold, their lungs need to be supported. By failing to recognize this concept, modern medicine completely disregards the importance of the body type, potentially helping some patients but sooner or later harming others. It is probable that most pharmaceutical side effects are based on body type mismatching. Nonsteroidal anti-inflammatory drugs (NSAIDs), such as ibuprofen, aspirin, and naproxen, may irritate the stomach wall. According to Sasang medicine, Yang Type A's are prone to stomach irritation due to excess heat and stomach acid buildup. NSAIDs can cause further irritation of the Yang Type A's excess stomach heat, possibly resulting in stomach ulcers after prolonged use. Other body types without the propensity for stomach heat issues, however, may not be as susceptible to such conditions.

The treatment of other ailments, such as indigestion, also varies according to body type. The weak stomach and spleen of Yin Type B's often lead to indigestion, while an overactive liver may be the source of indigestion for Yin Type A's, who are born with a stronger liver. The hyper-absorption of the Yin Type A's liver causes it to get congested easily, interfering with the digestive process. In many cases the symptoms of indigestion manifested by the Yin Type A and the Yin Type B may be identical, making it challenging but nevertheless crucial to determine the body type differences between them. The Sasang practitioner usually refers to a combination of body shape, tongue and pulse diagnosis, and/or a clinical questionnaire to determine body type. Treating the weakened spleen of the Yin Type B with the Yin Type A's liver-supporting herbs can be compared to arresting an innocent bystander while the villain gets away with murder. The Sasang approach allows us to fine-tune our strategy in overcoming illness by yanking it out by the root, rather than simply cutting off the branches.

HOW TO USE THIS PART

This part includes ten common conditions frequently encountered in the clinical setting.

Stress	Digestive Issues
High Blood Pressure	Weight Loss/Gain
Headaches	Joint Pain
Common Cold	Allergies
Lack of Sleep	Vision Problems

Each subsection offers both general and body type–specific tips on how to improve your health. Remedies for each body type are also provided with preparation instructions. Some will need to be ordered from online sources, since they are not readily available at the supermarket or health food store. In such cases I include the brand name and website, when available. If a website is not listed, the herbal product can still be found by conducting a quick Internet search. I've included this information not to promote the business of these manufacturers but to provide you with the most direct and easily accessible sources.

Several of the herbs specified in this part can also be purchased in seed form. For those who are interested in gardening, this method allows you to develop an intimate relationship with each herb as you watch it grow. Make sure that the plant is properly identified before purchasing it. I recommend that you engage in thorough research via literature or the Internet to familiarize yourself with each plant. Take a close look at the leaf configuration to make sure that it has the same design and structure as the herb you are looking for. Also, confirm with the nursery about the family, species, and edibility of each plant. Some plants may be of the same species but not the same family. Be careful! Just because a plant is the same species does not mean it is in the same family. Some plants of the same species may be poisonous and cause health problems. As long as you take these precautions, a powerful herbal experience awaits!

Each of the remedies provided in the following sections may have other properties beyond the ailment they are listed under. Be sure to check out the subsection titled "Common Uses" for each herb. You may also consult the index to look up each symptom by name and body type. When choosing this method, make sure to avoid herbs that do not match your body type. Familiarize yourself with each herb and its associate body type by reading through the whole section, rather than hastily choosing it based on your symptom. Sasang medicine places emphasis on the body type–specific energetic function of each herb, rather than its symptomatic function. Some herbs help the energy flow upward to strengthen the upper body; others help it flow downward to bolster the function of the lower body. An herb that is used for headaches may also be used in some cases for neck and shoulder pain, based on its energetic function. Once you get to know the energetic function of each herb, it is easier to apply it properly. Read through the entire section to become familiar with how each herb works according to body type.

The "Herbal Friends" boxes provide lists of herbs that interact nicely together. Herbal friends, also known as "pair herbs" in Eastern medicine, either complement or counteract each other's function. Pair herbs that complement each other mutually enhance their respective properties. Pair herbs that counteract each other moderate unwanted side effects from their partner, making them safer for ingestion. In the Eastern medicine clinic, it is common to have several pair herbs mixed into a single formula. Sasang medical formulas consist of about ten to fifteen different herbs. Each herb within a formula has both unique and combined (paired) functions. While single herbs are helpful for certain conditions, it is often challenging for them to do the whole job on their own. The use of pair herbs in Eastern medicine coincides with its philosophical emphasis on symbiosis and the premise that a sum is even more powerful and effective than the totality of its parts.

If a remedy is recommended for a particular ailment but is not listed under your body type, you should avoid it. Ingesting herbs for body types other than your own could lead to uncomfortable and possibly health-damaging side effects. If you experience indigestion after consuming any of the herbs listed in this section, discontinue the herb immediately. According to Sasang medical theory, herbs that match your body type should be easily digested. If you experience symptoms such as bloating, excess gas, lack of or excessive appetite, and/or bowel movement issues after taking an herb, chances are it does not match your body type.

Finally, make sure to read the "Caution" section provided for each herb to avoid interactions and other side effects. Herbs that do not contain a Caution section are, to the best of my knowledge, relatively safe with no known side effects. However, even if the herb is deemed safe, like any other food or herb, it should not be consumed in excess.

The dosage section offers information regarding appropriate dose ranges. Also, be aware that most extracts and tinctures contain traces of alcohol. If you are sensitive to even small amounts of alcohol, do not ingest an extract or tincture made with alcohol. Luckily, not all extracts contain alcohol. Make sure to read product labels carefully before purchasing any herb, herbal extract, or tincture. Non-alcohol-containing tinctures often have glycerin among their ingredients; these tinctures are included in this section, when they're available.

Most naturopaths and herbal practitioners in the United States may be familiar with the common uses of herbs in this section. Since Sasang medicine has yet to be popularized in the West, few practitioners are familiar with this particular herbal approach, which is often quite different. If you have any specific questions regarding the use of the herbs in this section, visit my website at sasangmedicine.com to contact a Sasang professional. See also the Useful Resources at the end of the book. And now, let the adventure begin. To your health!

Dealing with Stress

Stress is one of the most detrimental conditions of modern society. It can be considered a silent killer that saps our energy and health little by little. Unlike an acute injury, psychological stress does not produce pain; it lingers right below our internal radar. Over 70 percent of those who seek treatment at my clinic suffer from illnesses that can be traced to stress-related factors. Stress itself reduces immune activity by stimulating the excess release of a hormone called adrenaline (aka epinephrine), which helps us cope with emergency situations. It speeds up and stimulates our senses and muscle strength as if we were in a constantly threatening situation. Excess release of adrenaline into the bloodstream eventually leads to extreme adrenal fatigue and chronic pain as our body tightens itself up constantly preparing for battle.

Most of my patients seek to rid themselves of stress entirely. Stress itself is not what causes an imbalance of energy; it is how we respond to stress that determines the extent of the damage it causes. With the right tools we can actually transform stress into positive energy that could help us grow stronger and become wiser. Stress on the body helps our bones grow, while emotional stress helps our minds grow.

Since each body type is affected by stress in its own way, overcoming stress is not a one-size-fits-all process. When attempting to deal with stress, it is important to know your body type's innate stress response. Following are some general tips that may help you cope with stress no matter which body type you are.

General Tip #1: Breathe and Let It Go

The first step to overcoming stress is to stop fighting it! Let whatever stressful situation you encounter pass through without getting stuck in your mind or body. If you feel stressed out, try taking a deep breath. When breathing in imagine that you are sending the air past your heart and deep into your lower body. The heart stores our emotion, and suffers the most from the accumulation of stress. When breathing out imagine that you are exhaling the stress from your body.

General Tip #2: Exercise

Exercise is a wonderful way to relieve stress because it helps the body release endorphins. Endorphins are our "happy" hormones, promoting an elated emotional response. Since the body loves routine, a regular and consistent workout is very helpful in reducing and coping with stress.

General Tip #3: Make Time for Yourself

Yang, in Asian philosophy, corresponds to control, while Yin corresponds to passivity. It is easier for Yang types than Yin types to feel that they are in control of stressful situations. Yin types are inclined to escape from stress while Yang types attempt to face it head-on. While both approaches have their merits, neither should be taken to an extreme. It is crucial not to let stress control your life or feel that you always have to be in control of it. Take time away from a busy schedule to engage in fun things that promote your health and well-being.

General Tip #4: Do Abdominal Breathing

Have you ever watched the tummy of sleeping toddlers as they breathe in and out? You can see it rise and sink with each breath. As we get older and face the stresses of daily life, our breathing gets shallower and shallower. With stress and age, the energy within the body also has a tendency to rebel upward, causing tension in the shoulders, hot flashes, and neck pain. Uprooted energy inside the body can be compared to a tree that is so focused on growing that it forgets to nourish its roots. The hectic pace of modern life causes many of us to become excessively task-oriented. This makes it harder for our roots to stay strong. Deep breathing helps promote the harmonious flow of energy throughout the body by encouraging uprooted energy to flow downward again. According to Eastern medicine, the root of the body's energy resides in the kidneys. Adrenaline is released from the adrenal glands above the kidneys when we are stressed or in danger. Breathing helps nourish the kidneys, thus helping our roots stay strong even in stressful situations.

Try this exercise to maintain harmonious balance and flow.

ABDOMINAL BREATHING EXERCISE

- Start by lying down facing upward.
- Place both hands, palms facing downward, directly below your belly button.
- Push your lower abdomen in and out to feel which muscles you use when you breathe.
- Now start to breathe very slowly while engaging the same muscles, but this time use your breathing to push your abdomen in and out.
- When you breathe in, imagine the air filling your lower abdomen, pushing it upward. Exhale by slowly releasing the pressure in your lower abdomen.

Abdominal breathing is particularly beneficial for Yin Type A's, who are born with weaker lungs. This can keep the lungs stronger, thus helping the other organs function efficiently.

General Tip #5: Take Calcium and Magnesium

In Eastern medicine minerals are said to help calm the mind and ground the spirit, thanks to their "heavy" nature and ability to encourage the downward flow of energy. The energy of the digestive system naturally flows downward, from mouth to anus. However, if we get stressed or sleep-deprived, the energy of the digestive system has a tendency to rebel upward, adding to our woes. Minerals, such as magnesium and calcium, help to reestablish the natural flow of downward energy. Both are necessary to balance and harmonize the body's energy. Magnesium helps the body absorb and utilize calcium, while calcium helps the body absorb magnesium. Sound familiar? This relationship is similar to that of Yin and Yang, which support and balance each other. It is recommended to take up to 350 mg of magnesium and 1,000 mg of calcium per day. You can get 1,000 mg of calcium by consuming 100 grams of raw sesame seeds, 300 mg by drinking a glass of milk, and 350 mg by eating six ounces of yogurt. Other sources of calcium and magnesium are dark leafy greens and beans.

STRESS AND YIN TYPE A

Yin Type A's are born with weaker lungs. In Sasang medicine the lungs correspond to grief and sadness. Therefore, Yin Type A's may have a "Woe is me" reaction to stress and simply feel sorry for themselves. Weaker lungs also cause Yin Type A's to breathe shallowly when they're stressed, so they have to constantly be aware of the need to inhale deeply.

The stronger liver of the Yin Type A leads to a constant desire for relaxation and comfort. When stress gets in the way of comfort, Yin Type A's often seek to escape it entirely or search for a comfortable solution.

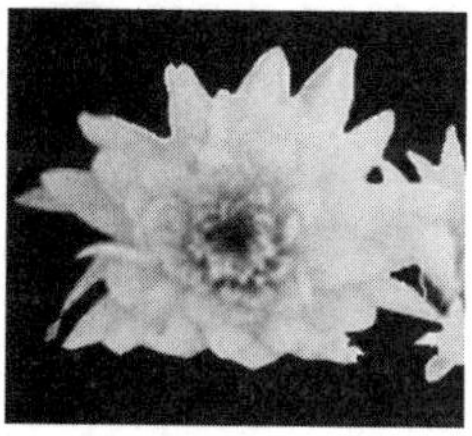

Chamomile (*Matricaria Recutita*)

Since this herb supports the function of the lungs, it is an important herb for Yin Type A's. Chamomile calms the lungs and can therefore be used to help calm them in times of stress. Taken about an hour before bedtime, it can also alleviate insomnia. Chamomile is known to have several other very useful functions. It contains flavonoids and tannins, which help soothe stomach irritability and fight off infections, such as staphylococcus. The energy from an unsettled stomach can easily rebel upward and bombard the heart, which resides directly above the stomach. Since the heart is the seat of emotion, an unsettled stomach often leads to anxiety and stress. Therefore, chamomile's ability to calm the stomach may calm our emotions as well.

Common Uses of Chamomile in Sasang Medicine

For relief of stress, indigestion, insomnia, sinus inflammation, sinus congestion, vision-related ailments (blurry vision, stigmata, cataracts, glaucoma)

Sources of Chamomile

Chamomile in tea bag form is readily available in most supermarkets. It can also be obtained online from manufacturers such as Traditional Medicinals (traditionalmedicinals.com). This company offers a product made from pure organic chamomile alone or combined with lavender. Lavender is also known for promoting relaxation and a good night's sleep.

Preparation and Dosage of Chamomile

In tea bag form, chamomile is a safe herb that can be ingested throughout the day. Serving chamomile tea warm enhances its calming effects and ability to soothe the digestive system.

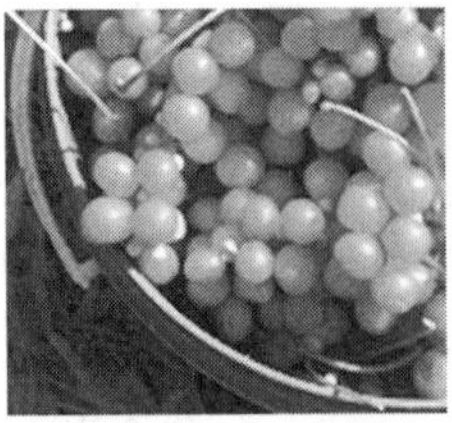

Schizandra Fruit (*Schisandrae Chinenses*)

Schizandra is used often in the Sasang medical clinic. In Korean it is called "five flavors herb" because it is one of the few herbs that have all five flavors. The taste of an herb determines its characteristics. Bitter herbs, for example, support the function of the heart, sweet herbs support the function of the spleen, salty herbs support the function of the kidneys, sour herbs support the function of the liver, and acrid herbs support the function of the lungs. With its five flavors, schizandra supports the function of all the body's organs, but is especially good at nourishing and supporting the function of the heart, lungs, and kidneys. It is an excellent herb to help alleviate the Yin Type A's stress, insomnia, or fatigue.

In the Sasang medical clinic, schizandra is used in combination with up to fifteen herbs in complex formulas geared to the needs of each patient. By itself schizandra can still be beneficial to your overall health.

Common Uses of Schizandra in Sasang Medicine

To alleviate stress, insomnia, palpitations, anxiety, dry skin, dry eyes, dry nasal passages, dry mouth, fatigue

Sources of Schizandra

Schizandra can be found online in capsule, tincture, or extract form. Manufacturers include Nature's Way (naturesway.com), Paradise (paradiseherbs.com), and Nature's Answer (naturesanswer.com). It does not matter which form of schizandra you ingest as long as you follow the manufacturer's dosage guidelines carefully.

Preparation and Dosage of Schizandra

Dried schizandra fruit: Boil ½ ounce of Shizandra with 2 cups of water. Let it simmer on low flame for fifteen to twenty minutes or until the water becomes a light brownish color. One cup of schizandra tea can be taken up to three times a day. If you purchase schizandra extract, capsules, or tincture, be sure to follow the manufacturer's dosage guidelines carefully.

Caution

Schizandra is generally a safe herb, but it should not be ingested if you are prone to getting hot or you are currently running a fever.

STRESS AND YIN TYPE B

Social fear and anxiety are among the greatest sources of stress for Yin Type B's, so it's important for them to challenge their fears and make a sincere effort to meet and share their thoughts with others. This brings out the Yin Type B's ability to love and show compassion for others.

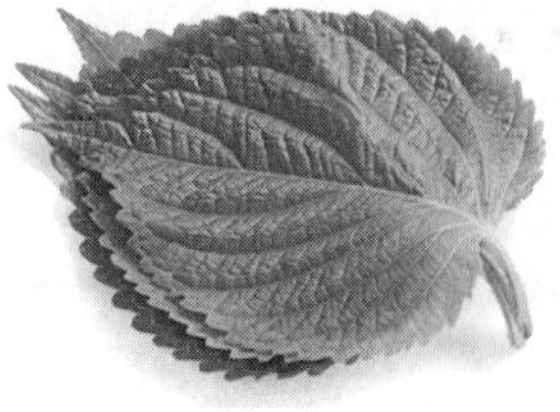

Perilla Leaf (*Folium Perillae Frutescentis*)

This herb is commonly prescribed for Yin Type B's to clear the lungs and sinuses of obstruction and phlegm accumulation. It is related to mint and has similar properties. In Japan and Korea it is commonly used in cuisine to wrap meat, sushi, or vegetables. As a tea it soothes and calms the mind and spirit. Most relatives of the mint family also have a calming effect, reduce phlegm, and alleviate sinus issues. Keep in mind that each herb travels to a different organ, making it beneficial for one body type but not others. Perilla travels to the Yin Type B's weakest organ, the spleen.

Common Uses for Perilla Leaf in Sasang Medicine

To relieve stress, chest and nasal congestion, coughing, indigestion

Sources of Perilla Leaf

For the gardener seeds can be purchased from companies such as Kitazawa Seed Company (kitazawaseed.com). For others without a green thumb, perilla oil supplements can be purchased in capsule form from Source Naturals (iherb.com). Perilla oil is made from the seeds of the perilla plant. The seeds and the leaves have similar healing properties. However, the seeds are slightly better at relieving nasal and chest congestion, while the leaves are slightly better at relieving stress.

Preparation and Dosage of Perilla Leaf

If raw leaves are used, boil three to five leaves per two cups of water, then simmer on the lowest flame for fifteen minutes. If you're consuming the extract, follow the dosage guidelines provided by the manufacturer.

STRESS AND YANG TYPES A AND B

Yang types rarely "feel" their stress because they are so focused on getting things done that stress often goes unnoticed! It is very difficult for Yang types to slow down, even though it is key to preserving their health. Although Yang types may not be aware of stress, they often experience it and it can sometimes take a serious toll on their health. If left untreated, chronic stress among Yang Type A's may cause injury to the kidneys, their weakest organ. In the case of Yang Type B's, stress may injure the liver, their weakest organ.

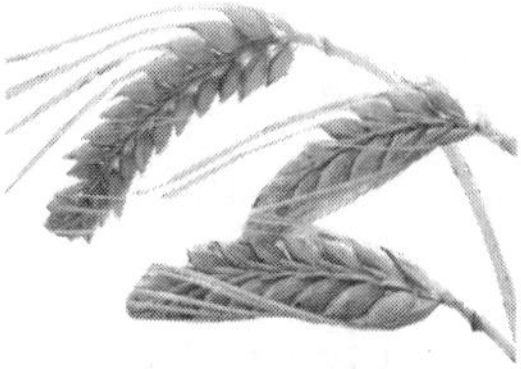

Roasted Barley Tea (*Hordeum vulgare*)

Roasted barley tea is a popular beverage in Japan and Korea, where it can even be purchased from vending machines! In wintertime roasted barley tea is consumed warm. In the summer it is boiled, refrigerated, and then drunk cold. Barley itself has a very cold nature. In Eastern theory Yang corresponds to heat while Yin corresponds to cold. Roasted barley tea effectively cools the excessive heat of Yang types, which is often brought on by stress. Recent studies have shown that roasted barley tea may also have oral antibacterial effects, thus inhibiting tooth decay!*

Common Uses of Roasted Barley Tea in Sasang Medicine

For relief of stress, chronic fever, stomach inflammation, anxiety, overheating, hot flashes, diabetes

*For example, see Papetti, Adele, Carla Pruzzo, Maria Daglia, Pietro Grisoli, Alessandro Bacciaglia, Barbara Repetto, Cesare Dacarro, and Gabriella Gazzani, "Effect of Barley Coffee on the Adhesive Properties of Oral Streptococci" *Journal of Agricultral and Food Chemistry* 55, no. 2 (2007): 278–84.

Sources of Roasted Barley Tea

Roasted barley tea can be purchased on the Internet. The Japanese brands House and Marubishi sell barley tea on amazon.com. The Korean company Dongsuh also offers barley tea on the same website. The Japanese name for roasted barley tea is *mugi-cha* and the Korean name is *bori-cha.*

Preparation and Dosage of Roasted Barley Tea

Roasted barley tea usually comes in small cheesecloth bags. The bags are boiled in water but the tea itself is served cold, thus enhancing the cooling characteristics of barley. In both Korea and Japan, barley tea is often mixed with water and consumed throughout the day.

Caution

The cold nature of roasted barley tea may lead to diarrhea among Yin types. If you develop diarrhea after drinking barley tea, you may be a Yin type. In this case stop ingesting barley tea and retake the body type test or contact our Sasang medicine team through our website at sasangmedicine.com for further guidance.

Did You Know?

A company called Bob's Red Mill (bobsredmill.com) produces barley flour that can be used as a baking ingredient or as a thickener for soups and sauces. While this form of barley is not as cooling as chilled barley tea, it is still worth a try.

Reducing High Blood Pressure

Like stress, high blood pressure may also be considered a silent killer because symptoms are either slow to manifest or not apparent at all. Even though some of us are genetically prone to high blood pressure, this condition does not automatically affect us. The onset of high blood pressure is, in most cases, due to factors like emotional stress, unhealthy eating, and overwork. Therefore, cultivating our emotional and physical well-being is an essential component in the prevention and reduction of high blood pressure.

High blood pressure affects each body type differently, since we each have different stronger and weaker organs. When the body and/or mind are under stress, pressure tends to build up around the strongest organ, blocking the flow of energy to the weaker organs. A buildup of pressure around the stronger organ also interferes with the circulation of energy and blood throughout the entire body. A blockage of blood and energy often leads to a buildup of cholesterol in the arteries.

The discovery of your stronger and weaker organ is the first step toward balancing high blood pressure. Only after taking this step can you proceed to enhancing the flow of blood and energy throughout your body. This section will serve as a map to help guide your energies in the right direction.

The following general tips can be implemented by all body types in order to help prevent and treat high blood pressure.

General Tip #1: Monitor Your Pressure Frequently

A blood pressure monitor could be your best ally when it comes to fighting high blood pressure. Monitor your pressure at set times throughout the day in order to get an idea of how your blood pressure ebbs and flows according to the time of day and your mood. The first blood pressure reading should be done as soon as you get up in the morning, the second should be taken after lunch, and the third should be done before bedtime. Knowing when your readings are higher and lower offers insights into the cause of high blood pressure. If your blood pressure is high first thing in the morning, sleep issues may be the culprit. If it is high after lunch, digestion may be an issue. If it is high right before bedtime, the accumulation of stress throughout the day may be the cause.

General Tip #2: Adjust Your Habits around High Pressure Times

We get so used to the stresses of daily life that it becomes difficult to know when our blood pressure rises. This is why General Tip #1 is an important step in dealing with the blood pressure issue. The next step is to take action once you figure out when your blood pressure has a tendency to be on the rise, which can be done by addressing sleep, digestion, or the accumulation of stress (refer also to "Getting Better Sleep" pages 298–306 and "Maintaining a Healthy Digestive System" pages 307–24).

General Tip #3: Breathe!

The stresses of daily life often cause us to breathe shallowly. As time goes by, shallow breath contributes to slowly increasing blood pressure levels. Take the time to reflect on your breathing. If you find yourself taking short gasps of air, then make a conscious effort to breathe deeply. Our breath can be used as a tool for staying in balance at any time. It is the very first thing that we do when we're born, and the very last thing we do before we die. The breath is an essential part of staying alive.

If we breathe efficiently, breathing can enhance our overall health and prolong our life.

General Tip #4: Do Not Ignore the Signs and Symptoms of High Blood Pressure

If you have chronic headaches, nausea, dizziness, palpitations, and/or vision-related issues, it is time to get your blood pressure checked. If these symptoms are minor, then try purchasing a blood pressure monitor and check your pressure daily for a few weeks to discern patterns and trends. If these symptoms are acute, see a doctor.

General Tip #5: Control Your Weight

Excessive weight gain is one of the leading factors underlying high blood pressure (see "Shedding Those Extra Pounds," pages 325–45, for tips on losing weight).

General Tip #6: Avoid Extremes

For some people blood pressure has a tendency to jump up and down throughout the day. A difference of up to ten points of systolic or diastolic pressure is usually not alarming, unless your blood pressure is significantly high to begin with. Fluctuating blood pressure of more than ten points at a time, on the other hand, can lead to serious strain on the heart. In such cases consult with your doctor, even if you are already taking blood pressure medication.

General Tip #7: Consult Your Doctor

If you are currently taking blood pressure medication, consult your doctor before supplementing with herbs.

HIGH BLOOD PRESSURE AND YIN TYPE A

Yang refers to active energy while Yin is a reflection of sluggishness. Thus, the energy and blood of Yang types tends to flow more quickly and more efficiently than that of Yin types. Among the four body types, Yin Type A's are most prone to getting high blood pressure due to a sluggish circulatory system, which also contributes to a higher rate of cardiovascular and stroke-related issues. There are also more cases of genetically related blood pressure issues among Yin Type A's than among the other types.

Why are Yin Type A's so prone to high blood pressure? The Yin Type A's strongest organ, the liver, is in charge of absorbing and eliminating toxins from the body. Its ability to absorb is naturally stronger than its ability to eliminate toxins. Yin Type A's therefore succumb to excess absorption of toxins in the body, contributing to the accumulation of pressure. It can really get stuffy in there!

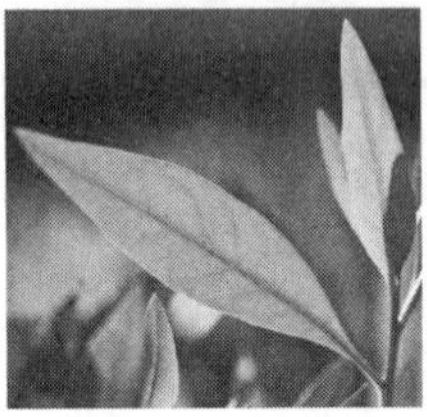

Green Tea (*Camellia Sinensis*)

In the West green tea is highly touted for being rich in antioxidants, which are said to scavenge and destroy those nasty free radicals. According to Eastern medicine, green tea helps circulate the energy of the liver to detoxify and clean the body. As we have mentioned before, the Yin Type A's have a tendency to develop congestion in the liver, so it is important to keep their liver functioning smoothly. Drinking two to three cups of green tea daily may help reduce or prevent high blood pressure.

Common Uses of Green Tea in Sasang Medicine

To assist with high blood pressure, circulatory issues (cold extremities, numbness of the extremities, weight gain), indigestion

Sources of Green Tea

Green tea is readily available in supermarkets throughout the United States. The quality of green tea varies tremendously. In China the price difference for one pound of green tea varies from about $3 to $300. The higher price does not necessarily signal a better-quality product. Manufacturers such as Yamamoto Yama, Yogi, and Bigelow offer relatively good-quality green tea that is readily obtainable and affordable. Organic varieties are also available. Green tea is the mature leaf of the camellia sinsensis plant. Matcha, another type of green tea, is made from immature leaves of the same plant. It is significantly more expensive than other green tea, but much more effective in promoting circulation.

Preparation and Dosage of Green Tea

Steep a single tea bag in a cup of hot water. Wait about three minutes before consuming the tea so that it soaks thoroughly into water. Drink up to three cups of warm tea daily. Green tea is best if ingested after meals to aid in digestion.

Caution

Green tea contains about one-third to one-half the amount of caffeine as coffee. Although the amount of caffeine is significantly less in comparison, it may still interfere with sleep if it's ingested close to bedtime. While green tea promotes circulation, the caffeine content may aggravate high blood pressure in some people. If you already have high blood pressure, monitor it consistently for the first few weeks while starting a green tea regimen. You might also try decaffeinated green tea.

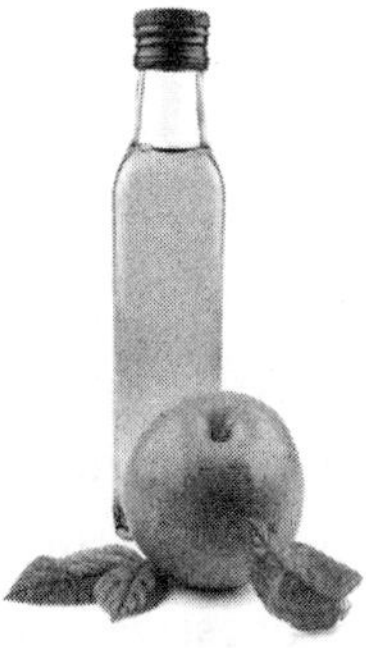

Apple Cider Vinegar

In Eastern medicine vinegar is often mixed with other herbs to promote blood flow. When treating the Yin Type A's joint pain, vinegar is often mixed with turmeric. Both the turmeric and the vinegar enhance each other's effectiveness when treating joint pain. Vinegar can also be consumed with water to help prevent and reduce high blood pressure. There are more than twenty different types of vinegar, each derived from different sources. Vinegars produced from cider have a higher acetic acid content, which is said to have cholesterol- and blood sugar–reducing effects.

Common Uses of Apple Cider Vinegar in Sasang Medicine

To alleviate high blood pressure, circulatory issues (cold extremities, numbness of the extremities, weight gain), indigestion

Sources of Apple Cider Vinegar

Naturally fermented apple cider vinegar is available at most supermarkets.

Preparation and Dosage of Apple Cider Vinegar

Add two tablespoons of apple cider vinegar to one cup of water. Stir well and drink it up. Take two doses a day for optimum efficiency. A teaspoon of honey can be added to moderate the sour flavor of the apple cider vinegar.

Caution

Apple cider vinegar is very acidic, aromatic, and potent. This is how it helps get energy flowing better throughout the body. However, this property may cause burning of the tongue and throat in some individuals. Make sure to dilute vinegar with a substantial amount of water when starting an apple cider vinegar regimen. The ratio under Preparation and Dosage should be adjusted appropriately to avoid a burning sensation.

HIGH BLOOD PRESSURE AND YIN TYPE B

The weaker digestive system of Yin Type B's may be the culprit in numerous seemingly unrelated health issues. High blood pressure, for instance, is due to stagnation of the Yin Type B's digestive system. The accumulation of inefficiently digested food eventually puts pressure on the heart and blood vessels. To treat the Yin Type B's blood pressure–related issues, it is necessary to address the digestive system.

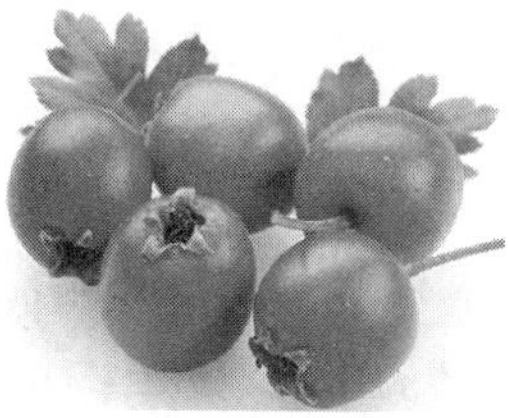

Hawthorn Berry (*Crataegi Fructus*)

The color of an herb tells a lot about its function in Eastern medicine. Each organ of the body has its own energetic color. The heart, for example, corresponds to the color red. The bright red color of the hawthorn berry therefore signifies its association with the heart. Once ingested hawthorn berry immediately travels to the heart to support its function. Both modern science and traditional Eastern medicine value the use of the hawthorn berry for disorders such as high blood pressure and cardiac arrhythmia. Hawthorn berry also supports the digestive system of Yin Type B's, and it is particularly helpful in cases of indigestion from excessive meat intake.

Common Uses of Hawthorn Berry in Sasang Medicine

To alleviate high blood pressure, circulatory issues (cold extremities, numbness of the extremities, fat accumulation), indigestion, anxiety, stress, nervousness, insomnia, and vision-related issues

Sources of Hawthorn Berry

Hawthorne berry extract can be purchased from manufacturers such as Nature's Way (naturesway.com), Nature's Answer (naturesanswer.com), and Now Foods (nowfoods.com).

Preparation and Dosage of Hawthorn Berry

Follow the dosage guidelines listed by each manufacturer.

Caution

Hawthorne berry may interfere with the action of other medications, such as digoxin (for heart-related issues) and phenylephrine (used as a decongestant). Be sure to consult a professional before using hawthorn berry if you are taking heart or allergy medication.

HIGH BLOOD PRESSURE AND YANG TYPE A

According to Sasang medicine, high blood pressure results from stagnation and heat accumulation, which have a tendency to affect the strongest organs of the body. The stomach and spleen, which are the strongest organs of the Yang Type A, play a significant role in digesting and metabolizing foods. The overactive digestive system of Yang Type A's can easily overheat, causing the stomach energy to rise upward, bombarding the heart. Symptoms such as high blood pressure and anxiety result when the heart is assaulted by energy from the digestive system. The blood pressure of Yang Type A's will usually rise suddenly in response to anger, their predominant temperament.

While the Yin Type B's hypertension is also related to the digestive system, it is a result of digestive weakness, rather than excessive strength. A stronger digestive system does not necessarily mean a healthier one, however. Excessive digestive strength, as seen in the Yang Type A, can be as much of a hindrance as weakness in the digestive tract.

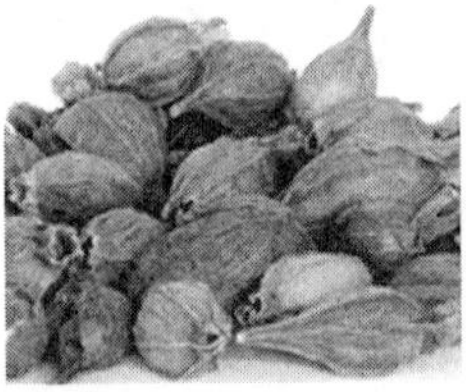

Gardenia (*Gardenia Jasminoides*)

In Eastern medicine gardenia is used to clear heat from every nook and cranny of the body. It is especially effective in clearing heat from the digestive system. Yang Type A's have a tendency to accumulate heat in the stomach, which can easily spread to the rest of the body. Bacterial infection, inflammation, and accumulation of pressure are also correlated with excessive heat in the body. Hence, gardenia is effective in reducing the Yang Type A's high blood pressure, among other heat-related issues.

Common Uses of Gardenia in Sasang Medicine

To alleviate high blood pressure, indigestion, anxiety, stress, nervousness, insomnia, inflammation of the muscles and joints, fever, hot flashes, bladder infections

Sources of Gardenia

Gardenia extract can be found at stakich.com. For the avid gardener, seeds may be purchased from Tropical Oasis on amazon.com. This plant is definitely worth the effort to cultivate for its beauty and fragrance. The fruits (flower bulbs) are collected in the fall and are sun-dried before use as a tea.

Preparation and Dosage of Gardenia

Follow the dosage guidelines listed by each manufacturer. If the raw herb is used, prepare tea by boiling up to six bulbs in two cups of water. Let the tea simmer for fifteen minutes. Drink half a mug of warm tea up to three times a day.

Caution

While gardenia fruit is very effective in reducing blood pressure, it is known to interfere with the effects of antihypertensive medication. Be sure to consult with a professional before ingesting this herb if you are taking antihypertensive medication. Discontinue use in cases of loose stools or loss of appetite. This herb is very cooling and should not be ingested by Yin types, because they have cooler energy in comparison to Yang types.

HIGH BLOOD PRESSURE AND YANG TYPE B

Yang movement is upward while Yin movement is downward. The excessive upward-moving energy of Yang Type B's inhibits the flow of energy and blood downward to the lower body. Their energy has a tendency to accumulate in the upper body, potentially leading to high blood pressure. This accumulation of energy also contributes to prominent upper-body features, such as a thick neck, pointy ears, and a pointy head. It also results in lower-body weakness and clumsiness. Treatment of the Yang Type B's high blood pressure involves rounding up all the excess upper-body energy and encouraging it to flow downward.

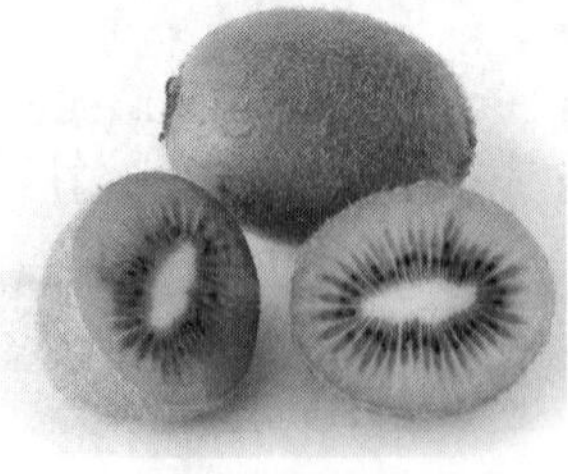

Kiwi Fruit

Because they have so much Yang energy floating around, Yang Type B's must always guard against high blood pressure. Kiwi has a cool nature, which helps to bring energy from the upper body down to the Yang Type B's weaker lower body. Drinking a glass of kiwi fruit juice or eating a kiwi or two is another effective way to reduce the Yang Type B's heat accumulation and hence avoid high blood pressure. Kiwi also clears heat from the digestive system and bladder, promoting the smooth flow of urination.

Kiwi is a unique fruit in many ways. One kiwi has 75 percent of the recommended daily allowance of vitamin C and almost as much potassium as a banana. The skin is filled with antioxidants and the seeds are a significant source of omega-3 fatty acids. Kiwi also significantly reduces platelet aggregation, making it a possible remedy for excessive blood clotting.* Even though kiwi is particularly good for Yang Type B's, like most other fruits, it can be enjoyed in moderation by all the body types.

Common Uses of Kiwi Fruit in Sasang Medicine

To address high blood pressure, circulatory issues (cold extremities, numbness of the extremities, fat accumulation), indigestion, common colds, sinus and lung congestion, painful/scanty urination

Sources of Kiwi Fruit

Kiwi fruit can be found in most supermarkets throughout the United States all year round.

*For more on this, see Duttaroy, Asim K., and Aud Jørgensen, "Effects of Kiwi Fruit Consumption on Platelet Aggregation and Plasma Lipids in Healthy Guman Volunteers" *Platelets* 15, no. 5 (August 2004): 287–92.

Preparation and Dosage of Kiwi Fruit

Eat two kiwi fruits a day to alleviate high blood pressure. One kiwi fruit a day can help to prevent colds and support the digestive process.

Getting Rid of Headaches

The head can be compared to a lighthouse that illuminates the way for blood and energy to navigate through the darkness of our body. The structure and color of the eyes, nose, face, and tongue help the Eastern medical practitioner to understand what is going on in other parts of the body.

In Sasang medicine headaches are a reflection of energy blockage somewhere in the body. Since each body type is equally prone to energy blockage, they are also equally prone to getting headaches. Have you ever wondered why headache medication works for some but not for others? On the surface headache symptoms may seem identical, despite our body type. However, each type has its own areas where energy tends to get blocked, making it necessary to address headaches according to body type, not just symptoms.

The location of a headache also offers insight to its source. A frontal headache, for instance, usually indicates digestive upset. One-sided headaches are usually a result of stress and fatigue, which affect the energy of the liver. Occipital headaches, felt in the back of the head, may simply be a result of tension in the shoulders. They may also be a sign of eye or bladder strain. Some people may experience this type of headache after lower-back issues, since tension and pain have a tendency to work their way up the spine. Still others may experience headaches as a result of serious trauma or illness. If you have recently suffered a significant head injury, it is important to consult a medical professional. Moreover, if headaches are chronic, despite your decision to try herbs or other natural remedies, then it may also be advisable to consult a professional.

General Tip #1: Breathe Away Those Headaches

Deep breathing can help improve almost any health condition by restoring the balance and harmony of bodily energy. When breathing in imagine the air going past the lungs and flowing deep within the abdomen. This will help the excessive energy flowing around the head to slide downward, restoring a natural flow. When breathing out imagine ridding yourself of all tension and discomfort.

General Tip #2: Check Your Pillow Height

A pillow that is too low or too high may be the cause of chronic headaches. Is it time to change your pillow? The average pillow may last as little as one month before it starts to lose its fluff. Before buying a new pillow, experiment with different heights by folding towels, one by one, underneath the one you already have. It is often a challenge to figure out what pillow height works best for you. If you are battling with the pillow-height scenario, start with a single folded towel and work your way upward to see which height works best. Side-sleepers may try folding a washcloth under each side of their pillow to increase height and avoid tilting their head to the side when sleeping.

General Tip #3: Inspect Your Mattress

An old mattress may contribute to numerous avoidable health problems. As the years go by, mattresses begin to lose their spring or begin to sink in the areas where they're most used. Have you flipped your mattress within the past few years? As a rule of thumb, it is a good idea to flip your mattress after two years of use. This may help avoid chronic neck, back, and headache problems.

General Tip #4: Stretch It Out

The circulation of blood and energy in the body decreases significantly while we are sleeping, since we hardly move at all. A good stretching routine in bed right before we sleep or first thing in the morning can keep the body limber and prevent muscle and body aches (see pages 219–22 for a few practical and effective stretches).

General Tip #5: Eat Softer, Easier-to-Digest Foods

Eating foods that are easier to digest helps reduce stress on the digestive system. According to Eastern medicine, humans (and all other animals) have twelve major energy channels that flow from each organ to the surface of the body. The stomach energy channel flows from the stomach to the forehead. Thus, if the stomach is in distress, the forehead may start to ache. In many cases frontal headaches can be avoided by eating softer and easier-to-digest foods.

General Tip #6: Check Your Vision

The occipital cortex, located in the back of the head, controls vision and focus. Headaches centered here are often caused by excessive eyestrain. When using the computer or reading a book, try to give your eyes a break every half hour by simply closing your eyes for a few seconds or getting up and walking around a bit. If headaches persist for more than a few days, it is advisable to get your vision checked, purchase reading glasses, or get your current pair adjusted.

HEADACHES AND YIN TYPE A

Headaches suffered by Yin Type A's are due to either sinus congestion from their weaker lungs or energy stagnation around their stronger liver. Sinus congestion will cause excess pressure in the sinus cavity, leading to headaches. Stress, trauma, high blood pressure, eyestrain, and other factors cause congestion of the Yin Type A's liver energy. When in balance the liver energy flows upward and downward smoothly. If it's unbalanced, the congested liver can cause excessive energy to flow rebelliously toward the head, resulting in the accumulation of pressure and pain. If liver energy rebels upward, it can cause other symptoms, such as tinnitus (ringing in the ears), nausea, hot flashes, excessive stomach acid (acid reflux), and/or acne.

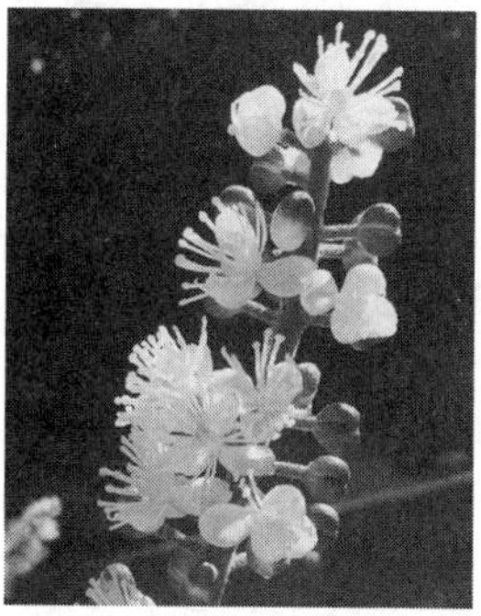

Black Cohosh Tea (*Rhizoma Cimicifugae*)

In Sasang medicine black cohosh is primarily prescribed for its ability to clear heat and congestion from the liver. It is thus used to treat headaches and other signs of liver congestion from heat, such as tinnitus, nausea, hot flashes, excess stomach acid, acne, and fever. This herb could help prevent these symptoms as well as alleviate them and is especially beneficial for Yin Type A's, born with a stronger and easily congested liver. Black cohosh is also used to treat sore throat and sinus congestion, making it suitable for use whether headaches are due to lung weakness and/or liver stagnation.

Common Uses of Black Cohosh in Sasang Medicine

For relief of headaches, throat issues (sore or swollen throat, tonsillitis, swollen glands), coughing, hot flashes, stomach acid, acne, tinnitus, nausea, sinus congestion (with other heat signs, such as fever, sore throat, hot flashes, etc.)

Sources of Black Cohosh

Black cohosh is readily available because of its common use for hot flashes and postmenopausal symptoms, and is carried by Nature's Way (naturesway.com) and Planetary Herbals (planetaryherbals.com).

Caution

Black cohosh is a cold-natured herb. If you cannot drink cold fluids without getting a stomachache, having diarrhea, indigestion, or sneezing, then black cohosh may not be suitable for you. These symptoms will occur after ingesting black cohosh if there is not enough heat in the body. Very high doses of black cohosh may cause a slower heart rate, lower abdominal cramps, dizziness, tremors, or joint pain. Women who are pregnant should consult a professional before ingesting this herb.

Herbal Friends

For a stronger effect in reducing headaches or other heat-related issues of Yin Type A's, take equal amounts of black cohosh extract with kudzu root extract (see kudzu root on pages 313–15 for more information).

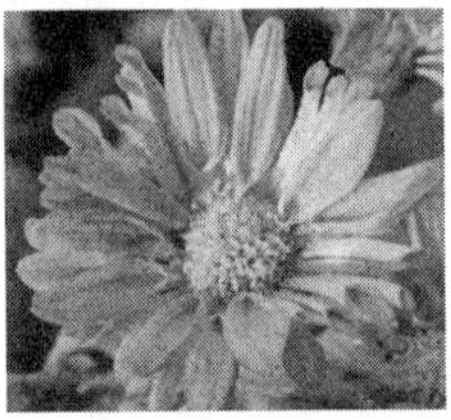

Chrysanthemum Tea (*Flos Chrysanthemi Morifolii*)

Occipital headaches are often caused by excess neck tension and/or eyestrain. Chrysanthemum is very useful for eyestrain or chronic muscle inflammation, common among Yin Type A's. The lightweight character of floral remedies makes them beneficial for the upper body. Since we are all part of Mother Nature, it is common for us to treat illness using herbs that have human characteristics. Chrysanthemum was traditionally thought to look like a glistening, wide-open human eye; hence it has been used for thousands of years to treat vision-related problems. Chrysanthemum is also used to treat and prevent sinus headaches.

Common Uses of Chrysanthemum Tea in Sasang Medicine

To treat headaches (occipital and sinus), vision disorders (blurry vision, cataracts, glaucoma, focal issues, itchy eyes, floaters, failing vision)

Sources of Chrysanthemum Tea

Chrysanthemum tea can be purchased from manufacturers such as Mighty Leaf (mightyleaf.com) and Tea Spring (teaspring.com).

Preparation and Dosage of Chrysanthemum Tea

Steep three to five flowers in one cup of hot water. Let the tea sit for four minutes until the water turns light yellow. Drink warm. The leaves may also be chewed after finishing the tea to enhance its effect. Up to four cups a day may be consumed.

Caution

Studies have showed that chrysanthemum is a relatively safe herb when ingested orally. However, if you are taking this herb within the recommended dose range and experience indigestion or allergy-related symptoms (such as sinus inflammation, rash, or runny nose), you may be allergic to chrysanthemum or it might not correspond with your body type.

HEADACHES AND YIN TYPE B

Yin corresponds to cold, while Yang is associated with heat. With so much Yin, Yin Type B's often succumb to cold-related issues. Coldness has a tendency to impede circulation and contract the blood vessels, leading to headaches and other circulatory issues. Cold may also interfere with the digestive system of Yin Type B's and/or contribute to frequent colds. Excess cold Yin within the body will also chase heat Yang away, causing it to escape upward and produce headaches. No matter how cold Yin Type B's may feel, their head will often feel warm or hot to the touch.

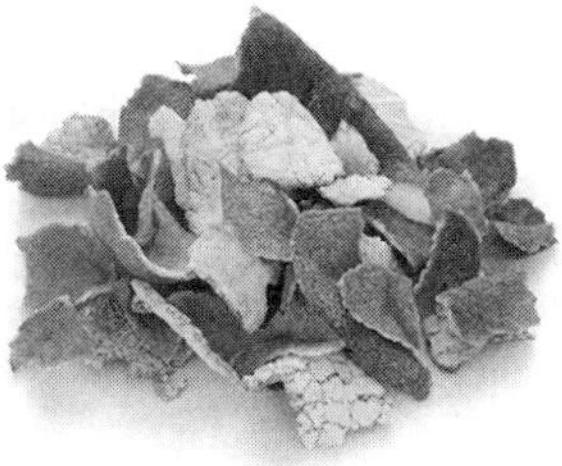

Tangerine Peel (*Citrus Reticulate*)

A weakened digestive system may be the source of the Yin Type B's frontal headache, which can occur anywhere along the face or forehead. With indigestion the Yin Type B's stomach energy will rebel upward, making its way to the forehead and causing excessive pressure. Stomach energy naturally flows downward, but, in distress, its energy will flow upward, causing frontal headaches, nausea, hot flashes, and/or acne. Tangerine peel tea is an excellent choice to address these situations because it helps the energy of the digestive system flow smoothly.

Common Uses of Tangerine Peel in Sasang Medicine

Tangerine peel tea is also an effective remedy for sinus congestion and phlegm buildup. This herb could help prevent as well as alleviate indigestion, phlegm, and headaches.

Sources of Tangerine Peel

Tangerine peel in tea bag form may be acquired from TerraVita, located on zooscape.com, and in concentrated powder form at Plum Flower on mayway.com.

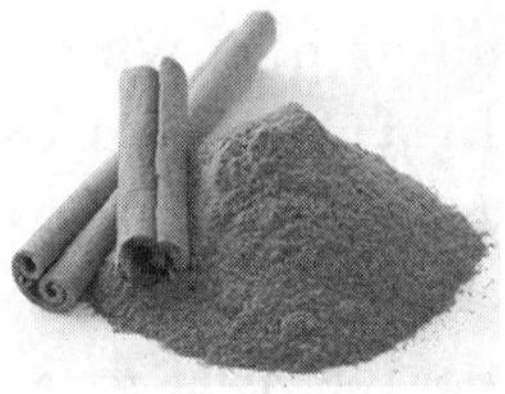

Cinnamon Tea (*Cortex Cinnamomi Cassiae*)

Cinnamon is referred to as *gui pi* in Chinese. *Gui* means "to restore." The spleen and stomach are in charge of digestion and transforming food into energy. This warm-natured herb therefore warms up and restores the energy of the digestive system, the Yin Type B's weakest and coldest area. It also helps restore the flow of energy downward and away from the head. Cinnamon is often used to prevent and alleviate most types of Yin Type B headaches. Recent studies suggest that cinnamon is also effective in the treatment of type 2 diabetes and yeast infections, the reduction of lymphoma or leukemia cancer cell proliferation, and blood clotting.* It is rich in fiber, calcium, and iron. Now doesn't that sound like a pretty cool (but warm-natured) herb?

*For more on this, see "Natural Home Remedy—Cinnamon," http://naturalhomeremedies.co/cinnamon.html.

Common Uses of Cinnamon Tea in Sasang Medicine

To alleviate headaches, circulatory issues (numbness, tingling, and/or coldness of the extremities), joint and muscle inflammation, lower-back and knee pain, sensitivity to cold

Sources of Cinnamon Tea

Raw cinnamon bark can be purchased from most supermarkets and natural food stores. Suppliers such as Nature's Answer (naturesanswer.com), Solaray (solaray.com), and Gaia (gaiaherbs.com) offer an extract form of cinnamon in capsule form.

Preparation and Dosage of Cinnamon Tea

Raw cinnamon bark is prepared by boiling three (two- to three-inch) bark slices with two cups of water. Let simmer on the lowest flame for fifteen minutes and drink it while it's still warm. The exact amount of cinnamon may vary, depending on your taste preference. For capsules refer to the manufacturer for dosage guidelines.

Herbal Friends

The ginger and cinnamon duet is a match made in heaven. Together, they join hands in alleviating colds and stomachaches and in warming the body and promoting general circulation. Boil three slices of fresh ginger with the above dosage of cinnamon for an extra kick!

HEADACHES AND YANG TYPE A

Much like headaches suffered by Yin Type B's, Yang Type A headaches often originate from an imbalance in the digestive system. However, the Yang Type A's headaches come from an overactive digestive system, while the Yin Type B's headaches come from an underactive, weaker digestive system. The overactive digestive system of the Yang Type A causes stomach heat accumulation that rises upward and bombards the head, leading to frontal headaches due to excess Yang, which often produces a pounding and full sensation. It is certainly possible but less common for Yang Type A's to get headaches in other parts of the head. The Yin Type B's headaches, on the contrary, arise from deficient Yang, which floats upward to escape excessive Yin. This headache is often dull and achy, without the pounding and full sensation that may occur from excess Yang in the Yang types.

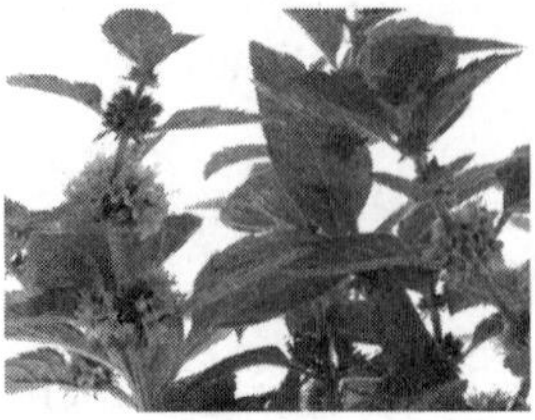

Field Mint (*Mentha Arvensis*)

Field mint soothes and cools the stomach energy of Yang Type A's. It also has a calming effect on the mind, alleviating stress and anger, and promoting sleep. Field mint is also beneficial for any kind of Yang Type A headache. Chilled field mint tea makes for a refreshing drink in the summer or simply when you need to cool down. Mint contains a significant amount of iron and vitamin D. Vitamin D deficiency has been linked with seasonal affective disorder (SAD), a form of depression brought on by a lack of sun exposure. Field mint may also help to pick up your mood on a gloomy day.

Common Uses of Field Mint in Sasang Medicine

For relief of headaches, throat disorders (swollen and sore throat, tonsillitis, swollen glands), stress, anxiety, insomnia

Sources of Field Mint

Mint tea is sold at most supermarkets, but can also be found in tincture and capsule form at health food stores. Keep in mind that most tea bag sources combine mint with ingredients that may or may not agree with your body type. Mint is also available in tincture and capsule form. While mint itself is readily available, field mint, also known as wild mint, is not as easy to find. In our clinic we import field mint directly from China. Field mint grows wild in open fields throughout the United States and Canada. While field mint may have the strongest effect, other types of mint can be substituted.

Preparation and Dosage of Field Mint

Insert a tea bag into a mug of hot water. Let the tea bag steep in the water for two minutes before drinking. If field mint leaves are available, boil 9 grams per two cups of water and let it simmer for fifteen minutes on the lowest flame. Strain out the leaves before drinking. Up to four cups of mint tea can be consumed in a day. Drink chilled for best cooling effect.

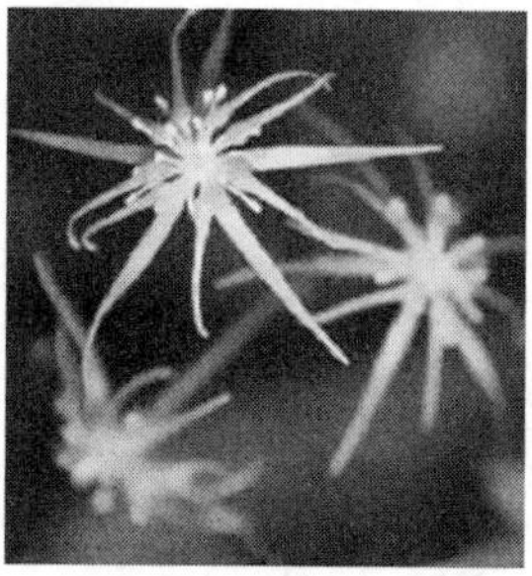

Canker or Coptis Root (*Rhizoma Coptidis*)

Canker (or coptis) root received its name as a traditional mouthwash for treating canker sores. In Eastern medicine canker sores are said to be a result of excess heat from the stomach that rebels upward, causing inflammation of the gums. Coptis root is a rich source of berberine, which has a strong anti-inflammatory effect. This property is so strong that both Eastern and Western herbalists have traditionally used it for exactly the same reason. Modern science has discovered several other benefits of berberine, including its efficacy in treating diabetes and certain cardiovascular conditions.

Common Uses of Canker or Coptis Root in Sasang Medicine

For relief of headaches, stomachaches, indigestion, acid reflux, a sensation of fullness in the chest or epigastric area

Sources of Canker or Coptis Root

An extract of coptis can be purchased online from Herb Pharm (herbpharm.com) and Thorne Research (thorne.com).

Preparation and Dosage of Canker or Coptis Root

Follow manufacturer's guidelines.

Caution

Canker or coptis root is very bitter and cold-natured, making it difficult to digest for most Yin type individuals. I recommend consuming it together with mint to dilute the bitter taste. This herb is contraindicated during pregnancy.

HEADACHES AND YANG TYPE B

Yang Type B's have the most Yang energy of all the body types. In general Yang energy moves upward, while Yin energy moves downward. Therefore, the Yang of the Yang Type B is always on the verge of explosion. The upward movement of Yang can be so extreme that Yang Type B's may lose consciousness and fall to the ground when exerting themselves. In less severe cases, Yang Type B's may develop chronically debilitating headaches.

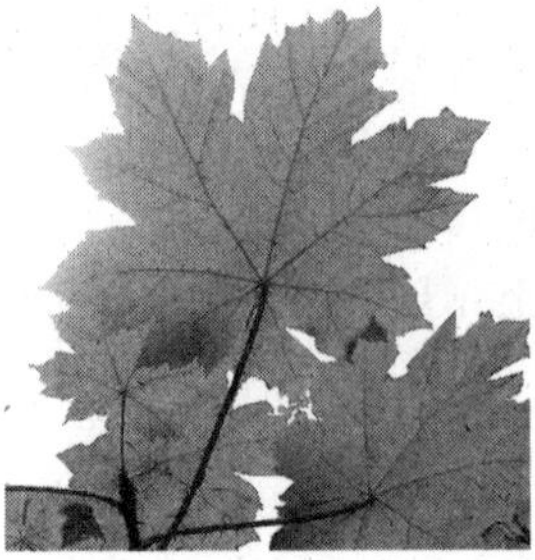

Devil's Club (*Oplopanax horridus*)

One of the most spectacular sights when hiking the mountains of the Pacific Northwest is the majestic devil's club. Its humongous leaves kneel down and pay tribute to a stem filled with bright white flowers bursting out from the center, indicating its profound medicinal power. Devil's club gets its name from the prickly appearance of its thorny stem, resembling a devil's club. For thousands of years, the local Native American population made use of devil's club for its healing properties. As a plant native to East Asia, it also plays a major role in Sasang medicine: it grounds the excessive Yang of the Yang Type B. Like its cousin, ginseng, it has the ability to support and strengthen the immune system and has been traditionally used to combat pneumonia, tuberculosis, tumor growth, and diabetes.

Common Uses of Devil's Club in Sasang Medicine

To address immunodeficiency (common colds and allergies), headaches, paralysis or weakness of the lower extremities, soreness/numbness of the muscles, cramps and spasms of the legs

Sources of Devil's Club

Devil's club is available from manufacturers such as Herb Pharm (herb-pharm.com) and Alternative Health and Herbs (herbalremedies.com).

Preparation and Dosage of Devil's Club

Follow manufacturer's suggested dosage guidelines.

Caution

The prickly spine of devil's club may cause topical allergies if touched. Devil's club also has the potential to lower blood sugar levels and should be used with caution while consuming medications for diabetes. Devil's club is not recommended for use during pregnancy or breast-feeding.

Overcoming Common Colds

As the name implies, common colds are commonly experienced by all body types. The occasional cold is actually a means by which our body cleanses itself and forces us to slow down (if we listen to it). Common colds can also give the body's immune system a good workout, making it stronger in the long run. However, frequent and long-term colds signify that the body's immune system has been compromised and is in need of support.

The occurrence of a cold is a sign that the body is actively fighting off an intruder, and is usually marked by sneezing, runny nose, shivering, headaches, and/or body aches. While this is perhaps the most miserable state of a cold, it is a sign that the body's defense system is still intact. If these symptoms disappear and you are feeling stronger, then you are on the road to recovery. If you are still exhausted, coughing up a storm, running a fever, constipated, or have a swollen throat, the cold may actually be getting worse. These symptoms are nevertheless milder than the initial stage of a cold and often trick us into thinking that we are getting better! A skilled Sasang practitioner is well versed in prescribing remedies according to the different stages of a cold.

Following are a few common tips in the treatment and prevention of common colds.

General Tip #1: Jewish Penicillin

Now wait a second, who ever thought that there were Jewish remedies in Sasang medicine?!? Chicken soup (or "Jewish penicillin," as my grandma referred to it) is another remedy that crosses cultural boundaries because it provides warmth and protein to a cold-infested system without causing indigestion. The digestive system is capable of feeding the lungs, giving the lungs the energy to fight off intruders. Hence, the liquid protein contained in chicken soup, can serve as a perfect, easy-to-digest source of fuel. Don't forget to add lots of garlic and scallions to the mixture, which also help fight off common colds.

General Tip #2: Go for Warm and Soft Foods

When the system is under attack, most of its energy travels to the exterior of the body, forming a shield. With so much focus on the exterior, there is little energy left to support the digestive system. Therefore, it is important to ease up on the digestive system by consuming warm (cooked) and soft foods, such as soups or stews. Stay away from heavy and oily foods in order to give your body the chance to focus on the cold and not the digestion of too much oil.

General Tip #3: Spice It Up!

Spices are helpful when it comes to getting over the early stages of a cold. You can add spicy foods, such as rosemary, black pepper, garlic, onions, and ginger, to a pot of soup to get things going in the right direction. In Easrern medicine spicy foods and herbs help disperse and eliminate unwanted toxic energy and ward off oncoming colds.

General Tip #4: Stay Warm

There are several places on the body through which bacteria can get in and cause havoc. Most of these places are located on and around the nape of the neck. It is important to stay inside and rest as much as possible after catching a cold. However, if you need to get out, make sure to place a thick scarf around your neck. For those of you who, like myself, love to break rules, this does not mean going outside with just a scarf and nothing else on!

General Tip #5: Stay Low and Let It Flow

While our body's energy focuses on the exterior to ward off bacteria, it is important for our mind to focus internally and take time out of a busy schedule to heal. A busy and stressful schedule interferes with recovery, confusing the immune system. The production of phlegm, sweat, and other gooey substances is a reflection that the body is trying to cleanse itself of bacteria. Make sure to encourage flow by blowing your nose frequently, expectorating excess phlegm, and drinking plenty of water. Only use anti-expectorants if absolutely necessary because they can further suppress the phlegm inside your lungs.

COMMON COLDS AND YIN TYPE A

The weaker lungs of Yin Type A's may lead to frequent or difficult-to-overcome colds. In fact, chances are that if you have difficulty overcoming or contract frequent colds, you are a Yin Type A. Other body types have stronger lungs and tend to get over colds more quickly, even if it makes them absolutely miserable for a few days. If another body type has difficulty recovering from a cold, it is usually because of overall deteriorating health. In this case the lungs get weaker only after other organs lose their strength. Not all Yin Type A's get frequent colds or have difficulty overcoming them. Even though their lungs may be weaker than the other organs, a healthy Yin Type A can still avoid getting colds. The goal of Sasang medicine is to enhance health by cultivating the strength of our weaker organs. Yin Type A's can keep their lungs strong by eating and exercising according to their body type.

Once they catch a cold, Yin Type A's must take the steps necessary to prevent it from getting worse, since they are more prone than the other body types to getting long-term colds, pneumonia, or bronchitis. The herbs included in this section are intended to help you overcome and prevent an early-stage cold from getting worse. These herbs can also be used even if you feel the slightest hint of an oncoming cold.

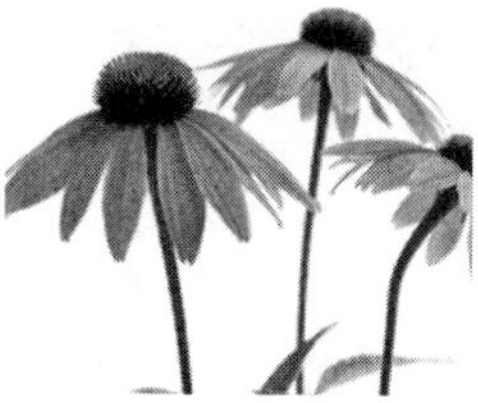

Echinacea Tea
(*Asteraceae*)

Echinacea is an herb that supports the function of the lungs and the immune system. Consuming echinacea in the early stage of a cold may keep it from getting worse. However, echinacea is also known to help, but to a lesser degree, once a cold has progressed into the heat stage (causing sore throat, fever, coughing, and/or sinus infection). In such cases other herbs that clear excess heat (such as black cohosh or kudzu root—further explained on pages 277–78 and 313–15, respectively) are added. If you are a Yin Type A who is experiencing a runny nose, chills, and/or body aches, echinacea may be the herb of choice. One study of ninety-five people with early symptoms of cold and flu found that those who drank several cups of echinacea tea every day for five days recovered sooner than those who did not.* Echinacea contains high concentrations of polysaccharides, which are known to play a role in stimulating the immune system.

Common Uses of Echinacea Tea in Sasang Medicine

To prevent and treat early-stage common colds

Sources of Echinacea Tea

Child Life (childlife.net) offers a sweet orange-flavored echinacea extract for children. Adults can purchase echinacea from manufacturers such as Yogi Tea (Echinacea Immune Support, yogiproducts.com) or Herb Pharm (Super Echinacea, herb-pharm.com).

Preparation and Dosage of Echinacea Tea

Dosages and preparation vary according to the manufacturer and product concentrations. Refer to the manufacturer's recommendations for

*For more on this, see "Echinacea," http://umm.edu/health/medical/altmed/herb/echinacea.

proper dosage. Make sure to take into consideration age-related dosages when giving echinacea to children.

Caution

Echinacea is a relatively safe herb when ingested, although there have been rare cases of nausea, abdominal pain, diarrhea, itchiness, and rash occurrence after intake. If you are taking this herb within the recommended dose range and experiencing any of these symptoms, you may be allergic to echinacea or it may not correspond to your body type.

Herbal Friends

For a stronger effect in preventing and/or addressing the early stages of the Yin Type A's common cold, take three cups of echinacea tea with up to 1,000 mg of vitamin C daily.

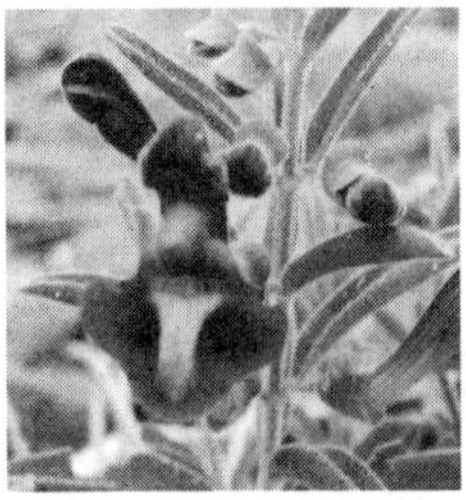

Skullcap Root (*Radix Scutellariae Baicalensis*)

In Sasang medicine skullcap root is used for clearing a variety of heat-related issues from the body. The accumulation of heat within the body can manifest as inflammation, hot flashes, anger, excessive appetite, or infection. Heat is often the result of illness penetrating further into the body after you contract a common cold. In most cases the early stage of a cold is marked by chills and sensitivity to cold. This is a sign that the body is trying to "shut out" a pathogen by contracting the skin pores. The second stage is marked by heat, which manifests as fever, coughing, and/or sore throat. If there is already a significant amount of heat hanging around inside the body before you catch a cold, the first sign of a cold may be indicated by heat-related symptoms—a sign that you have jumped right into the second stage of a cold. Skullcap root is appropriate for use during the second stage of a cold to alleviate heat-related symptoms.

Common Uses of Skullcap Root in Sasang Medicine

To alleviate sinus inflammation, throat soreness and inflammation, hot flashes, fever

Sources of Skullcap Root

Skullcap root extract is available from manufacturers such as New Chapter (newchapter.com) and Nature's Way (naturesway.com).

Preparation and Dosage of Skullcap Root

Follow manufacturer's specific dosage instructions.

Caution

There are over three hundred varieties of skullcap root! Baikal scullcap is the variety used in Eastern medicine, which is in the mint family. It is important not to confuse this herb with North American skullcap (*Scutellaria lateriflora*), which has different characteristics and could contain unhealthy toxins.

Herbal Friends

For a stronger effect in clearing heat from the body and preventing further progression of a common cold for Yin Type A's, take equal dosages of skullcap root together with kudzu root (refer to pages 313–15 for further information about kudzu root).

COMMON COLDS AND YIN TYPE B

Since Yin corresponds to cold, both Yin types are more prone than Yang types to getting common colds. Even though the lungs are not the Yin Type B's weakest organ, the Yin Type B's tendency toward coldness may trigger the onset of a cold. Sufficient heat is needed to support the body's immune system. Without heat the immune system does not have ability to "burn off" a cold. Healthy Yin Type B's are able to keep themselves warm through exercise and eating according to their body type. Unhealthy Yin Type B's are often emaciated and too cold, suffering from aches and pains as a result. Cold also inhibits digestion. Since Yin Type B's are born with a weak digestive system, their common colds are often accompanied by a lack of appetite and indigestion.

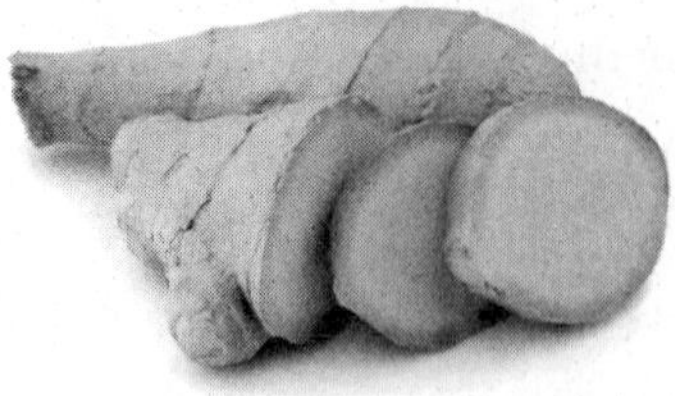

Ginger Tea (*Zingiber officinale*)

Ginger is perhaps the most beneficial medicinal herb for Yin Type B's because it effectively warms and supports the digestive system, their weakest link. Overcoming illness is much easier if Yin Type B's maintain a relatively healthy digestive system. When their digestion goes south, a Pandora's box full of health issues may arise. By promoting healthy digestion, ginger can also help strengthen their immune system; bolster energy and circulation; reduce joint pain, nausea, fatigue, infection, swelling, athlete's foot, and mouth sores; and even refresh the mind! It is a great herb to have around all the time if you are a Yin Type B. Drinking ginger tea up to four times a day helps prevent these ailments and helps keep the body working in harmony.

Common Uses of Fresh Ginger Tea in Sasang Medicine

To alleviate common colds, most types of digestive issues (bloating, gas, lack of appetite, diarrhea, constipation, fullness, nausea), infections, inflammation, joint pain, mouth sores, athlete's foot (applied topically), sadness, anxiety, seasickness, morning sickness, and to promote weight loss

Sources of Fresh Ginger Tea

Fresh gingerroot can be purchased at most supermarkets. It can also be purchased as an extract from olivenation.com or in tablet form at planetaryherbals.com.

Preparation and Dosage of Fresh Ginger Tea

In Eastern medicine fresh ginger is often used for common colds and indigestion because of its highly aromatic properties. These aromatic properties help disperse pathogens and undigested foods. Peel the skin of fresh gingerroot and thinly slice about one inch of the root. Boil two cups of water with five slices of fresh gingerroot and let the tea simmer for ten minutes on the lowest flame. Drink up to five cups a day warm. You can add more water if the ginger tea is too strong. It is also possible to add more ginger if you prefer a stronger taste. Adding honey helps to moderate the strong taste of ginger. Store the remaining gingerroot in the refrigerator to retain freshness.

Caution

If you are not a Yin Type B, this herb could cause irritation and excess acid accumulation in the stomach. If you experience such a reaction, discontinue use and retake the Yin Yang Body Type Test. If you are still not sure of what body type you are, log onto sasangmedicine.com to consult with a professional.

Herbal Friends

For a stronger effect in treating the common cold and indigestion, take one dose of ginger together with one dose of cinnamon (see dosage guidelines on page 281). Other herbs, such as perilla leaf, can also be added to help clear congestion from the lungs and sinuses and promote digestion (see dosage guidelines on page 260).

COMMON COLDS AND YANG TYPE A

Yang corresponds to heat while Yin is associated with cold. The common cold contracted by Yang types is often due to the accumulation of heat. The warmth of the summer generally prevents Yin types from getting colds, but Yang types often get colds in the summer, giving rise to heat-related symptoms, such as fever, rash, throat swelling, excessive sweating, and extreme thirst for cooler fluids. However, Yin types can get colds in the summer, just as the Yang types can get colds in the winter.

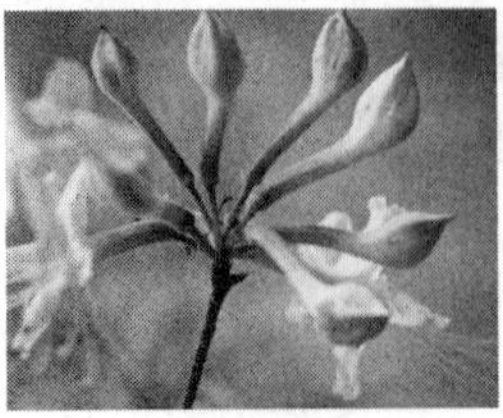

Japanese Honeysuckle (*Lonicera japonica*)

After getting up with a sore throat one morning, I decided to chew on a Japanese honeysuckle flower petal that I happily located in a park near my home. I immediately felt it getting to work on my throat and offering a soothing effect that lasted for hours. The sensation I felt was likely due to the fact that honeysuckle contains chlorogenic acid, which is known to have powerful antibiotic and antioxidant effects. Pharmaceutical antibiotics have a tendency to disturb the natural balance of bacterial flora in the body. However, the antibiotic effects of honeysuckle in its natural form are much gentler on the system because they help restore the natural balance of the body. This herb has an antibiotic effect on a wide range of bacteria, such as staphylococcus aureus, streptococcus B-hemolytic, Escherichia coli, vibrio cholera, salmonella typhi, diplococcus pneumoniae, diplococcus meningitidis, pseudomonas aerurginosa, mycobacterium tuberculosis, and bacillus dysenteriae. Honeysuckle is a helpful remedy for the Yang Type A's common cold accompanied by a sore throat.

Common Uses of Japanese Honeysuckle in Sasang Medicine

To relieve common colds with heat signs (sore throat and/or inflamed throat, fever, sweating), inflammation, pus-related skin disorders, sinus congestion (with heat signs such as fever, sweating, throat inflammation)

Sources of Japanese Honeysuckle

Not only are the flowers of Japanese honeysuckle beautiful, but they also emit a pleasant fragrance. Gardeners can purchase this medicinal plant online from Nature Hills Nursery (naturehills.com). You may also be able to buy this popular shrub at your local nursery. Japanese honeysuckle can also be purchased as a dried herb from Tea Spring (teaspring.com). Forest Rx (frx.com) carries a powdered extract of this herb.

Preparation and Dosage of Japanese Honeysuckle

Raw Herb Preparation: Boil two teaspoons of dried Japanese honeysuckle flowers in two cups of water. Let it simmer on a low flame for fifteen minutes. Drink up to three cups a day warm. For dosage directions regarding Japanese honeysuckle powdered extract, follow manufacturer's instructions.

Caution

Japanese honeysuckle has a very cold nature and is a strong natural antibiotic. It is therefore not recommended for use during pregnancy and when you have no heat-related symptoms. It is also not recommended for Yin types, who often succumb to cold-related issues.

Herbal Friends

Yin qiao jie du pian (in English: Honeysuckle and Forsythia Clear Toxin Formula or Cold Signoff) is a very popular remedy for sore throat and fever due to a common cold; it can be purchased as "Cold Signoff" at activeherb.com. It works quickly to soothe a sore throat and alleviate the symptoms of a cold. Most of the herbs in this formula are Yang Type A–category herbs, with the exception of a few for the Yin Type A and Yin Type B. Since this formula is only to be used short term and it is very effective, I decided to include it here. With the help of forsythia and others, such as burdock root and mint, this formula can offer significant cold relief for Yang Type A's. Yin Type A's with heat-related cold symptoms may also benefit from this formula. Since this formula does not precisely suit either the Yang Type A or the Yin Type A, only short-term use is recommended.

COMMON COLDS AND YANG TYPE B

Yang is quick-moving and forceful while Yin is slow-moving and gentle. The common cold of the Yang types tends to progress quickly, while Yin type colds often hang around in the early stages for a while. Healthy Yang Type B's will overcome a cold before they even realize they've contracted it! If their health is compromised, a cold may work its way deep into the body before they know it. Yang Type B's may even collapse from exhaustion before recognizing that they have a cold. Rather than rush to the finish line, Yang Type B's need to reflect inward and keep on the lookout for potential health-related issues.

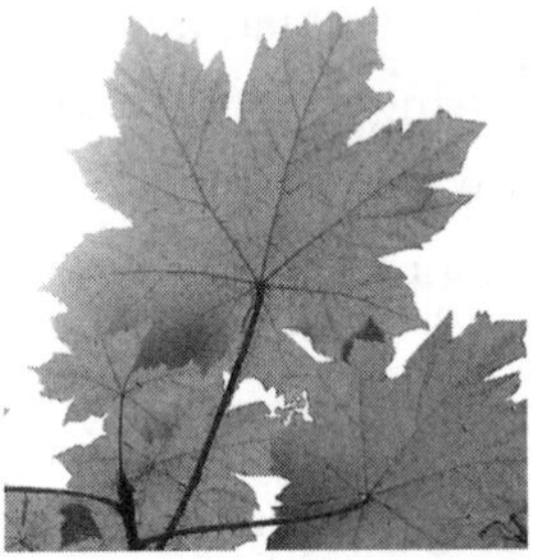

Devil's Club (*Oplopanax horridus*)

The use of devil's club for Yang Type B headaches was mentioned on pages 284–85. This herb is effective in relieving symptoms of the common cold as well. In Sasang medicine devil's club is an important herb for Yang Type B's because it strongly roots the rebellious upward movement of excessive Yang. Once Yang is grounded, the energy and blood can circulate much more efficiently throughout the system. Devil's club is therefore a wonderful match for the Yang Type B's overall health. As a cousin of ginseng, it also has the ability to support and strengthen the lungs and immune system and was traditionally used to fight off pneumonia, tuberculosis, tumor growth, and diabetes.

Common Uses of Devil's Club in Sasang Medicine

To address immunodeficiency (common colds and allergies), headaches, paralysis or weakness of the lower extremities, soreness/numbness of the muscles, cramps and spasms of the legs

Sources of Devil's Club

Devil's club is available in extract from manufacturers such as Herb Pharm (herb-pharm.com) and Alternative Health and Herbs (herbalremedies.com).

Preparation and Dosage of Devil's Club

Follow manufacturer's dosage guidelines.

Caution

See page 285 for devil's club cautions.

Getting Better Sleep

Lack of sleep is an issue that can affect all four body types equally. More often than not, everyday stress is a factor in sleep disturbances, making it difficult for the mind to slow down at night. While most of us would associate too much stress, light, or sound with a lack of sleep, there are several not-so-obvious factors that may also figure in this issue. The energy of an unsettled digestive system, for instance, may rebel upward against the heart, causing anxiety and/or insomnia. Consistent pain or the urge to urinate may also interrupt sleep. Sympathetic dog or cat owners may have trouble sleeping if they give their pets bed privileges. The same goes for having a partner who snores! Aside from getting rid of your partner or pets, there are others ways of addressing this issue. This section provides general tips and body type–specific methods for overcoming insomnia.

General Tip #1: Hit the Sheets before 11:00 p.m.

According to Eastern medicine, the energy of the body shifts from organ to organ every two hours. From 11:00 p.m. to 1:00 a.m., the body's energy is concentrated around the liver, which is responsible for creative thinking and focus. If you are suffering from a lack of sleep, the onset of creative thinking and focus right before going to bed only makes matters worse. Eventually, the body will become fatigued and lethargic during the day. Getting to bed before creative thoughts creep into your mind may contribute to deeper sleep and more energy the following day.

General Tip #2: A Bed Is for Sleeping!

Some of us love to do absolutely everything, aside from sleeping, while in bed. However, the more active you are in bed, the less your body associates the bed with sleep. If you are having trouble sleeping and like to read, jump up and down, have pillow fights, or play hide-and-seek in bed, try reserving these activities for another comfortable place in your home. Reserving your bed simply for rest, and, of course, making love, can often help improve sleep.

General Tip #3: Focus on Your Breath

Counting sheep may work for some people, but others may just keep on counting until they have accounted for every sheep on the planet. Instead, try to focus on the feeling and sound of slowly inhaling and exhaling while you lie in bed. Not only does focusing on your breath help to relax your body, it also assists in clearing your mind of accumulated daily clutter.

General Tip #4: Repeat the "Just Let Go" Mantra

If you can't shut down your mind before bed, this tip is for you. While in bed try repeating the words *Just let go* over and over again. Every time a thought knocks on the door of your consciousness, repeat to yourself, *Just let go*. This can be used in conjunction with General Tip #3.

INSOMNIA AND YIN TYPE A

The inherently weaker lungs of Yin Type A's play a major role when it comes to insomnia. When we are healthy, the lungs help to supply ample amounts of blood and energy to the heart. Weaker lungs may have trouble transferring enough energy to the heart. According to Eastern medicine, our heart is where the emotions are stored. Sleep depends on a sufficient supply of blood and energy reaching the Yin Type A's heart, which in turn helps them relax and feel emotionally balanced. When the lungs are in relatively good shape, they have little difficulty getting us to sleep at night. After dealing with chronic stress, physical and/or emotional trauma, or illness, the lungs may gradually become weaker, initiating the vicious cycle of insomnia. For the same reasons, weaker lungs may also contribute to the onset of heart palpitations, feelings of anxiety, and being easily awakened at night.

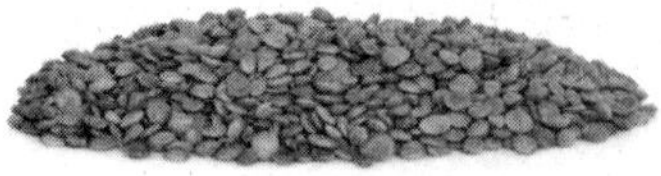

Sour Jujube Seed (*Semen Zizyphi Spinosae*)

Sour jujube seed is commonly used in Eastern medicine to calm and soothe the heart and mind. These little red seeds nourish and support the function of the heart and lungs and are one of the most effective herbs to treat the Yin Type A's insomnia. They are used in a variety of herbal formulas for this reason. Sour jujube seeds contain substantial amounts of flavonoids, alkaloids, and saponins, the combination of which likely contributes to their strong calming effects.

Common Uses of Sour Jujube Seed in Sasang Medicine

For relief of insomnia, anemia, anxiety, nervousness, stress, calming an unsettled fetus, night sweats, thirst, palpitations

Sources of Sour Jujube Seed

Even though sour jujube is readily available in China and Korea, it is difficult to obtain as a raw herb in the United States. It is, however, part of a popular and easy-to-obtain formula that helps with sleep called Suan Zao Ren Tang (Sour Jujube Decoction). This formula can be purchased from Chinese Herbs Direct (chineseherbsdirect.com) and Vita Living (vitaliving.com).

Preparation and Dosage of Sour Jujube Seed

Follow the manufacturer's recommended dosage instructions.

Caution

Consult a professional if you are taking other medications for sleep before trying sour jujube. When combined with other sleep medications, it may cause excessive drowsiness.

INSOMNIA AND YIN TYPE B

By nature Yin Type B's have a tendency toward nervousness and fearfulness, which can easily contribute to a lack of sleep. The Yin Type B's weaker digestive system may stagnate, causing energy to rebel upward and bombard the heart, which can result in anxiety and/or insomnia.

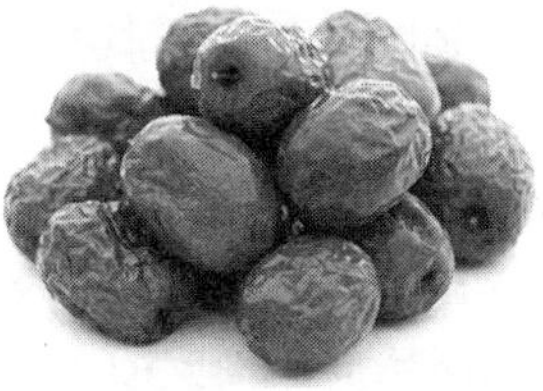

Chinese Jujube (*Fructus Zizyphi Jujubae*)

Chinese jujube, a sweet-tasting fruit often used in Chinese dishes, is said to nourish the heart and blood. In Eastern medicine herbs that support the heart also alleviate insomnia. The true value of Chinese jujube, though, comes from its ability to support the weaker digestive system of the Yin Type B. By balancing the digestive system, Chinese jujube can promote heart function. Chinese jujube is often used in Eastern medicine to balance and harmonize the properties of other herbs in a formula. Recent studies have suggested that Chinese jujube may be able to slow the progression of leukemia and increase the flow of oxygen to the heart.*

Common Uses of Chinese Jujube in Sasang Medicine

To alleviate insomnia, indigestion, anemia, a restless and unsettled fetus, visual impairments (blurry and weak vision, floaters), anxiety, stress, lack of energy

*For example, see Tulika, Mishra, Khullar Madhu, and Bhatia Aruna, "Anticancer Potential of Aqueous Ethanol Seed Extract of Ziziphus mauritiana against Cancer Cell Lines and Ehrlich Ascites Carcinoma" *Evidence-Based Complementary and Alternative Medicine* 2011: http://dx.doi.org/10.1155/2011/765029 (accessed July 22, 2014).

Sources of Chinese Jujube

There are many ways to acquire Chinese jujube. For the gardener purchasing a Chinese jujube tree might be the method of choice. Willis Orchard Company (willisorchards.com) and Ty Ty Nursery (tytyga.com) offer mail-order Chinese jujube trees, which grow rapidly in almost all climate zones throughout the northern United States. These trees are also referred to as *li jujube* trees. Chinese jujube is also available in bulk or in extract form from manufacturers such as Active Herb (activeherb.com) and Chinese Herbs Direct (chineseherbsdirect.com).

Preparation and Dosage of Chinese Jujube

Raw Chinese jujube: Thinly slice three dried fruits and boil in two cups of water. Let simmer for thirty minutes on the lowest flame. If the water level sinks rapidly, add another half a cup and then monitor it. If the water level continues to sink, lower the flame or discontinue boiling. Drink one cup up to four times a day for insomnia. Avoid drinking this directly before bedtime so you aren't awakened for a trip to the bathroom at night.

Caution

Chinese jujube can cause fullness and distention of the digestive system in body types other than the Yin Type B. If you experience these symptoms consistently when ingesting Chinese jujube, stop immediately. It is sometimes very difficult to determine your body type. Try taking the Yin Yang Body Type Test again or log onto sasangmedicine.com to contact a professional.

INSOMNIA AND YANG TYPE A

The overactive nature of the Yang Type A's digestive system can easily lead to insomnia. The digestive energy of healthy Yang Type A's smoothly flows downward to support the kidneys, their weakest organ. However, it does not take much for the digestive system to go into overdrive, causing upward-moving, rebellious energy to bombard the heart.

Stress, illness, anger, or trauma will likely affect the digestive system of Yang Type A's.

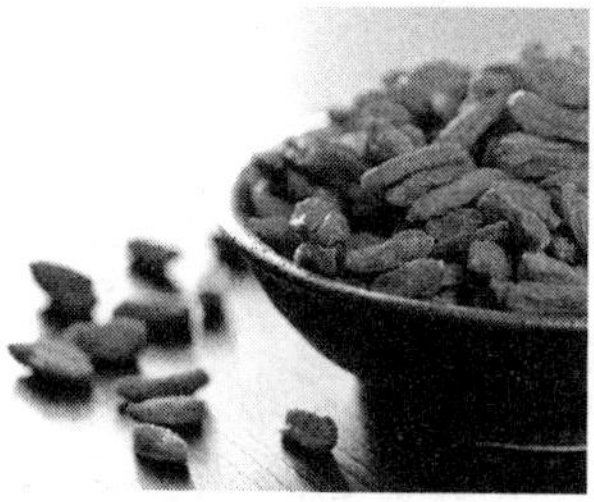

Chinese Wolfberry/Goji Berry (*Lycium Chinenses*)

It seems as if almost every herb mentioned so far in this book has had its own time in the media spotlight of best natural remedies, and wolfberry is no exception. Throughout the web, manufacturers claim it can cure one disease or another. Some even refer to it as a superfruit that cures all ills. There is no doubt that wolfberry plays a significant role in the Eastern medical clinic. However, it is impossible to say that this or that herb is superior to others, since they all contribute in their own way toward balancing and harmonizing the body's energy, depending on our constitution. Wolfberry is nonetheless a very helpful herb for Yang Type A's because it nourishes and strengthens the kidneys, their weakest organ. In Sasang medicine the kidneys help ground the energy of the body, thus preventing the rebellion of the Yang Type A's energy upward. Upward rebellion of energy may lead to insomnia, poor vision, headaches, and chronic sinus issues. Herbs that support the kidneys also strengthen the bones. Wolfberry can therefore also be used for bone-related issues in Yang Type A's. Several recent studies have reported positive effects of wolfberry in the treatment of macular degeneration, cancer, cardiovascular, and inflammatory diseases.*

*For example, see Bucheli, Peter, Karine Vidal, Lisong Shen, Zhencheng Gu, Charlie Zhang, Larry E. Miller, Junkuan Wang, "Goji Berry Effects on Macular Characteristics and Plasma Antioxidant Levels" *Optometry and Vision Sciences* 88, no. 2 (2011): 257–62; Luo, Qiong, Zhuoneng Li, Jun Yan, Fan Zhu, Ruo-Jun Xu, and Yi-Zhong Cai, "*Lycium barbarum* Polysaccharides Induce Apoptosis in Human Prostate Cancer Cells and Inhibits Prostate Cancer Growth in Xenograft Mouse Model of Human Prostate Cancer" *Journal of Medicinal Food* 12, no. 4 (2009): 695–703; and "Side Effects and Benefits of Wolfberry (Juice)" www.zhion.com/herb/Wolfberry_goji_berry.html (accessed June 22, 2014).

Common Uses of Wolfberry in Sasang Medicine

For treating insomnia, vision disorders (blurry vision, weak vision), fatigue, anxiety, osteoporosis/osteopenia

Sources of Wolfberry

Wolfberry (goji), also called Himalayan goji, is currently available in just about any health food store in powder or capsule form. You can purchase wolfberry in its original form online from manufacturers such as nuts.com and navitasnaturals.com. Wolfberry juice is available from healingnoni.com and dynamichealth.com.

Preparation and Dosage of Wolfberry

Raw wolfberry is another fine example of the culinary use of herbs. It can be sprinkled on salads or mixed with nuts, granola, or yogurt. In China it is often stirred into soup to add a slightly sweetened flavor. Herbs that are also enjoyed as foods are safe for ingestion in higher dosages.

Caution

Diabetics should monitor their blood sugar levels carefully when ingesting wolfberry, since it is a fruit and contains sugar. Wolfberry may reduce the effects of Warfarin and other blood thinners, so if you are taking a blood thinner, consult a medical professional before adding wolfberry to your diet.

Yang Type A's should not consume wolfberry if they are experiencing heat-related symptoms, such as fever, sensitivity to heat, excessive appetite, or pounding (as opposed to dull) headaches, because this herb is slightly warm-natured.

INSOMNIA AND YANG TYPE B

The mind of Yang Type B's is constantly on the go, making sleep a common issue for them. For Yin Type A's, the inability to get to sleep is a sign of weak lungs. However, the opposite is true for Yang Type B's, who often have way too much energy circulating around the lungs and heart. While having so much upper-body energy may sound like a good thing, it actually leads to congestion and blockage. The body relies on a smooth flow of lung and heart energy to sink into a deep sleep. Utter exhaustion through overactivity is sometimes the only way that Yang Type B's get to sleep.

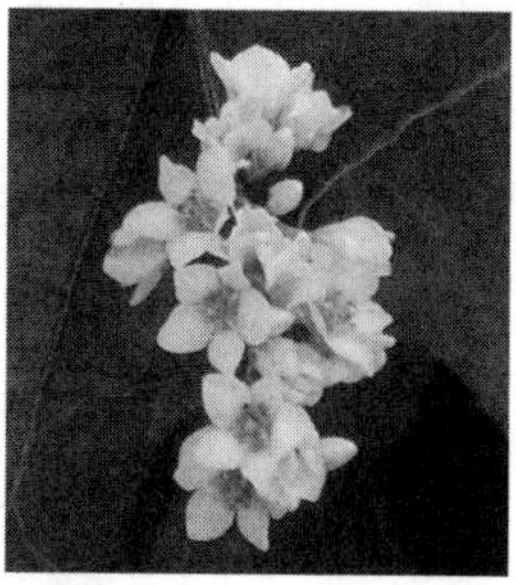

Buckwheat (*Polygonum fagopyrum*)

Buckwheat is a cold-natured herb that helps calm the excessive Yang energy of Yang Type B's. In the summer buckwheat tea is often used to hydrate and cool the body. Buckwheat's cool nature soothes and relaxes the mind to promote sleep. It also helps with other excessive Yang conditions, such as headaches, acne, and high blood pressure.

Buckwheat is one ingredient in the drug Rutin, which is used to treat high blood pressure and injury due to radiation (excessive Yang exposure).

Common Uses of Buckwheat in Sasang Medicine

To alleviate insomnia, high blood pressure, headaches, acne, unsettled emotion (anger, frustration, stress), fever, sensitivity to heat

Sources of Buckwheat

Buckwheat comes in several forms. Buckwheat noodles, also called soba in Japanese, are a popular summertime delicacy in Japan and Korea, where they are boiled in water, chilled, and eaten with a soy-based sauce. Buckwheat noodles are available from Annie Chun (anniechun.com) or Eden Foods (edenfoods.com). Buckwheat flour for baking can be purchased from Bob's Red Mill (bobsredmill.com) and is often used as a gluten-free substitute for wheat flour. A very popular drink in Asia, buckwheat tea can be purchased from Tea Spring (teaspring.com).

Preparation and Dosage of Buckwheat

Buckwheat noodles: A recipe for preparing buckwheat noodles can be found on anniechun.com.

Buckwheat tea: Boil two teaspoons of dried buckwheat in two cups of water. Let simmer on the lowest flame for five minutes. Buckwheat tea bags can be boiled or steeped in warm water to make a soothing after-dinner tea. Buckwheat tea can be chilled or cooled to room temperature and consumed in place of water throughout the day.

Caution

Since buckwheat is used as food, it is generally considered a safe herb. However, its cooling effect may cause diarrhea or indigestion for Yin types whose cool and/or cold-natured digestive systems benefit from warm or hot-natured herbs.

Did You Know?

Despite its name, buckwheat is not related to wheat (which is a type of grass). Instead it is closely related to rhubarb, sorrels, and knotweeds, making it safe for those who are gluten-sensitive.

Maintaining a Healthy Digestive System

Digestive issues, such as bloating, gas, constipation, and/or diarrhea, may affect any body type. Yet of the four body types, the Yin Type B and the Yang Type A have the most digestion-related issues. The Yin Type B's weaker digestive system often leads to indigestion, while the stronger digestive system of the Yang Type A results in overactive stomach energy, with issues related to stomach acid. Even though Yang Type B's rarely feel any digestive discomfort, they tend to vomit frequently if they're sick. Otherwise, there will rarely be any accompanying signs of digestive discomfort, such as bloating, gas, or stomach pain. Most Yin Type A's have a natural flair for eating, which they can easily overdo.

According to Sasang medicine, indigestion results from too much cold or heat accumulation in the digestive system. Heat accumulation occurs after excessive intake of warm-natured foods or if the body has a tendency to overheat in general. Cold accumulation is a result of eating too many raw, chilled, or cold-natured foods, such as salads, pork, and ice cream. See table 4.1 on page 308 for a list of warm- and cold-natured foods. Cold accumulation may also occur if the body is prone to feeling cold. The appetite often increases when indigestion is heat-induced because heat enhances metabolism. Indigestion due to cold results in a lack of appetite because the cold freezes up the digestive system and slows down the metabolism.

TABLE 4.1. WARM- AND COLD-NATURED FOODS

Warm-Natured Foods	Cold-Natured Foods
Spices (ginger, garlic, onions, cinnamon, cardamom, turmeric)	Milk and other dairy products
Chicken, beef	Pork, fish, shellfish
Tea and warm fluids	Cold fluids, smoothies, green veggie drinks
Thoroughly cooked foods	Chilled foods
Soups and stews	Raw foods

Since Yang corresponds to heat, Yang types have a tendency to overheat. When heat accumulates Yang types don't necessarily feel hot. Heat can get "trapped" inside the stomach, while other areas may still feel cool or cold. Yang types may simply notice increased appetite, bad breath, and/or an unsettled feeling in the chest. Increasing the intake of cold-natured foods and decreasing the consumption of warm-natured foods can help dissipate heat in the digestive system. Yin types, on the contrary, are often affected by cold. When cold accumulates it may not necessarily make Yin types feel cold. Cold can get "trapped" inside the stomach while other areas feel warm or hot. When affected by cold, the Yin types may simply experience a lack of appetite, general discomfort, or lethargy. Increasing the intake of warm or hot-natured foods and reducing consumption of cool or cold-natured foods can therefore help support the Yin type's digestive system.

General Tip #1: Simplifying Your Food Intake

If you experience symptoms such as gas, bloating, or stomachaches, try taking a short break from eating solid foods. These symptoms are an indication that your digestive system is stressed out and in need of some time off. Try skipping a meal or consuming warm and soft foods, such as soups, stew, porridge, and rice. You might also try to avoid eating too much or too quickly. If you experience these symptoms after eating, try to lighten up, skip meals, or eliminate certain foods from your diet altogether.

General Tip #2: Drink Tea after Meals

If you suffer from chronic indigestion, drinking tea after meals may resolve this issue. The stomach needs a certain amount of heat to digest foods efficiently. Tea provides the stomach with a little extra warmth for this purpose.

General Tip #3: Eat More Frequent Smaller Meals

Diabetics are often advised to consume smaller, more frequent meals to avoid excess insulin excretion from the pancreas after eating. This method also helps supply a consistent level of energy throughout the day, without overwhelming the digestive system. When living in Japan, my host family chose to eat four to five smaller meal portions throughout the day and I felt more overall energy and less digestive distress as a result.

Try preparing three six-ounce zipper bags every morning. Fill the first zipper bag with veggies, the second with nuts and grains, and the third with fruit. Eat small portions from each bag throughout the day.

General Tip #4: Don't Skip Breakfast!

Many of us do not have the time to prepare breakfast in the morning before we rush off to work. Eating on the run will eventually lead to fatigue, since our body is forced to focus on external activity, rather than absorbing energy from food. Eventually, we become more and more addicted to the pick-me-up effects of substances like caffeine, which inevitably wear us down even further.

Breakfast is the most important meal of the day. It helps to warm up the digestive system and recharge our batteries. Overwhelming the body with heavy foods or underwhelming it with a simple cup of coffee and bread is not enough to provide the energy we need. Make the time to prepare yourself a healthy breakfast. The healthier your breakfast is, the less your body needs to rely on caffeine. Also, you may want to try drinking tea instead of coffee in the morning to give your body extra warmth and herbal support.

General Tip #5: Acupressure Points

Eastern medicine is based on the principle of *qi,* or life force, which flows within all living and nonliving things. This force flows to and from each organ and from head to toe along meridians, also known as energy channels. Qi also flows from the organs outward to the surface of our body where hundreds of acupuncture points exist. These points, also referred to as "access points," help to regulate the smooth flow of life force throughout the body. There are also several acupuncture points on the body that promote digestion. Acupuncture points can be stimulated by the insertion of a needle or massaged while applying pressure with your finger. When pressure, instead of a needle, is applied, the above points are often referred to as acupressure points. Our body depends on the smooth flow of life force to keep us healthy and in balance. However, the flow of this life force may stagnate in response to stress, indigestion, and physical and/or emotional trauma. Here are a few effective ways to help calm an upset stomach, alleviate bloating, and/or help the intestines do their job.

THE "MEETING OF THE VALLEY" ACUPRESSURE POINT

* Locate the "meeting of the valley" on the hand directly in between the thumb and the pointer finger, this is the fourth point on the large intestine meridian, starting from the tip of the pointer finger.
* Gently rub your finger along the inside ridge of the thumb until it meets the second finger. This soft and fleshy point can help the flow of bowel through the intestines, soothe an unsettled digestive system, and clear the sinuses.
* Massage in a circular motion with the tip of the thumb while applying medium to heavy pressure.
* Repeat this step as often as needed.

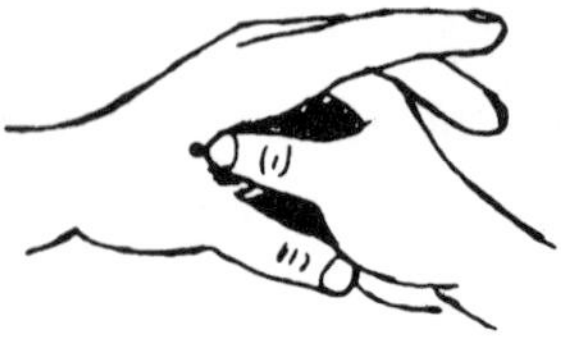

Figure 4.1. Meeting of the Valley acupressure point

THE "INNER COURT" ACUPRESSURE POINT

* Follow the outside corner of the toenail downward along the second toe until you reach a crease between the second and third toe. This is the second point on the stomach meridian starting from the tip of the second toe. The "Inner Court," located at this junction, can promote healthy stomach function in cases of acidity, gastritis (swelling of the stomach wall), bloating, distention, and lack of appetite.

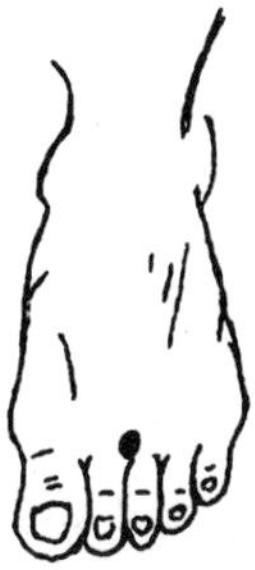

Figure 4.2. Inner Court acupressure point

* Inhale and exhale slowly while applying pressure to this point with your index finger.
* Repeat this step as often as needed.

General Tip #6: Let Go of Stress

Emotional stresses are often the culprit in indigestion. A fight with a loved one, for instance, may leave us with a bad feeling in our gut. Some situations in life are often too hard to digest! Since the stomach digests not only food, but also our daily experiences, holding on to negative or unnecessary thoughts may lead to digestive discomfort. A healthy digestive system can eliminate unnecessary by-products and absorb optimum energy from food. A healthy mind can eliminate unnecessary thoughts while accepting new experiences and ideas. Try to let go of negative thoughts and grudges against others and/or yourself. A Japanese philosopher named Nichiren once said, "Suffer what there is to suffer and enjoy what there is to enjoy. Regard both suffering and joy as mere facts of life."

General Tip #7: Rest after Lunch

Have you ever felt lethargic after eating lunch? For centuries in China, it was customary to take a nap after lunch to recharge the body for the remainder of the day. Although we may not think about it much, it takes a lot of energy to digest food. The body has difficulty exerting itself on a full stomach. Taking time after lunch to relax and recuperate can benefit the mind and body immensely. It is not necessary to sleep after lunch. Simply lying down, breathing deeply, meditating, or relaxing is enough to replenish the body.

General Tip #8: Listen to Your Digestive System

When was the last time you asked your stomach if it liked a meal? Most of us are guided by what our taste buds tell us about food, rather than how our stomach or intestines feel about what we consume. The reaction of our stomach and bowels is the best indication of whether or not a particular food is a good match for our body. It is sometimes difficult, however, to detect whether or not our digestive system enjoyed a particular food. A negative reaction may cause issues such as losing the urge to poop or minor belching. Other signs and symptoms may be more obvious, such as excess fullness, bloating, and diarrhea, which warn us against eating a certain food or drinking a certain drink. Listen to your digestive system after eating a meal to see whether or not it is happy. Try to avoid foods that cause the above-cited issues as much as possible because your body may be resistant to them.

INDIGESTION AND YIN TYPE A

In Sasang medicine the liver plays a major role in facilitating the digestive process. The stronger liver of Yin Type A's helps them enjoy a variety of foods without experiencing digestive discomfort.

While having a stronger liver may sound appealing, it often gets Yin Type A's in trouble because they have difficulty knowing their food intake limits. For Yin Type A's, food can be either a great source of energy or the culprit behind failing health. With such a strong liver, Yin Type A's rarely have any indication that they are eating foods that harm them. They may even find excuses to eat this or that food, even though common sense suggests otherwise.

Excess intake of unhealthy foods can lead to congestion and inflammation of an overactive liver, which also results in liver heat accumulation, and that may eventually bring on constipation, diarrhea, stomachaches, and the like.

Another source of indigestion for Yin Type A's comes from the influence of a common cold. The Yin Type A is born with weaker lungs, which are in charge of the immune system. In Sasang medicine the lungs and stomach have a strong influence on each other. The lungs provide oxygen for the digestive system to carry out its function. The digestive system, in turn, sends the energy it gets from food back to the lungs.

If Yin Type A's catch a cold, the lungs can easily get fatigued, resulting in digestive problems. This type of cold may be accompanied by other symptoms, such as a stuffy nose, a sinus headache, chills, and a runny nose. Otherwise, it may manifest simply as a stomach cold with no other symptoms except indigestion.

Cold weather usually causes the former symptoms while excessive intake of cold-natured foods causes the latter. Food poisoning and food allergies may also fall into this category.

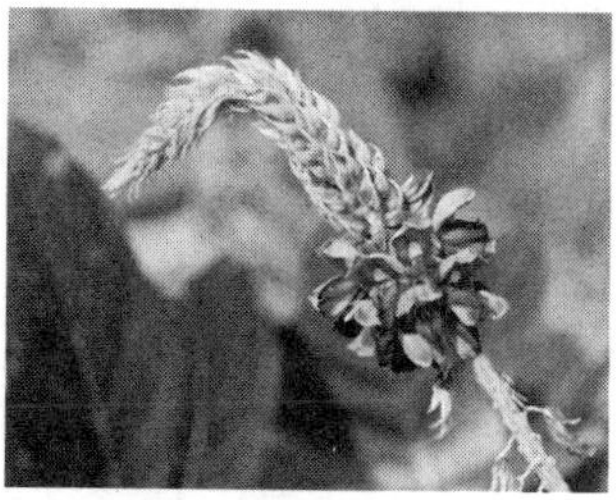

Kudzu Root (*Radix Peurariae*)

This herb is one of the few in Sasang medicine that has the dual function of moistening and clearing heat from the liver. Excessive use of most herbs that clear internal heat also tend to cause side effects like skin dryness and indigestion. Kudzu root, by contrast, is a gentle but effective herb that is almost always used in cases of Yin Type A liver heat. The liver plays a central role in the digestive process; it absorbs and eliminates toxins from food and drink. An overactive liver is good at absorbing toxins but poor at getting rid of them. The accumulation of toxins in the liver leads to inflammation and heat buildup in the body. Recent studies suggest that kudzu is effective in reducing alcohol addiction.* Traditionally, kudzu root has also been used as a hangover remedy. It contains a number of useful isoflavons, such as daidzein, which acts as an anti-inflammatory, a natural antibiotic, and a preventive for various forms of cancer.

Did You Know?

Kudzu was originally introduced into the southeastern United States for its ability to prevent erosion from riverbanks and irrigation ditches. However, once introduced, it proliferated like wildfire, spreading for thousands of miles in all directions and killing everything in its path! It eventually earned the title of the "vine that ate the South." Rather than fearing its wrath, many Americans have incorporated it into their diet. An often-admired elderly but youthful woman, known as the "Kudzu Queen of North Carolina," credits her good health to daily intake of kudzu roots and leaves.

Common Uses of Kudzu Root in Sasang Medicine

For relief of indigestion due to heat accumulation (acid reflux, dry stools, and/or feverishness), swelling of the eyes, neck pain and headaches located in the back of the head, shoulder muscle spasms, excessive thirst, high blood pressure, fever, anger, constipation and/or diarrhea due to heat, dysentery, alcohol addiction, hangover

*For example, see Lukas, Scott E., David Penetar, Jeff Berko, Luke Vicens, Christopher Palmer, Gopinath Mallya, Eric A. Macklin, David Y. Lee, "An Extract of the Chinese Herbal Root Kudzu Reduces Alcohol Drinking by Heavy Drinkers in a Naturalistic Setting" *Alcoholism Clinical and Experimental Research* 29, no. 5 (May 2005): 756–62.

Sources of Kudzu Root

Kudzu root extract can be purchased from manufacturers such as Vitacost (vitacost.com) and Nature's Way (naturesway.com). The starch from kudzu root can be used to thicken soups, sauces, and pudding, and can be purchased in powder form from Florida Herb House (floridaherbhouse.com). It's also available in the Asian/international food sections of most natural food stores.

Preparation and Dosage of Kudzu Root

Follow the manufacturer's instructions for dosage and cooking.

Herbal Friends

Kudzu root is often combined with other herbs to complement and balance the function of clearing heat. It is commonly used with skullcap root and/or Chinese lovage root to clear heat from the liver to aid indigestion (due to heat) and counter swelling of the eyes, headaches, excessive thirst, fever, high blood pressure, and/or anger. The dosage of kudzu root in this case is twice that of the other herbs. Skullcap root is available from New Chapter (newchapter.com) and Nature's Way (naturesway.com). A powdered extract of Chinese lovage root is available from Efong by typing "Gao Ben" in the amazon.com search engine (*Gao Ben* is the Chinese name for Chinese lovage root).

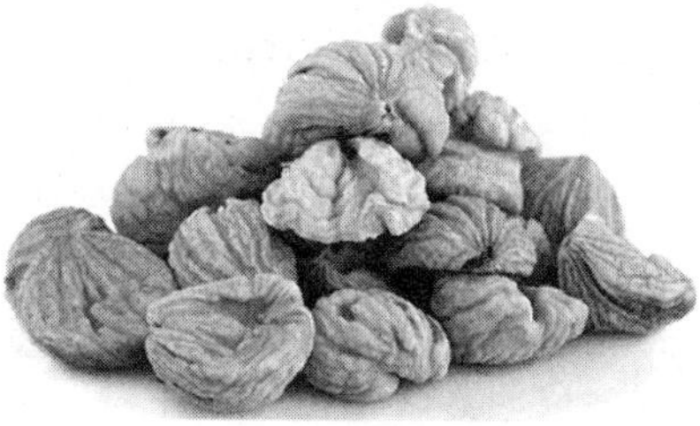

Chestnuts (*Castanea*)

Eating roasted chestnuts beside an open fire during Christmas may be the only time we pay any attention to them in the West. In the Sasang medicine clinic, however, chestnuts are frequently prescribed for indigestion from cold accumulation in the body, which is signaled by sensitivity to cold, a lack of appetite, watery dark brown/tarry stools, and sensitivity to the cold. Chestnuts make an excellent nutritious snack because they are high in minerals, vitamins, and phytonutrients, while still keeping a low-calorie/low-fat profile. They are also gluten-free, making them a good option for those with gluten sensitivities.

Common Uses of Chestnuts in Sasang Medicine

For relief of indigestion, diarrhea (usually with darker brown or tarry stools, indicating the influence of cold), abdominal fullness, lack of appetite, nausea, malnutrition

Sources of Chestnuts

Roasted, dried, and powdered chestnuts can be purchased by the pound from nuts.com.

Did You Know?

Fresh chestnuts are the only nut that contains vitamin C! One hundred grams of chestnuts contain 65 percent of the recommended daily allowance.

Preparation and Dosage of Chestnuts

Roasted chestnuts are peeled and ingested directly from the shell. Chestnut powder (also known as chestnut flour) can be used as a gluten-free white flour alternative for baking. After being soaked and peeled, dried chestnuts also become a yummy ingredient for a variety of healthy dishes to be found on recipe.com. A tea made of dried chestnuts is prepared by boiling four chestnuts in two cups of water, then simmering the tea on the lowest flame for thirty minutes. Drink two to three warm cups per day to relieve diarrhea and indigestion.

Herbal Friends

Chestnuts are often used with other herbs to address digestive issues due to cold. Job's tears is a close herbal friend of chestnuts, and they are almost always seen together in Sasang herbal formulas. Job's tears also alleviates diarrhea with indigestion, while strengthening the digestive system and clearing phlegm from the lungs. Chestnuts and Job's tears also help in treating common colds with indigestion. Job's tears is available in powder form from Veggie Land (veggielandbrea.com). The powder can be added to yogurt, soymilk, oat milk, or soups for increased flavor and health benefits.

INDIGESTION AND YIN TYPE B

Indigestion is a common issue among Yin Type B's, since they are born with a weaker spleen, which regulates the digestive system. As a result they tend to be very picky about food, because one wrong move could lead to serious digestive issues. Fussy Yin Type B's manage to stay healthy by avoiding foods that disagree with them.

The digestive system in Yin Type B's is a direct reflection of how healthy they are. Some healthier Yin Type B's can enjoy just about any type of food. However, when they get sick, the digestive system is usually to blame. Even when they are feeling well, it is important for Yin Type B's to support the stomach and spleen with foods and herbal supplements associated with their body type.

Each organ of the body has a different temperature. The warmer organs, such as the lungs and stomach, warm up the body, while the cooler liver and kidneys cool it down. Yin Type B's stronger kidneys tend to keep the body on the colder side most of the time. Since the stomach and spleen need warmth to break down foods, internal coldness can easily cause digestive issues. If Yin Type B's ingest too many raw or cold-natured foods, their stomach and spleen function will be impaired, leading to symptoms such as bloating, gas, stomachaches, and lack of appetite. This situation can sometimes get worse and cause vomiting, high fever, swollen glands, or even loss of consciousness.

Not all Yin Type B's suffer from Yin induced cold-related issues. They may also be afflicted with Yang induced heat-related issues, such as high blood pressure, headaches, fever, and/or hot flashes. In such situations it may seem as if they need to stay cooler or ingest cold-natured foods. Yet, unlike the other body types, heat-related symptoms in Yin Type B's are actually caused by cold lurking deep in the body, pushing Yang and heat helplessly outward. When it comes to addressing these situations, things can get a bit tricky. First of all how do we know for sure if a symptom is the result of heat or cold lurking in the body? Unlike the other body types, Yin Type B's rarely desire to drink cold fluids, no matter how hot or feverish they feel, because they always get sick from too much cold. By contrast heat-related symptoms often make the other body types thirsty for cold fluids. The ability and desire to drink cold fluids signal an extremely healthy Yin Type B, who by nature is colder at the core.

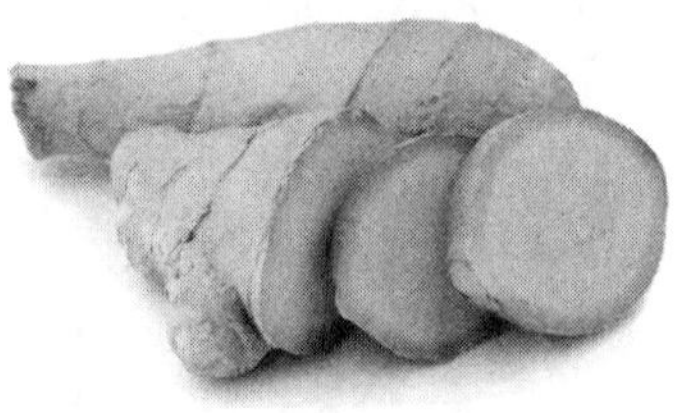

Ginger
(*Zingiber officinale*)

For Yin Type B's, ginger warms and supports the digestive system. Since the digestive system is the source of most Yin Type B health issues, ginger can be used to alleviate practically any health concern. The strong dispersing qualities of ginger also make it an effective herb for chasing away pathogens and other immune-related issues. To promote digestion dried ginger is usually more effective than fresh ginger, while fresh ginger is more effective for colds. If you have a cold and are experiencing indigestion, either type would suffice. The active ingredients in ginger, called oleoresin and terpenes, help kill unwanted bacteria and regulate bowel movement.

As a Yin Type B myself, I keep ginger within arm's reach at all times. I find myself drinking ginger tea several times a day when the weather cools down in late autumn. Not only does it help prevent the onset of a cold, it also gives me a boost of energy.

Common Uses of Ginger in Sasang Medicine

To remedy common colds, most types of digestive issues due to cold (bloating, gas, lack of appetite, diarrhea, constipation, fullness, nausea), infections, inflammation, joint pain, mouth sores, athlete's foot (topically), sadness, anxiety, seasickness, morning sickness

Sources of Ginger

Ginger is readily available in most supermarkets in fresh or tea bag form. Certain tea companies like to add licorice root for sweetness or lemon for more zest. These ingredients are also Yin Type B–compatible and therefore support the digestive system. Dried pure ginger can be purchased from floridaherbhouse.com.

Preparation and Dosage of Ginger

Drying ginger: Remove the outer skin from the fresh gingerroot, then cut it into very thin slices. Place the slices on a paper towel or other absorbent material that won't contaminate the ginger. Let it sit in a sunny and/or dry area until the ginger hardens, which takes about twenty-four hours, and pat the slices with a clean paper towel to remove any excess moisture.

Fresh ginger: Break (usually easy to do) or cut off about one inch of the gingerroot and peel off the dry skin with a knife, a spoon, or a stiff brush. Slice it into approximately five pieces and discard the peel.

To prepare dried or fresh ginger: Boil two cups of water with five slices of dried or fresh ginger and let it simmer for ten minutes on the lowest flame. Drink up to five cups a day, warm. You can add more water if the ginger tea is too strong, or add more ginger if you prefer it stronger. If you are using fresh ginger, store the remaining root in the refrigerator to retain freshness. If you decide to use ginger extract capsules, follow the dosage instructions provided by the manufacturer.

Caution

Ginger can easily cause stomach irritation for the other body types. Yet, this is rarely an issue for Yin Type B's, who often shock the other body types with how much ginger they can consume! Because it is so hot, ginger may nevertheless irritate the stomach of even a Yin Type B if taken in excess or on an empty stomach. Try taking a little break or reducing the dosage if you notice an uncomfortable burning sensation and/or acid reflux.

INDIGESTION AND YANG TYPE A

The indigestion of the Yang Type A is caused by heat accumulation in the stomach. This heat comes from an overactive stomach and spleen, which are the strongest organs of the Yang Type A. When things are in balance, the Yang Type A's stomach energy flows downward, as it sends digested foods toward the intestines. When the stomach is unsettled, its energy rebels upward toward the mouth, leading to bad breath, swollen gums, bloating in the upper abdomen, frontal headaches, fullness in the chest, and/or excessive appetite. The Yang Type A benefits from herbs that cool and soothe the stomach and spleen.

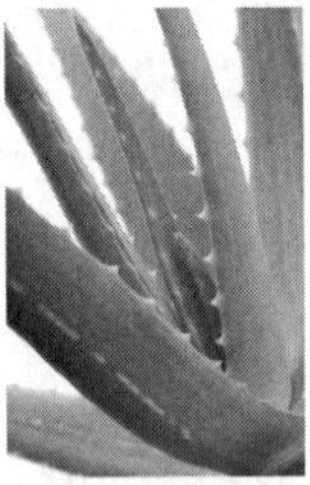

Aloe Vera Juice

Aloe vera has a powerful effect on reducing the Yang Type A's indigestion, which stems from stomach heat. Its antimicrobial properties make it useful in treating parasitic infection. Aloe vera juice is a relatively safe and very effective drink that can be ingested frequently and can be used topically to accelerate the healing of burns, bruises, and cuts.

Common Uses of Aloe Vera in Sasang Medicine

To alleviate indigestion due to heat, which may cause heartburn, headaches, dizziness, bloodshot eyes, insomnia, irritability, constipation, and parasitic infection (roundworm and ringworm)

Sources of Aloe Vera

Pure aloe vera juice can be purchased online from Lily of the Desert (lilyofthedesert.com) or Aloe Life (aloelife.com) or most health food stores. Other forms of aloe vera are also available on the market, including in pill form from Source Naturals (sourcenaturals.com).

Caution

Aloin, a component of aloe vera, stimulates the movement of fecal material. Hence, too much stimulation of the bowel can lead to diarrhea and further indigestion. Some manufacturers remove this component when processing aloe vera. Aloin may be beneficial for Yang Type A's, whose constipation comes from excessive stomach heat. If diarrhea occurs after drinking aloe vera juice, try reducing your intake or find another aloe-based product.

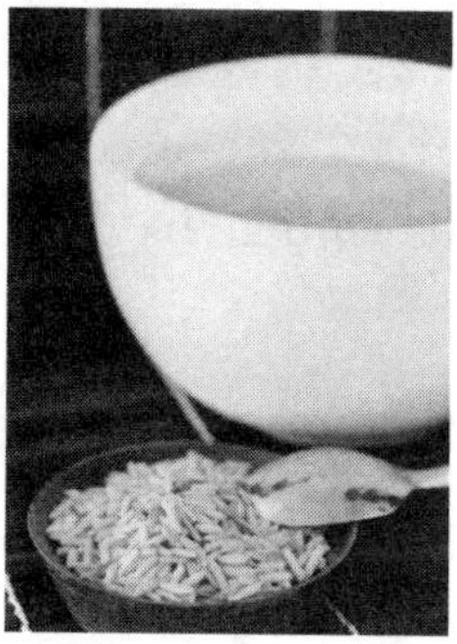

Korean Shikye (Fermented Rice) Drink

Shikye is another wonderful example of how Korean culture has integrated herbal medicine into daily life. This fermented beverage is often consumed after meals to promote digestion. It has a slightly sweet taste and is very soothing to drink, even for Yin types! Shikye is especially beneficial for Yang Type A's because it is made of barley malt, whose cold nature cools stomach heat. Shikye is usually ingested cold for this reason. In Korea shikye is often consumed after meals, regardless of body type because the fermentation process itself gives shikye its ability to promote digestion.

Preparation and Dosage of Korean Shikye (Fermented Rice) Drink

Ingredients

1 cup barley malt
2 cups Asian (Japanese or Korean) glutinous rice
1 cup of sugar (or to taste)
2 tablespoons of pine nuts
6 cups water

Soak the barley malt in water for two to three hours. All the malt should sink to the bottom. Meanwhile, cook the rice, according to package directions, in a rice cooker or in a pot. Pour the water from the malt mixture into a bowl, taking care not to stir up the malt. Discard the malt. Pour the malt water over the cooked rice and cook it over low heat for four to five hours. Another option is to keep the rice and malt water warm in your rice cooker for four to five hours. A few rice grains should float to the surface at the end. Add sugar and boil the mixture for fifteen to twenty minutes. Serve cold after meals with a few pine nuts as garnish.*

INDIGESTION AND YANG TYPE B

Yang Type B's rarely experience what other body types may consider indigestion, such as bloating, gas, or stomach pains. This does not necessarily indicate the absence of digestive issues. The inability of Yang Type B's to detect digestive issues partially stems from their tendency to lose touch with their body. With such busy minds, they rarely have time to think about or do anything to promote their health! When the digestive system is distressed, Yang Type B's will simply vomit up practically everything they eat. Since there are no other signs of digestive

*This recipe, from maangchi.com, is one of Maangchi's many delicious Korean recipes listed on her site.

distress, Yang Type B's rarely heed this symptom and manage to keep going. If this situation lingers, their general health can take a turn for the worse.

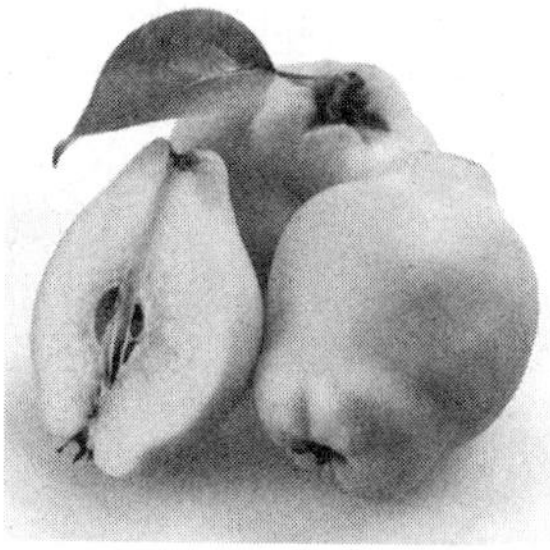

Chinese Quince Fruit (*Cydonia oblonga*)

Quince is a fruit with a taste somewhere in between that of a pear and an apple when mixed with honey or sugar. It is seldom consumed fresh because of its very astringent and bitter taste. In Sasang medicine the dried fruit (including the peel) is often used to treat indigestion, lower-body weakness, and lower-back and knee-joint pain. Quince is a good source of vitamin A, fiber, and iron.

Common Uses of Chinese Quince Fruit in Sasang Medicine

To alleviate indigestion, vomiting, joint pain of the lower body, weakness of the legs and hip area, swelling of the legs, knees, and/or ankles

Sources of Chinese Quince Fruit

Quince fruit tea mixed with honey is often sold in Korean markets. If you do not live near a Korean market, try ordering it from posharp store.com. Gardeners can purchase quince trees from Willis Orchard Company (willisorchards.com). A delicious quince fruit spread can be purchased from Made in Oregon (madeinoregon.com). You can find quince fruit extract at theherbdoc.com.

Preparation and Dosage of Chinese Quince Fruit

Quince can be consumed often as a tea or as jam. Check out recipe.com for several do-it-yourself quince recipes. For quince fruit tea, follow the preparation instructions on the label. Quince fruit extract should be ingested according to the manufacturer's suggestions.

Did You Know?

The Croatians traditionally planted a quince tree when a child was born to symbolize fertility, love, and life. It was also a ritual offering during weddings in ancient Greece. Hence it was called the "fruit of love, marriage, and fertility."

Shedding Those Extra Pounds

According to the Centers for Disease Control and Prevention, obesity has risen dramatically in the past decade. The American population in 2010 displayed the highest rates of obesity ever—33.8 percent.* Obesity is perhaps the most significant health issue of our time and is linked to heart disease, high blood pressure, stroke, diabetes, and other life-threatening conditions.† While it would be difficult to pinpoint one particular reason why weight gain has become so widespread, it is likely due to a combination of reasons, such as food intake quality and quantity, eating on the go, and stress.

In Eastern medicine obesity is referred to as a "phlegm dampness accumulation disorder," in which phlegm and dampness accumulate in the body. There are two types of phlegm accumulation in the body: visible and invisible. Visible phlegm refers to the icky stuff that we can cough up, feel in the back of our throat, or blow out of our nose. Invisible phlegm is the accumulation of fat, cysts, and/or tumors in the

*From Centers for Disease Control and Prevention, "Adult Obesity Facts," www.cdc.gov/obesity/data/adult.html.

†For more on this, see National Heart, Lung, and Blood Institute, "What Are the Health Risks of Overweight and Obesity?" www.nhlbi.nih.gov/health/health-topics/topics/obe/risks.html.

body. Excess fat tissue accumulates as a result of insufficient digestion of foods. This may be due to a weakened digestive system, stress, anxiety, and/or eating incompatible foods. Each of the body types has its own food requirements, based on the needs of their internal organs. Consuming foods that do not benefit our body type eventually leads to a weakened digestive system. Making correct food choices can be challenging because there are so many different ideas of "healthy food." Most of us would assume that eating too much chocolate, for example, could have negative effects on our health, but research helps us find excuses to eat more by stressing its antioxidant and other health-inducing properties.* Culture also plays a significant role in our food choices. It is common in the United States for people to eat deep-fried foods that place a burden on the digestive system. A balanced diet, according to Sasang medicine, consists of choosing food according to our body type and not necessarily what our taste buds wish us to eat.

Fat accumulation is an issue that can affect anyone, but usually occurs in different areas of the body, according to body type. Yin Type B's tend to gain weight in the buttocks area, while Yang Type A's generally gain weight in their thighs and arms. Yang Type B's have a tendency to gain weight in the neck, chest, and shoulder area, while Yin Type A's usually gain weight in their abdominal area. The abdomen can store abundant amounts of fat and fluid, making it an area of the body that is hard to conceal. Since the strong liver of Yin Type A's is exceptionally good at absorption, it is often difficult for them to shed those extra pounds. Knowing your body type and how to keep your body in balance gives you an advantage in the battle against weight gain.

TESTING FOR OBESITY

There are several methods you can use to determine your healthy weight range. The National Heart Lung and Blood Institute, for instance,

*For more on this, see Verna, Roberto, "The History and Science of Chocolate" *Malaysian Journal of Pathology* 35, no. 2 (December 2013): 111–21.

offers a free BMI calculator on its website (www.nhlbi.nih.gov/health/educational/lose_wt/BMI/bmicalc.htm). For those of you who have a flair for math, the body mass index (BMI) can be calculated using the equation below:

$$\text{BMI} = \frac{\text{mass (lbs)} \times 703}{(\text{height (in)})^2}$$

According to the above calculation, if your BMI is equal to or less than 18.5, then you are considered underweight. If it is above 25 but less than 29.9 then you are considered overweight. A BMI of 30 or greater is considered obese. A healthy BMI range is from 18.5 to 24.9.

The BMI is not the most accurate method of testing obesity, since each of us has our own body shape, bone density, and muscle mass accumulation. It therefore tends to be less accurate when used with children, the elderly, and athletes who tend to vary greatly in muscle and bone mass.

Another approach is simply to ask your doctor to do an assessment during your next checkup. Family doctors, naturopaths, and nurse-practitioners can usually give you adequate information regarding your healthy weight range.

PREVENTING WEIGHT GAIN

In order to avoid the buildup of toxins, fat, and fluid in the body, it is necessary to keep things circulating as much as possible. When the circulation of blood and energy in the body slows down, there is a much greater chance of fat accumulation. Here is a list of ten tips that can enhance circulation and help you lose weight.

General Tip #1: Eat the Right Foods

Consume foods that are easily metabolized for your body type. Yin Type A's, for instance, benefit from eating foods that promote lung function. Most of us may not necessarily associate the lungs with metabolism or losing weight. However, for Yin Type A's, the lungs play a central role because they help send oxygen to the digestive system. Without oxygen the stomach would not be able to break down food efficiently and the intestines would not have the strength to eliminate stools. Stagnant stools can be compared to a clogged sink that threatens to overflow. When our "pipes" get clogged, we gain weight, and experience a buildup of toxicity.

General Tip #2: Balance Exercise and Rest

Both rest and exercise are indispensable when it comes to staying healthy. Each body type has its own specific requirements in these areas. Yin types tend to be more sedentary, while Yang types tend to be overactive. Regardless of your body type, you need to strike a balance between exercise and rest. While it is important to exercise regularly and stay active in order to keep your energy and blood flowing efficiently, try to avoid pushing your body too hard. While it is important to rest in order to replenish your energy, living a sedentary life may add to fat accumulation.

General Tip #3: Keep Those Bowels Moving!

Most of us would get excited as we engage in a conversation about vacation, retirement, or money. My clients never fail to chuckle when I get excited about healthily flowing poop. In Sasang medicine the bowels tell a lot about our health. Healthy bowel movement is a sign of a healthy body as it eliminates the by-products of food and emotion efficiently. Excess stress or food intake may cause sluggishness. Eating foods that are not associated with your body type may also cause stagnation of the bowel. Lack of water intake, eating too late at night, eating meals off schedule, or ignoring the impulse to go to the bathroom all contribute to bowel issues as well. Drinking approximately thirty-two ounces of water a day should help keep things moving nicely through the intestines. Eating meals around the same time each day also helps prepare the intestines for a good bowel movement. There is less chance for fat or other types of accumulation when the body's "back door" is working effectively.

General Tip #4: Be Wary of Too Much Stress

Are you eating right for your body type and still gaining weight? If so, stress may also be a contributing factor when it comes to weight gain. Heavy workloads, relationship issues, and/or financial situations all put pressure on the digestive system, reducing metabolic efficiency. Exercise is a fantastic way to reduce stress because it increases the body's endorphin levels. Endorphins are naturally occurring hormones in the body that play a major role in helping us feel happy. Other methods of reducing stress are taking the time to breathe deeply and slowly, letting go of stubborn thoughts and emotions, sexual intercourse, masturbation, reading an interesting book, and setting time aside for your well-being. While these methods are helpful, none of them should be taken to extremes. Eastern medicine emphasizes the need for moderation and balance, no matter what path we take.

General Tip #5: Establish Balanced Eating Habits

Weight gain is not just a result of food quantity. Many people gain weight even if they eat smaller meal portions. How we eat is also an important factor in the process of losing weight. If we are always in a rush and eat our meals quickly, there is much less chance that it will get digested efficiently. Some of us like to watch TV, engage in heated conversation over meals, or run around with food in our mouths! These activities can easily distract the digestive system, leading to inefficient digestion. Eating slowly and being mindful of the eating process not only contributes to healthy digestion, it also helps us savor each bite.

General Tip #6: Follow a Routine

Have you ever wondered why your dog is even more reliable than an alarm clock when he is hungry? My cute, but annoying, little dog jumps onto my bed and salivates all over the place at exactly 6:32 every single morning. At one point I even hid the clock, which I assumed he could somehow read, under my bed, hoping that this would solve the problem. I later realized that my doggie actually has a clock of a different kind, called a circadian clock. This clock is a gift (or curse!) from nature. It gives him an accurate sense of time, based on hunger and sleep patterns. Humans also have an internal circadian clock that may not work as well as that of other animals, but is still capable of reminding us when to perform certain functions. If you eat breakfast at 8:00 a.m. every day, the body will eventually look forward to this time for food intake. Fifteen minutes earlier the body will start to increase saliva and digestive juices to get ready for food intake. Eating on schedule prepares the body for digestion. Preparation helps the body digest food much more efficiently. The same holds true for routine exercising, working, sleeping and waking, taking naps, and having sex. Going to the bathroom at similar times every day also helps with bowel flow.

General Tip #7: Go Light on Breakfast

We all need a little time to get ready in the morning as the body transitions out of sleep mode. The digestive system is no exception to this rule; it prefers to get going gradually, instead of jumping right out of bed. Starting the day with a light and warm breakfast helps to kick-start the digestive system. Soup, oatmeal, porridge, and congee are great options for a healthy and easy-to-digest breakfast because they are warm and soft. Oily foods, on the other hand, are overwhelming for a sleepy digestive system and will slow it down even further. Contrary to some other dietary approaches, the Sasang approach cautions the Yin Types again eating higher amounts of protein first thing in the morning. Consuming protein-heavy foods, such as sausage and bacon, as part of your first meal of the day could result in a sluggish digestive system and prompt weight gain. If you are a Yin type, rather than eliminating protein altogether from your morning, try adjusting your intake of protein according to your activity levels. A protein shake or drink directly before or after a workout, for example, may offer an extra boost. Exercise is the most efficient way to break down protein and transform it into energy.

General Tip #8: Eat Dinner Early

Night corresponds to Yin while day is Yang. During Yin time the body slows down as it gets ready for rest and replenishment. During Yang time the body naturally gets ready for movement, digestion, and elimination. It is much more challenging for our body to break down foods later in the evening. It is best to eat dinner before 7:00 p.m. to ensure efficient digestion and assimilation of nutrition.

General Tip #9: Drink Tea after Meals

The digestive system relies on warmth to break down foods. Since Yin corresponds to cold, it is more difficult for Yin body types than Yang types to break down foods. If the stomach does not receive enough warmth, foods will stick around longer inside the body and eventually morph into fat tissue. Tea helps create enough warmth in the stomach to digest foods more efficiently. Try drinking tea directly after meals in order to promote the digestive process. Green tea, chamomile tea, ginger tea, or chai tea make good after-meal drinks for Yin types. Peppermint and barley tea are suitable for the Yang types.

General Tip #10: Go Easy on the Weights!

Weight lifting, if done in moderation, can be a wonderful way to stay in shape and keep your energy flowing. Heavy weight lifting, by contrast, is not conducive to losing weight and may even impair your long-term health. From the body's perspective, muscle and fat tissue are not all that different. Muscle mass, if not maintained, could easily morph into fat tissue, just as fat tissue can be transformed directly into muscle mass. Excess muscle or fat tissue makes it challenging for the heart to pump blood throughout the body, thus making it easier to gain weight. If your goal is to stay healthy and lose weight, try focusing on cardiovascular activities such as bike riding and swimming, and if you desire to lift weights, try more repetition with moderate weight.

Weight gain is usually due to a combination of issues, including indigestion, stress, and/or circulatory problems. Therefore, when approaching the weight gain issue, it is important to address its underlying causes, rather than seeking a quick fix. Losing weight usually requires an integrative approach that incorporates four essential components:

- Proper foods (those that are easily metabolized by your body type)
- Exercise (according to your body type)
- Supplements/Herbs for Proper Circulation
- Emotional Balance (making an effort to relax or meditate)

Try to incorporate each component consistently throughout the process. Not only will this list help you navigate toward permanent weight loss, but it will also help you enjoy the benefits of an overall healthy mind and body. Stay persistent and don't give up!

WEIGHT GAIN AND YIN TYPE A

Born with a stronger liver, Yin Type A's have the greatest tendency toward weight gain compared to the other body types, because they powerfully absorb toxins and other by-products from food. The Yin Type A body does not want to get rid of food and instead transforms it into body fat, more so than stool. When the mind and body are not in balance, Yin Type A's may also start to crave unhealthy foods, resulting in more weight gain. The inability to sweat efficiently is another challenge that many Yin Type A's face. This is also a reflection of too much absorption and the inability to release.

Yin Type A's benefit the most from performing cardiovascular exercise because it helps move their sluggish blood and stagnant energy. Cardiovascular exercises, such as brisk walking, light jogging, bicycling, swimming, hiking, and aerobics also help to strengthen the weaker lungs of Yin Type A's, forcing them to expand and contract to their utmost capacity. When the lungs are healthy, they circulate energy and help the body eliminate stool and sweat more efficiently.

Because of their propensity to absorb, Yin Type A's tend to gain fat and muscle mass more easily than other body types. Heavy weight lifting may lead to acute health issues for Yin Type A's by increasing their blood pressure and causing an energy blockage. From the standpoint of Eastern medicine, bulky muscles are actually large blockages of blood and energy! Moderate weight lifting, in combination with a focus on cardiovascular exercise, could significantly enhance their health.

How to Work Up a Good Sweat

Yin Type A's need to sweat regularly in order to release toxins and by-products from their body. If you are a Yin Type A who sweats a lot, this is a good sign that your body is making an effort to release toxins and by-products. Most Yin Type A's have trouble sweating and have to really work to get things flowing. Try these ideas to build up a good sweat: Wear thick clothing while doing cardiovascular exercises. Use a sauna regularly. *(Caution: After sweating, make sure to hydrate your body by drinking ample amounts of water. The sauna may easily dehydrate an elderly or frail person. If you feel queasy or uncomfortable while in the sauna, it is time to get out. Frail or elderly people may need to spend less time in the sauna or avoid the sauna altogether.)*

Yin Type A's often have issues with bowel flow because of their tendency toward excess absorption. They often suffer from irritable bowel syndrome, constipation, diarrhea, ulcerative colitis, leaky gut syndrome, Crohn's disease, diverticulitis, or other intestine-related issues. These issues are not always obvious. Constipation, for example, may still be an issue even if you have frequent bowel movements. The length of an adult's large intestine is approximately five feet and the small intestine is about twenty-two feet long! A lot of stool can be stored in such a long space. The intestines of Yin Type A's have a tendency to expand and store too much stool. As a result they may become constipated or have frequent bowel movements as the body attempts to rid itself of excess accumulation. Excess storage of fecal material could play a significant role in issues related to weight gain. To keep the bowels moving regularly, Yin Type A's should consume enough insoluble fiber in their diet and drink at least forty-eight ounces of water daily. The combination of insoluble fiber and water helps flush the intestines. Common sources of insoluble fiber are whole grains, nuts, seeds, cauliflower, and avocados. Protein, on the other hand, tends to stick around in the system longer than fiber. If consumed in larger amounts, protein can lead to constipation. Yin Type A's can benefit from limiting their intake of protein. Protein intake should correlate directly with activity levels. The more active you are, the more protein your body needs to repair the wear and tear on its tissues.

Stress may also cause an increase in appetite and weight gain for Yin Type A's. Under stress they may find themselves binge-eating or craving certain foods. Yin Type A's often need to reflect on their relationship with food and muster the courage to modify their eating habits. The regulation of stress levels has an important role to play in losing weight. Make sure to balance your day with ample exercise and enough rest to rid yourself of excess stress. See "Dealing with Stress" (pages 254–62) for more information about this.

There is no such thing as a perfect herb for losing weight. Losing weight takes a tremendous amount of persistence and patience. However, the incorporation of herbs and supplements is a great way to support this process. The following section includes supplements that help promote the Yin Type A's circulation and may interact with other medicines used for the same reason, such as blood thinners or aspirin. Make sure to consult a medical professional before using the following supplements if you are currently taking any pharmaceutical medications.

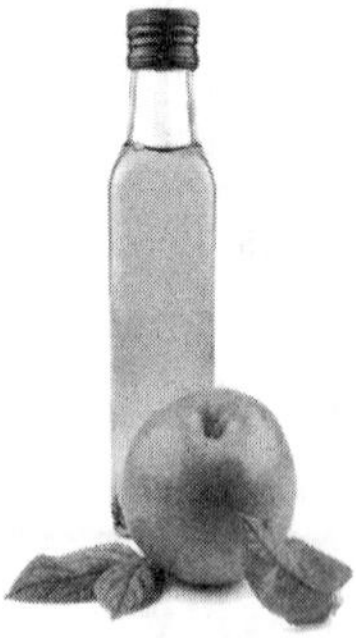

Apple Cider Vinegar

In Eastern medicine herbs are often soaked in vinegar to enhance their ability to promote blood and energy flow. This combination is also used to flush the liver of toxins and reduce the accumulation of by-products within the body. Vinegar can reduce the amount of serum triglyceride, which is the precursor of cholesterol. An active component of vinegar known as acetic acid (AcOH) is said to help reduce body fat. Modern research has also discovered that apple cider vinegar can prevent and reduce high blood pressure, as well as rid the body of several different types of unwanted bacteria.* From the standpoint of Eastern medicine, herbs that promote energy and blood flow are also effective in treating muscle and/or joint pain.

Common Uses of Apple Cider Vinegar in Sasang Medicine

To alleviate high blood pressure, circulatory issues (cold extremities, numbness of the extremities, weight gain), indigestion, joint pain

Sources of Apple Cider Vinegar

Apple cider vinegar is available at most supermarkets throughout the United States. Other types of vinegar are also readily available.

Preparation and Dosage of Apple Cider Vinegar

Add two teaspoons of apple cider vinegar to one cup of water. Stir well and then drink it up! Take two doses a day for optimum efficiency. A teaspoon of honey can be added to reduce the sour flavor of apple cider vinegar. According to one study, a daily intake of 15 ml of vinegar with one glass of water may help to reduce obesity caused by overeating.†

Caution

Apple cider vinegar is very aromatic and acrid and elicits a taste and smell unpleasant to many. The acetic acid in vinegar may cause burning of the tongue and throat in some individuals. Try adding a small amount of honey and increasing the amount of water if the taste is too strong or it burns your mouth. For most people the ratio listed in the

---

*For example, see Budak, Nilgün H., Elif Aykin, Atif C. Seydim, Annel K. Greene, and Zeynep B. Guzel-Seydim, "Functional Properties of Vinegar" *Journal of Food Science* 79, no. 5 (May 2014): R757–64.

†For more on this, see Kondo, Tomoo, Mikiya Kishi, Takashi Fushimi, Shinobu Ugajin, and Takayuki Kaga, "Vinegar Intake Reduces Body Weight, Body Fat Mass, and Serum Triglyceride Levels in Obese Japanese Subjects" *Bioscience, Biotechnology, and Biochemistry* 73, no. 8 (2009): 1837–43.

Preparation and Dosage section should be adequate to avoid burning. If excessive burning still occurs, reduce the amount of vinegar or discontinue it altogether. Some may have difficulty drinking apple cider vinegar on an empty stomach due to its acidity. If you experience an upset stomach after drinking vinegar on an empty stomach, try it after meals.

From the Clinic

A few years back, I gave a lecture about Sasang medicine at my local library. While I was giving the lecture, there was one Yin Type A woman who kept a very stern look on her face, as if to say, "What is this guy talking about?!" After the lecture I realized that she was the only one who crossed her name off the list of participants so that I would not contact her again.

Unexpectedly, she showed up at my clinic about a week later, looking very surprised. She told me that with her background as a medical doctor, she doubted that the Sasang approach would work. However, she decided to stop eating bananas and drank vinegar just to prove me wrong! During the lecture I had suggested that bananas were a Yang type food and therefore not beneficial for Yin body types. The next day she noticed a significant improvement in energy and overall digestion. She mentioned that weight gain, indigestion, and lack of energy had been an issue for her since childhood. Thinking that this may have been a fluke, she decided to continue drinking vinegar for a week longer and felt better as time went on. She even lost five pounds in that one week!

WEIGHT GAIN AND YIN TYPE B

Born with a weaker stomach and spleen, Yin Type B's are often afflicted with issues involving the digestive system. Most of them are aware of having a weaker digestive system and therefore avoid overeating or consuming foods that are not compatible with their body type. Yin Type B's also lose their appetite when they're sick or feeling stressed. Both of these contribute to the fact that Yin Type B's often appear skinny or emaciated.

Yin Moves Slowly While Yang Is Quick

The slow-moving nature of the Yin body types results in a sluggish circulatory and metabolic system. A sluggish metabolic system often leads to weight gain for Yin Type A's, but for the Yin Type B's it usually contributes to a lack of appetite, fatigue, and lethargy. Occasionally, however, a sluggish digestive system combined with the intake of incompatible foods may lead to excessive weight gain for Yin Type B's. Yin Type B's receive tremendous benefit from engaging in cardiovascular exercises, such as bicycling, jogging, swimming, brisk walking, and aerobics, because these exercises help warm up their cold system. Since they do not eat much when they're sick, unhealthy Yin Type B's often appear frail, and pale, while healthier Yin Type B's often look "pleasantly plump." If Yin Type B's experience sudden weight loss, it is usually a sign of illness, while weight gain is often a sign of improving health.

Yin Is Cold While Yang Is Hot

Yin Type B's have the least Yang energy of all the body types, contributing to cold-weather and cold-natured food sensitivities. The digestive function will slow down considerably after they ingest too many cold-natured foods or get too cold. Warmer foods, on the contrary, speed up the sluggish digestive system of Yin Type B's, giving them more energy. The Yin nature of cold fluids and cold weather steal energy away from Yin Type B's, who need ample amounts of Yang energy to survive.

An Abundant Amount of Yin Chases Away the Yang

Yin Type B's have an abundance of Yin and a lack of Yang energy. When it comes to stress and illness, too much Yin can cause trouble, leading to the stagnation and accumulation of energy in the body. An excess amount of Yin will naturally try to chase away and eliminate its opponent, Yang. Chronic stagnation of Yin may lead to issues such as weight gain, swelling, tumor growth, or other types of accumulation in the body.

Staying active is a great way to avoid the accumulation of Yin and keep the Yang energy flowing smoothly. However, with so little Yang, Yin Type B's must be careful about pushing themselves too hard. They need to cultivate their Yang as if it were still a tiny seedling. Excessive sweating, which pours down from the face like a faucet, is a sign that Yin Type B's are ill or have overworked themselves. In Sasang medicine this type of sweating occurs when Yang runs away from Yin and escapes through the skin pores. It is healthier for the Yin Type B to engage in short spurts of activity, rather than forcing themselves to continue too far past their limits. They benefit from slowing down or taking a break if they're fatigued. It is also important for Yin Type B's to consume protein shortly after working out to replenish their Yang energy.

Warm- and Hot-Natured Foods

Another way to increase Yang energy and warm the body is to eat warm- or hot-natured foods. This category of food is extremely beneficial for Yin Type B's, because it helps increase circulation, prevent colds, and support their overall health. Cool-natured foods, on the other hand, benefit Yang body types. If Yin Type B's eat too many cool-natured foods, they will eventually get indigestion, feel fatigued, and possibly gain weight. For a list of warm- and cool-natured foods, refer to table 4.1 on page 308.

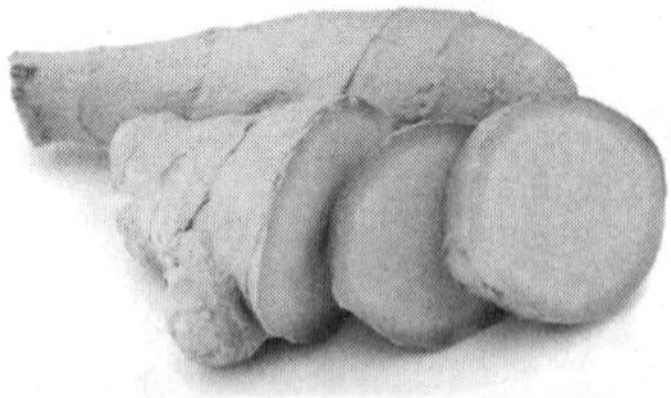

Dried Ginger (*Zingiber officinale*)

Ginger has been mentioned several times already because it is the most commonly prescribed and beneficial herb for Yin Type B's. I previously pointed out that ginger can be used for the common cold or in cases of indigestion. It can also be used to increase circulation and reduce the accumulation of Yin (or weight gain, in this case).

Recent studies have shown how that shogaol, the active ingredient in dried ginger, has the ability to enhance metabolism by stimulating the digestive process.* Shogaol's ability to regulate adipocyte (fat cell) activity and assist in the treatment of diabetes has also been documented.† Shogaols are present only in dried ginger, making it more effective than fresh ginger in supporting the digestive system and reducing fat tissue. Fresh ginger, on the other hand, contains gingerols, which are more effective in treating common colds. When ginger dries out, the gingerols naturally morph into shogaols.

Common Uses of Dried Ginger in Sasang Medicine

To alleviate weight gain, most types of digestive issues (bloating, gas, lack of appetite, diarrhea, constipation, fullness, nausea), infections, inflammation, joint pain, mouth sores, athlete's foot (topically), and emotional issues such as grief, anxiety, seasickness, morning sickness

Sources of Dried Ginger

Fresh gingerroot can be purchased at most supermarkets. Simply Organic (simplyorganic.com) sells dried ginger powder, which can be used as a condiment to spice up soups, salads, meats, and stews. Dried ginger can be purchased in bulk from manufacturers such as the Spice House (thespicehouse.com) or in capsule form from Puritan's Pride (puritan.com).

Preparation and Dosage of Dried Ginger

See page 319 for preparation and dosage of dried ginger. Follow manufacturer's dosage guidelines for intake of ginger extract capsules.

---

*For example, see Li, Yiming, Van H. Tran, Colin C. Duke, and Basil D. Roufogalis, "Preventive and Protective Properties of *Zingiber officinale* (Ginger) in Diabetes Mellitus, Diabetic Complications, and Associated Lipid and Other Metabolic Disorders: A Brief Review" *Evididence Based Complementary and Alternative Medicine* 2012: http://dx.doi.org/10.1155/2012/516870.

†See Rani, M. Priya, Mahesh S. Krishna, Keezheveettil P. Padmakumari, K. Gopal Raghu, and Andikannu Sundaresan, "*Zingiber officinale* Extract Exhibits Antidiabetic Potential via Modulating Glucose Uptake, Protein Glycation and Inhibiting Adipocyte Differentiation: an In Vitro Study" *Journal of the Science of Food and Agriculture* 92, no. 9 (July 2012): 1948–55.

Caution

Ginger can easily cause stomach irritation in the other body types. Yet this is rarely an issue for Yin Type B's, who often shock the other body types with how much ginger they can tolerate! Because it is so hot, ginger may nevertheless irritate the stomach of even a Yin Type B if taken in excess or on an empty stomach. Try taking a little break or reduce the dosage if you notice an uncomfortable burning sensation and/or acid reflux.

Herbal Friends

For a greater impact when it comes to enhancing metabolism and promoting digestion, try mixing one teaspoon of ground cinnamon and three dried cloves with one cup of ginger tea. This mixture is one of those rare Eastern herbal formulas that actually taste fantastic.

WEIGHT GAIN AND YANG TYPE A

Fat accumulation in Yang Type A's usually occurs in areas that can be easily concealed by clothing, such as the arms, thighs, and chest. This is how the Yang Type A's fatty tissue earned the name "bashful fat" in Korean. The abdomen, hips, and face are usually spared, making it difficult for others to notice the fat accumulation of the Yang Type A. Only after significant weight gain does the excessive fat start to show through clothing and extend beyond the arms, thighs, and chest of the Yang Type A. Yang Type A's with a few extra pounds may feel comfortable in a cooler climate, since they have so much Yang heat. In warmer climates, however, they tend to feel uncomfortable, fatigued, and usually sweat profusely.

Yang Moves Quickly While Yin Moves Slowly

The metabolic system relies on Yang energy to function efficiently. Since Yang Type A's have more Yang and thus a quicker metabolism than Yin types, they rarely have to worry as much about gaining too much weight. However, even Yang Type A's can gain too much weight, leading to a series of other health problems. The kidneys, which are responsible for water metabolism, are the weakest organ of the Yang Type A. The overweight Yang Type A often experiences issues related to water retention because it is the job of the kidneys to flush the system of excess water. Since most of the weight gain among Yang Type A's is due to water retention rather than fat tissue accumulation, their weight can fluctuate tremendously from one day to the next. It is common for Yang Type A's to notice swelling that comes and goes in their arms or legs after waking or eating.

Excess Yang Chases Yin Away

Like Yin Type B's, Yang Type A's also tend to get fatigued easily from exercise—but for the opposite reason, since Yang Type A's have plenty of Yang while Yin Type B's have plenty of Yin. The body is healthiest when there is a balance between Yin and Yang. Yin energy tends to be at risk when there is an excess of Yang because it can easily be pushed outward through the pores of the skin. When working out Yang Type A's easily sweat away their deficient Yin. Because Yin energy is responsible for nourishing our organs, muscles, and bones, Yang Type A's who engage in a vigorous cardio workout might experience fatigue and weakening of the muscles, organs, and bones. It is a good idea for Yang Type A's to slow down if they start to get fatigued and/or sweat profusely when working out.

Settling down and relaxing are usually the last thing on mind of Yang Type A's, since they love to stay in motion! Nevertheless, it is important for Yang Type A's to relax more often. The practice of yoga, tai chi, qi gong, and/or meditation is just as beneficial, if not more so, than a cardio workout for Yang Type A's, because these activities focus on relaxing the mind and body. It is also important for Yang Type A's to drink enough water when working out. Drinking ample amounts of water helps to replenish Yin and cool down Yang.

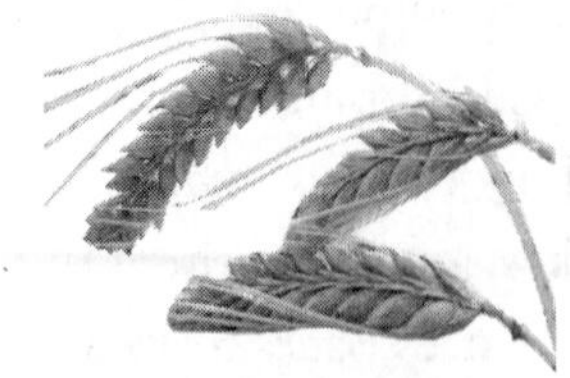

Barley
(*Hordeum vulgare*)

Barley was introduced earlier on page 261 for its stress-releasing properties. Barley has other valuable functions as well, and Yang Type A's should definitely keep it on hand. Its ability to regulate and harmonize the digestive function gives barley another moment in the Sasang medical spotlight. This function stems from barley's cold nature, which helps cool down the stomach heat of Yang Type A's. An unsettled digestive system might prevent the stomach from breaking down foods and processing them efficiently. Barley is rich in soluble and insoluble fibers. It contains a high amount of beta-glucan, a fiber that is known to help reduce cholesterol.

Common Uses of Barley in Sasang Medicine

To alleviate indigestion, weight gain, high cholesterol, stress, chronic fever, stomach inflammation, anxiety, overheating, hot flashes

Sources of Barley

There are several forms of barley available on the market. The Japanese brands House and Marubishi sell roasted barley tea bags on amazon .com. The Korean brand Dongsuh also offers roasted barley tea on the same website. The Japanese name for roasted barley tea is *mugi-cha* and the Korean name is *bori-cha*. These names may be helpful in your search for barley tea at Asian markets or online.

The other two forms of barley available in most supermarkets are pearl (or pearled) barley and hulled barley. The hulled form of barley is preferable because it retains the nutritious bran layer. Pearled barley, which is less chewy, can be used as a substitute for rice. It can be purchased from Honeyville (honeyville.com), while hulled barley can be found at Purcell Mountain Farms (purcellmountainfarms.com). Bob's Red Mill (bobsredmill.com) carries whole grain barley flour, which can be used in place of, or in conjunction with white, or wheat flour. In this form barley can be used to bake or as a thickener for soups.

Preparation and Dosage of Barley

Roasted barley tea usually comes in small tea bags. The bags are boiled with water and served warm or cold. In both Korea and Japan, roasted barley is often boiled and then chilled and consumed throughout the day in place of water. Chilled roasted barley tea is an efficient way to quickly cool the body down and keep it hydrated. Follow the directions on the package for boiling roasted barley tea. If you would like to use barley for cooking, check out recipe.com for some great ideas!

Caution

The cold nature of barley tea may lead to diarrhea in Yin types. If diarrhea occurs after drinking barley tea, it is possible that you may be a Yin type. In this case discontinue consumption of barley tea and retake the body type test or log on to sasangmedicine.com to contact a professional.

WEIGHT GAIN AND YANG TYPE B

Yang Type B's account for only 2 percent of the world's total population. With so few Yang Type B's, they are commonly mistaken for other body types. The other types may share similar psychological traits with Yang Type B's, making the body type differentiation process even more challenging!

Weight gain is one way to determine whether or not we are dealing with a genuine Yang Type B. If you come across someone with Yang Type B personality traits, take a good look at her abdomen, buttocks, chest, and neck. Don't stare too long, though, or you may be asking for trouble! A protruding abdomen would likely indicate that she is a Yin Type A. Larger buttocks without a protruding abdomen may be a sign of a Yin Type B. Broad shoulders and a developed chest without a protruding abdomen or buttocks may be a sign of a Yang Type A. If she has a thicker neck, pointy ears or a cone-shaped head, and/or upwardly slanted eyebrows, you may be dealing with a genuine Yang Type B! These characteristics often set Yang Type B's apart from the other body types, even though they can display similar personalities.

An Abundance of Yang

Yang Type B's have an abundance of Yang, making them reluctant to slow down and rest when necessary. This also makes it challenging for Yang Type B's to gain weight because they are constantly burning off extra calories. Yang Type B's need to keep themselves occupied while refraining from overwork. Pushing too hard can contribute to weight gain just as much as inactivity, because it derails the body's natural cycle. Yang Type B's benefit tremendously from taking short naps in the afternoon, eating at regular intervals, and getting enough sleep. It is also important for Yang Type B's to drink at least thirty-two ounces of water throughout the day to replenish their Yin and flush their system of toxins.

In conjunction with a balanced lifestyle, Yang Type B's should choose the foods that correspond to their body type and support the function of their weaker liver. When the energy of the liver is not flowing in harmony, the Yang Type B's health can take a turn for the worse. The liver plays a primary role in filtering waste from food products. Despite being so active, even Yang Type B's could gain too much weight as the result of an overwhelmed liver.

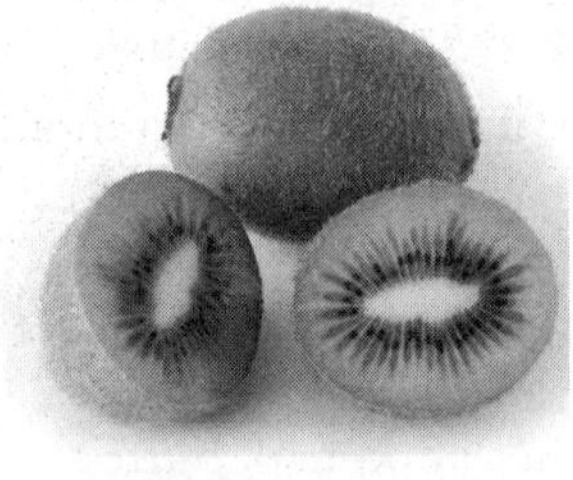

Kiwi Fruit

Kiwi fruit was introduced on page 272 for its ability to alleviate high blood pressure because it cools the excessive heat of the Yang Type B's liver. By reducing excess heat, kiwi also helps the liver eliminate food by-products and toxins from the body. Hence, it can play an effective role in the Yang Type B's weight loss program.

As noted one kiwi fruit has 75 percent of the recommended daily allowance of vitamin C and almost as much potassium as a banana. Kiwi skin is filled with antioxidants and the seeds are a significant source of omega-3 fatty acids.

Common Uses of Kiwi Fruit in Sasang Medicine

To alleviate high blood pressure, circulatory issues (cold extremities, numbness of the extremities, weight gain), indigestion, common colds, sinus and lung congestion

Sources of Kiwi Fruit

Kiwi fruit can be found in most supermarkets year-round.

Preparation and Dosage of Kiwi Fruit

Ingest two kiwi fruits a day to cool liver heat. One kiwi fruit a day can help prevent colds and promote digestion.

Joint Pain

Eastern medicine developed through the belief that there is no separation between people and nature. The observation of nature thus shed light on the biological processes of the human body. Rivers were equated with blood vessels and flowing water with blood circulation in the body. There is an ancient story in China of a man named Yu the Great, who prevented a major flood by diverting the Yangtze River, while his predecessors made several failed attempts at blocking water overflow by stacking up trenches. This story illustrates that Eastern medicine focuses on directing the flow of energy throughout the body, rather than blocking the signal of pain to the mind. The joints of the body can also be compared to a bend in a river, where water tends to accumulate and lose its momentum. Joints are areas where blood and fluid tend to slow down and accumulate, especially as a result of too much or too little exercise. Too much exercise makes our joints resemble a river bend that swells after a flood. A lack of exercise causes the blood and fluid to stagnate, like the murky pockets of water in a dried-out riverbed.

Most of us would be shocked to hear our doctor diagnose arthritis when we report joint pain. *Arthritis* literally means "inflammation of the joint(s)," which actually starts to occur in most people from the young age of thirty. Arthritic pain, though, does not necessarily occur after the onset of arthritis. Pain due to arthritis is usually detected earlier in individuals who lead either an excessively active or an excessively sedentary lifestyle. It also shows up in those who live in markedly warmer or colder climate zones. Since Yang types are sensitive to heat, their joints may start to hurt in warmer and/or dryer weather, while Yin types usually experience joint pain in cooler and/or damper weather.

So why do our joints swell? The simple answer is usage. The more we use our joints, the more energy and blood our body sends to them. Most doctors fail to tell their aching patients that swelling of the joints is actually a natural process. The pulling action of a muscle on the bone helps make it stronger. This pulling forms the "T" shape at the end of every bone, and is the result of the body's natural growth process. However, as we get older, our bones get weaker. In order to avoid fracturing, the joints absorb more calcium and continue to increase in size. This is when issues such as arthritis and bone-spur formation begin. Arthritis and bone spurs are the body's way of protecting us from injury. Pain arises when a joint gets too big and starts to press down on surrounding nerves and soft tissue.

This section offers several strategies for treating common joint-related issues, such as lower-back pain, knee pain, and shoulder pain. These remedies can also be extended to the treatment of joint pain elsewhere on the same limb. Herbs prescribed for shoulder pain, for example, are often used to treat wrist pain as well. Herbs prescribed for hip pain are often used for knee pain, too. Each remedy listed in this section will specify its primary area of focus.

Let's take a moment to review some helpful suggestions for keeping your joints healthy and happy. These extend beyond the boundaries of our body type and could be applied to almost every situation.

General Tip #1: Avoid Too Much or Too Little Activity

It is human nature to think that more is better. Exercise is no exception to this rule, so most avid runners show early signs of arthritis. Try exercising every other day, alternate between working out flexor and extensor muscle groups, or rotating your workout routine to avoid taxing the same joint. Lifting heavy weights can also cause joint injury. Try more repetitions of lighter weights to avoid placing a heavy load on the joints.

Inactivity is just as damaging to the joints as too much activity. Blood and energy tend to accumulate in the joints when the body is stationary for more than thirty minutes. This accumulation in the joints leads to inflammation and weakness. Those with jobs requiring prolonged use of a computer can benefit their joints by getting up and moving around a bit every thirty minutes, as movement helps circulate blood and energy through them. Exercise sends oxygen and essential nutrients to the bone and also helps prevent disorders commonly seen after menopause, such as osteoporosis or ostepenia.

General Tip #2: The Power of Stretching

Time seems to pass by so quickly, especially as we get older. Even finding the time to eat is often a challenge for many of us, let alone making the time to stretch in the morning or before and after exercise. Exercise is, nevertheless, a great way to keep our joints and muscles relaxed and free of pain. We spend plenty of time flexing our muscles throughout the day. But the muscles need to extend just as much as they need to flex. Stretching helps give our muscles and joints a break by reversing the direction of movement they typically follow during the day. Joint pain is often the result of too much flexion and a lack of extension. A balance between the two is the key to maintaining healthy joints. Check out pages 219–22 in the "Exercise according to Your Yin Yang Body Type" chapter for a few common stretches for your general health.

General Tip #3: Walking Is the Best Exercise

While at the gym yesterday, I read a sign claiming that pain is a form of weakness and stressing the importance of pushing beyond pain to enhance our health. Actually, we do not have to push ourselves too hard or work out vigorously to maintain optimum health. After the age of thirty, consistent but less arduous exercise is the key to staying healthy. The continuous push past our physical limitations when exercising eventually leads to arthritic pain as we age. Brisk walking, biking, and swimming are perhaps among the best exercises for strengthening the joints and improving our circulation. It is much easier on the knees than jogging or running but just as, if not more, beneficial. Work your way up to a thirty-minute to one-hour walk five times a week to maintain ample circulation and bone strength.

General Tip #4: Watch Those Cravings!

Food plays an important role in the health of our joints. Ingestion of excessively sweet or salty foods can result in joint inflammation and fluid retention. Deep-fried and oily foods tend to thicken the blood and impede circulation around the joints. Foods that are easier to digest also make it easier for the blood to flow to and through the joints.

General Tip #5: Hang Around

Our joints are constantly under pressure during the day while we are out and about. Standing, in and of itself, places a tremendous amount of pressure on practically every joint in the body. The knees and lower back get the worst of the abuse, since they hold most of our weight. In short our joints could always use a break. Hanging from a chin-up bar and swinging gently back and forth is one way to release the pressure on the joints. An inversion table is another way to "hang out."

General Tip #6: Don't Slouch!

When sitting the pressure on the lower back increases approximately 20 percent, compared to when we are standing. The rise of lower-back problems in modern society coincides with the increase in sedentary, computer-related jobs. Our body was not made to sit as long as many of us ask it to. Slouching can make matters worse, since we lose the natural "S" shape of the spine. The "S" shape is what helps it to absorb excess pressure, like the coiled shock absorbers in an automobile. If we are sitting in a slouched position, pressure on our lower back may increase by more than 100 percent! This can be compared to jumping on a small balloon, filled with water. Such excessive pressure would likely cause the balloon to pop, sending water in all directions. Luckily each gel-filled disk in our spine is encapsulated within a very hardy shell. However, years of ongoing pressure eventually cause the gel to get squeezed beyond its limits and to protrude outward. Maintaining good posture can save your spinal disks from extensive damage!

Caution: Most herbs that help with joint pain also promote circulation and should not be used in conjunction with blood thinners, such as Coumadin. They should also be avoided directly before or after surgery because of possible interference with other medications.

JOINT PAIN AND YIN TYPE A

Only with an ample flow of oxygen from the lungs can the heart circulate blood efficiently. The weaker lungs of Yin Type A's contribute to diminished overall circulation, eventually leading to an accumulation of blood and energy around the joints. This, in turn, leads to swelling and toxicity. To make matters worse, the stronger liver of Yin Type A's is much better at absorbing toxins from the bloodstream, but less efficient at eliminating them from the body. These toxins may leak back into the bloodstream and get lodged in the joints, causing additional swelling and discomfort.

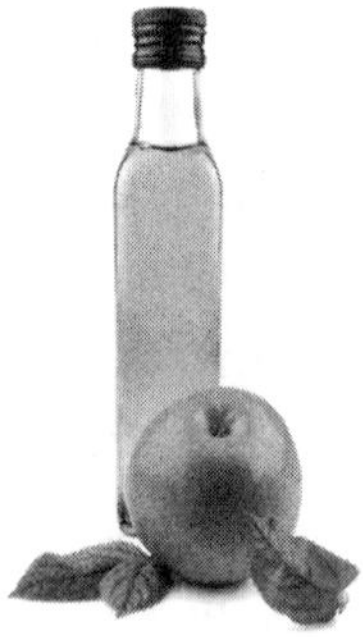

Apple Cider Vinegar

Sound familiar? Vinegar was introduced on page 267 for its ability to treat high blood pressure and weight gain in Yin Type A's. I would like to reintroduce it here as a remedy for joint pain as well. Vinegar is one of the most effective supplements for Yin Type A's when it comes to blood circulation. In Sasang medicine pain stems from stagnation of energy and blood flow. Pain is not an issue when energy and blood flow smoothly to and through the joints. Vinegar promotes joint health throughout the body because of its ability to send blood and energy to and through the joints. Pectin, a component of vinegar, helps absorb and flush the system of excess toxicity. The acetic acid in vinegar also helps to purify and cleanse the body.

Common Uses of Apple Cider Vinegar in Sasang Medicine

To address joint pain, high blood pressure, circulatory issues (cold extremities, numbness of the extremities, weight gain), indigestion

Sources of Apple Cider Vinegar

Apple cider vinegar is available at most supermarkets year-round.

Preparation and Dosage of Apple Cider Vinegar

See page 268, for preparation and dosage of apple cider vinegar.

Caution

Apple cider vinegar is very acidic, aromatic, and potent. This is how it helps get energy flowing better throughout the body. However, these properties may cause burning of the tongue and throat in some individuals. Make sure to dilute vinegar with an ample amount of water when starting an apple cider vinegar regimen. The above ratio should be adequate for most people.

Diary Entry:
Cathy—a 48-year-old Yin Type A

I have been suffering with arthritis pain of my hands and knees for several years. The pain was worse immediately after getting up in the morning. Dr. Wagman suggested that I try apple cider vinegar for my arthritis pain, after describing it as an important remedy for my body type. After the third day of taking apple cider vinegar I noticed that the pain in my hands and knees was gone! To be sure that this was not a fluke, I decided not to take the apple cider vinegar the following day, and the pain returned. I have been supplementing with apple cider vinegar every morning for three months now and have not noticed any recurrence of pain!

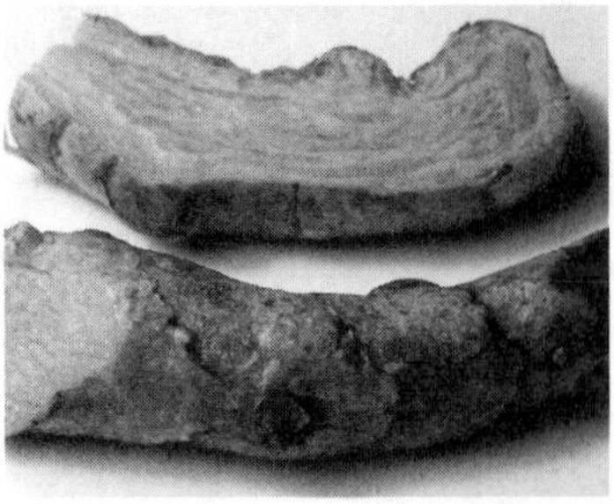

Turmeric (*Curcuma Longa*)

The use of turmeric in Indian (ayurvedic) medicine dates back to approximately 1900 BCE. As a sacred plant in the Hindu religion, it is often used in ceremonies. Turmeric's beautiful flowers and powerful medicinal function contribute to its significant role in Indian and Chinese history. Curcumin, the most active component of turmeric, is known to have an equal or greater effect than ibuprofen in relieving joint pain. Turmeric is especially useful for relieving joint pain in the upper body, such as the shoulders, neck, elbows, and hands. It also has anticancer and anti-inflammatory properties. According to Sasang medicine, turmeric enhances the flow of blood and energy circulation in the body, and when energy and blood are flowing harmoniously throughout the body, pain does not occur.

Common Uses of Turmeric in Sasang Medicine

To address upper-body joint pain (of the shoulder, neck, elbows, and/or hands), menstrual pain, traumatic injury that causes bruising, stiffness of the shoulder and/or arm

Sources of Turmeric

Turmeric (also known as curcumin) can be purchased from most supermarkets as a powder or condiment. Turmeric extract can be purchased in capsule form online from Puritan's Pride (puritan.com) and Nature's Way (naturesway.com). Curapro is a high-quality source of turmeric that can be purchased from euromedicausa.com.

Preparation and Dosage of Turmeric

Turmeric can be used as a condiment in soups, stews, and salads and is a component of curry powder, which is used in curries and other Indian dishes.

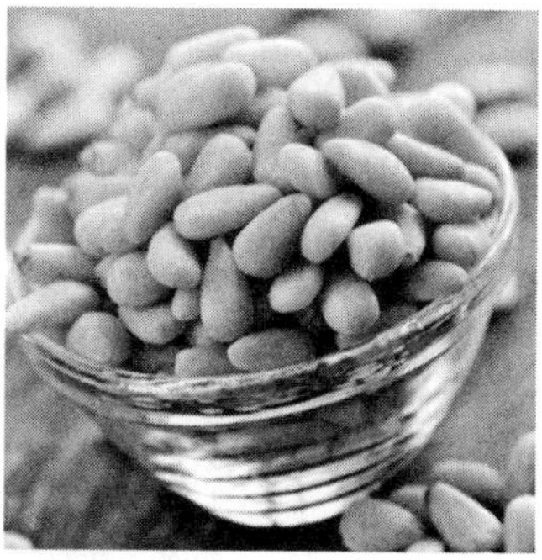

Pine Nuts
(*Pinus*)

Pine nuts are ingested to strengthen the bones, making them a suitable remedy for joint pain related to osteopenia or osteoporosis. Pine nuts are especially beneficial for joint issues occurring in the lower body, such as the lower-back, knee, ankle, or toe joints. Each pine nut has up to 35 percent of its weight in protein, therefore making it a great source of cellular energy. Pine nuts are also gluten- and cholesterol-free.

Common Uses of Pine Nuts in Sasang Medicine

To ease lower-body joint pain (ankles, knees, hips), osteoporosis, osteopenia, tooth decay, tooth pain, skin dryness, menstrual issues

Sources of Pine Nuts

Several varieties of pine nuts are available. European pine nuts, also called stone nuts, are slender and longer than the Asian variety. Despite a difference in shape, the two varieties are equally beneficial for the bones. Less expensive pine nuts can be purchased in bulk from nuts.com. Organic pine nuts are available from Woodstock Farms (woodstock-foods.com) and Trader Joe's natural food stores.

Preparation and Dosage of Pine Nuts

Pine nuts make a good snack and can also serve as a valuable ingredient in numerous delicious recipes: check out recipe.com. In Korea pine nuts are often sprinkled onto teas to add a pleasant, nutty taste. Try it with your favorite tea!

JOINT PAIN AND YIN TYPE B

In Eastern medicine stronger kidneys are equated with stronger bones. Since the kidneys are the strongest organ of Yin Type B's, those with this body type tend to have fewer long-term bone-related issues, compared to the other body types. The kidneys help "feed" the bones by supplying them with blood and energy. The bones of Yin Type B's are therefore stronger and less prone to fracture or arthritis than those of the other body types. The stronger bones of Yin Type B's often contrast with their frail-looking appearance. When the bones of Yin Type B's get weaker, it is a sign that their overall health is failing.

Yin Type B's are born with a weaker digestive system, which can eventually lead to the onset of arthritis and joint pain. The digestive system is a major source of strength for the bones because it provides them with energy from food. Herbs that have the dual function of promoting digestive health and supporting the bones are therefore used to assist Yin Type B's with joint pain.

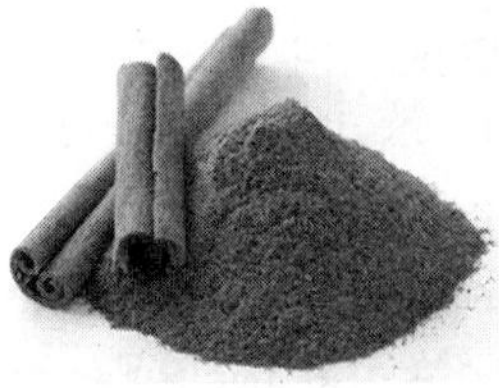

Cinnamon Tea (*Cortex Cinnamomi Cassiae*)

Cinnamon has the dual function of supporting the digestive system and strengthening the bones. The latter function stems from its ability to reinforce the kidneys, which are in charge of bone and joint health. Cinnamon is also rich in fiber, calcium, and iron, all of which help to strengthen the bones. In a Copenhagen University Hospital study, 200 patients with arthritis pain were given half a teaspoon of cinnamon powder with one tablespoon of honey every morning. Most patients showed significant relief of knee pain after one week. After one month 75 participants out of 200 who had been immobile before the study were able to walk without any pain at all.*

*From "Benefits of Cinnamon in Arthiritis," www.benefitsfromcinnamon.com/benefits/benefits-of-cinnamon-in-arthritis.

Common Uses of Cinnamon in Sasang Medicine

To address headaches, circulatory issues (numbness, tingling, and/or coldness of the extremities), joint and muscle inflammation, lower-back and knee pain, sensitivity to cold

Sources of Cinnamon

Cinnamon bark can be purchased from most supermarkets throughout the United States. Suppliers such as Nature's Answer (naturesanswer.com), Solaray (solaray.com), and Gaia (gaiaherbs.com) offer a capsulated extract form of cinnamon.

Preparation and Dosage of Cinnamon

Raw cinnamon bark is prepared by boiling three slices of two- to three-inch bark in two cups of water. Let the tea simmer on the lowest flame for fifteen minutes. More or less cinnamon can be added depending on your taste preference. If you're using capsules, refer to the manufacturer's dosage guidelines.

JOINT PAIN AND YANG TYPE A

As we have seen, the kidneys are responsible for supplying energy and blood to the bones. It is common for Yang Type A's, who are born with weaker kidneys, to feel chronic lower-back/knee pain and weakness. Older Yang Type A's are often plagued with excess curvature of the upper spine and/or arthritis of the lower back. To preserve the integrity of their bones, Yang Type A's must take every precaution. If you are a Yang Type A, consistent walking, stretching, and calcium supplementation will help do the trick. These methods are especially beneficial for postmenopausal Yang Type A women, who face the risk of osteopenia and osteoporosis.

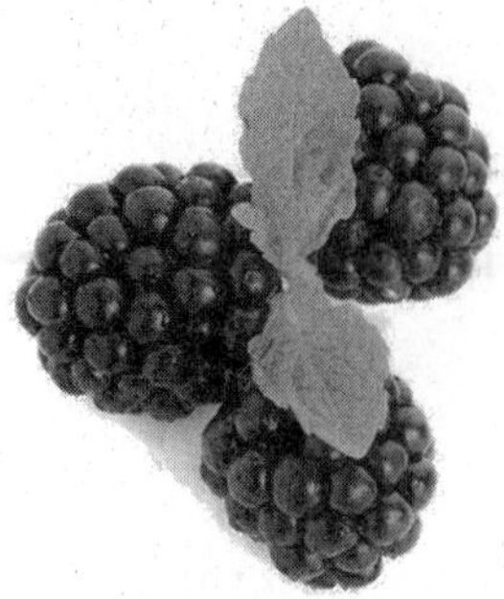

Blackberries
(*Rubus fruticosus*)

In my home state of Oregon, many of us are all too familiar with blackberries. This fruit, which was introduced on the East Coast in the early 1800s from Europe, traveled rapidly toward the Pacific Northwest, taking over fields and roadsides along the way! Most Oregonians view blackberries as a menace, rather than a medicine. However, blackberry is an invaluable medicine for Yang Type A's because it strengthens the kidneys, their weakest organ. Since the kidneys support the lower back and legs, this herb addresses chronic lower-back pain. Blackberry, which targets hips, knees, ankles, and toes, is very rich in nutrients, such as dietary fiber, vitamins C and K, folic acid, and manganese. It is ranked one of the best antioxidant foods by the National Institute of Health; antioxidants eliminate free radicals and help the body fight off infection.* The tiny black seeds in each blackberry are high in omega-3 and omega-5 fatty acids and protein. Lastly, blackberries have the highest concentration of phytoestrogens of any fruit. Phytoestrogens are a natural source of estrogen, which plays a major role in keeping the bones strong and the tendons flexible after menopause.

Common Uses of Blackberries in Sasang Medicine

To alleviate joint pain (hips, knees, ankles, and toes), bone pain, postmenopausal issues (osteoporosis, osteopenia), frozen shoulder (in Korean this is referred to as "fifty-year shoulder" because it traditionally occurs after or around menopause—at about age fifty—from a lack of estrogen)

*From "Top 100 High ORAC Value Antioxidant Foods," http://modernsurvivalblog.com/health/high-orac-value-antioxidant-foods-top-100.

Sources of Blackberries

Fresh blackberries are seasonally available fresh or frozen at most supermarkets. Off-season (winter) supplies are sometimes available in supermarkets along the West Coast. Dried blackberries are available all year-round from nuts.com. Freeze-dried blackberries, which can be easily dissolved in water, are available from Z Natural Foods (znaturalfoods.com).

Preparation and Dosage of Blackberries

A handful of fresh or dried blackberries a day can provide plenty of energy to the Yang Type A's kidneys. Three cups of blackberry tea a day can help prevent bone-related issues. Blackberry tea is prepared by boiling a handful of dried blackberries in two to three cups of water. Let the tea simmer for fifteen minutes and drink it cool or warm, depending on your preference. Blackberries also make a yummy ingredient or garnish in salads, oatmeal, or yogurt.

JOINT PAIN AND YANG TYPE B

Yang energy rises upward while Yin energy sinks downward. Joint pain and arthritic issues tend to develop in the weaker lower body of Yang Type B's. Yang also corresponds to activity while Yin corresponds to inactivity. When it comes to alleviating joint pain, it is important to establish a balance between activity and rest. The excess Yang energy of Yang Type B's makes it difficult for them to slow down and rest when they need to. Yang Type B's have to slow down and remember not to push their body too far, especially if they have joint issues.

Another challenge for Yang Type B's is that they have difficulty registering pain. Since their mind is always so active, they may not even realize that they're having arthritic issues! Yang Type B's rarely feel any discomfort when they are sick or experiencing trauma. A common cold, for example, can go from bad to worse without Yang Type B's taking notice. They simply push, push, and push until they're utterly exhausted.

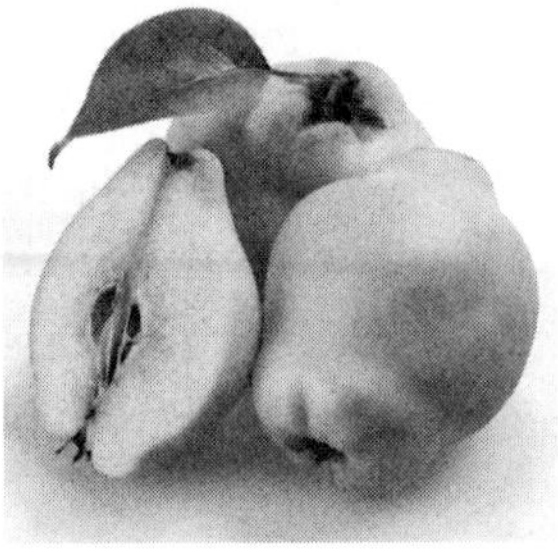

Chinese Quince Fruit (*Cydonia oblonga*)

See page 323 for a description of Chinese Quince Fruit.

Common Uses of Chinese Quince Fruit in Sasang Medicine

For relief of indigestion, vomiting, joint pain of the lower body, weakness of the legs and hip area, swelling of the legs, knees, and/or ankles

Sources of Chinese Quince Fruit

Quince fruit tea, mixed with honey, is often sold in Korean markets. If you do not live near a Korean market, try ordering it from posharpstore.com. Gardeners can purchase quince fruit trees from Willis Orchard Company (willisorchards.com). Made in Oregon (madeinoregon.com) has a delicious quince fruit spread, while quince fruit extract can be purchased from the Herb Doc (herbdoc.com).

The Pain Dilemma

The ability to ignore pain may sound appealing to most of us. However, pain is the body's way of signaling to us that something is wrong. Our ability to recognize pain allows us to take the necessary steps to improve our health situation. A broken leg would prompt most people to go to the hospital. Constant indigestion would likely cause us to make necessary changes to our diet and/or lifestyle. Yang Type B's are rarely aware of discomfort associated with illness or injury. Yin Type B's, by contrast, always seem to be plagued by one sort of pain or another. Which body type tends to be healthier? Despite the constant aches and pains of Yin Type B's, they tend to be healthier and live longer than Yang Type B's, simply because they can recognize pain.

When we are in the midst of a painful situation, it is often hard to see the light at the end of the tunnel. We may question whether or not it is possible to ever get better! Severe pain may cause us to think we are seriously ill. This is not necessarily the case. The extent of pain is not necessarily equivalent to the extent of injury or illness. Chronically debilitating illness often loses its ability to elicit a pain signal as time goes on. The level of pain depends solely on our level of sensitivity and the strength of our body's pain signal.

Most people spend a great deal of their energy avoiding pain. A recent study showed that one in five Americans misuse and often become addicted to pain-related pharmaceuticals, such as muscle relaxers, anti-inflammatory drugs, cortisone, or oxycodone.* Western medicine has developed efficient ways to mask pain through medication. While this approach may provide temporary relief, it could eventually make matters worse, because it shuts down the body's natural alarm system, giving us the illusion that we are better off than we really are.

Pain is the body's way of telling us that something is wrong. Severe illness could result if we simply ignore or suppress it. Listen to your body and try your best to address its concerns. If, no matter how you try, pain just keeps nagging its way into your comfort zone, perhaps the advances of Western medicine may be at least a temporary answer. Most of my patients, however, are surprised by how much they can accomplish by listening to their body and making a consistent effort to address the body's needs. It is my greatest hope that by introducing you to Sasang medicine, this book helps you navigate toward health and harmony.

---

*From "Substance Abuse and Addiction Health Center," *WebMD* www.webmd.com/mental-health/addiction/features/prescription-drug-abuse-who-gets-addicted-and-why.

Food and Airborne Allergies

Allergy treatment is nowhere to be found in Eastern medicine, despite its five-thousand-year history, filled with countless medical teachings and treatment strategies. If allergy symptoms are so common, why are they not mentioned? Let's take a look at a few possible explanations.

Centuries ago most people did not need to dead bolt their front doors, nor did they have to worry about protecting themselves from carbon dioxide or other pollutants that fill the air. The immune system of those living in contemporary society is often forced to be on high alert, as stress, fear, and mistrust become the norm. A constantly engaged immune system may eventually lose track of who is friend and who is foe. To further illustrate this point, imagine a situation in which every third person entering a palace intended to assassinate the emperor. The palace guards would quickly grow suspicious of everyone. This can be compared to an allergic reaction to pollen in the spring. Pollen itself does not pose a danger to the body, but other sensitivities cause the immune system to grow suspicious of everything it comes in contact with. When the immune system is constantly on high alert, our body will attempt to rid itself of danger by sneezing, tearing, or causing us to scratch out the "bad guys."

In ancient times work was less sedentary and required more time outdoors. In the modern era, most of us spend the majority of our time indoors, often exposing ourselves to dust, mildew, detergents, and other irritants, which may eventually confuse and overwhelm the immune system. Less physical activity may also lead to a greater accumulation of toxins in the body, and these too overwhelm the immune system.

According to Eastern medicine, both of the above scenarios—spending the majority of our time indoors and creating immune system hypersensitivity—could lead to an imbalance of *wei qi*, or "immune shield." The *wei qi* is a reflection of how we feel both emotionally and physically at any given moment. When the body is ill or stressed, the *wei qi* will naturally become more sensitive as it attempts to protect its vulnerable host. Although Eastern medicine does not mention "allergy" treatment per se, balancing the *wei qi* is effective in addressing practically any type of allergy-related symptom. The lungs, stomach, liver, and other organs all have their own "immune system," or *wei qi* affiliate. Each organ has its own immune-regulating function from the standpoint of both Eastern and Western medicine. Imbalance of one or more of these organs leads to an immune response.

While there are numerous external allergy triggers, such as pollen, mold, and fragrance, that may prompt the onset of allergies, Sasang medicine focuses mainly on addressing internal factors. Each of the body types has its own source of allergy symptoms, based on their weakest organ. Allergies are therefore addressed by supporting the weakest organ with foods, herbs, and/or supplements. To illustrate the Yin Type A's weaker lungs are the primary focus in allergy treatment, even if stomach allergies are present. When addressing allergies of the Yin Type B, treatment focuses on the weaker spleen. Allergy treatment for Yang Type A's bolsters their weaker kidneys. Finally, strengthening the weaker liver is a priority when treating the Yang Type B's allergies.

AIRBORNE ALLERGIES (TO DUST, POLLEN, MOLD, PET DANDER, AND/OR PERFUME)

Respiratory allergies are characterized by prolonged sinus congestion, sneezing, or coughing that is not associated with other common cold-related symptoms, such as fever and/or chills, fatigue, or excessive sweating. Symptoms may also be exacerbated by inhaling the scent of perfume, being outdoors, eating trigger foods, or entering a particular room or office. Allergy symptoms may become acute, causing difficulty breathing and even loss of consciousness. If you experience difficulty breathing, whether or not it is due to an allergic reaction, seek medical attention immediately.

It is common in the West to focus on elimination when it comes to treating allergies. Obviously, it is beneficial, if possible, to remove an allergy trigger from your immediate environment. However, this leaves us with the question of how and why the allergy occurred in the first place. Yin Type A's, for example, are born with weaker lungs, and since the lungs play a major role in immune activity, this weakness may lead to allergies and hypersensitivity. Even if Yin Type A's suffer from food allergies, it is still important to address the weakness of their lungs. Yin Type B's are born with a weaker digestive system, and even if Yin Type B's suffer from airborne allergies, it is still important to address the weaknes of their digestive system. The Sasang approach focuses on balancing the organs as a means of treating allergies. A balanced system does not overreact to its environment.

FOOD ALLERGIES AND SENSITIVITIES

A food allergy or sensitivity is an acute or chronic immune response to eating a particular food. Food allergy symptoms may not be as conspicuous as respiratory allergy symptoms. Chronic fatigue, bloating, and/or bowel issues (such as constipation and/or diarrhea) after eating certain foods may be signs of food allergies. I often see clients who experience chronic headaches due to food allergies. Food allergies may also cause acute symptoms, such as severe bloating, gas, stomach cramps, and/or vomiting. Knowing if you have food allergies is no easy task. The Eastern medical practitioner usually checks the pulse to determine how your digestive system is doing, but this is not the only method. The most effective way to determine if you have a food allergy is simply to listen to your stomach. A food allergy is nothing other than an overwhelmed digestive system. Our relationship with food is an excellent way to get to know our body type.

General Tip #1: Listen to Your Body

The body is our greatest source of information when it comes to food allergies. After eating a meal, listen to what your body is saying. Are you excessively fatigued? Do you feel bloated or have a lot of gas? Are you constipated or do you have diarrhea? Do your sinuses feel congested all of a sudden? If you answered yes to any of these questions, it is likely that your stomach may be reacting to recently ingested food. In some cases it may be easy to identify which food triggered such symptoms. In other cases it may be necessary to eliminate certain foods one by one until you are sure of what triggered your symptoms. However, elimination itself is not the only answer. Treatment in Sasang medicine often focuses on strengthening the digestive system with foods, herbs, and exercises that mesh with your body type.

An allergic reaction may also be due to how the food was prepared, the quality of the food itself, or how quickly you ate it. In such cases chewing food more slowly and making an attempt to consume good-quality foods may be the answer.

General Tip #2: Simplify Your Diet

Do you often feel bloated or uncomfortable after eating? Does your body seem to resist almost everything you eat? If so, it may be a good idea for you to simplify your diet and start from scratch. To accomplish this you may want to cook up a large bowl of soup while eliminating other foods from your diet. Each day add another ingredient to the soup, such as vegetables, meat, and condiments. After ingestion listen to your tummy and see if you are experiencing any distress. Are you still feeling bloated? Are your bowels flowing smoothly? If things go well, try expanding your meal by adding a side dish, such as rice. If you have only minor bloating or discomfort after meals, the solution may simply be to reduce your food intake per meal or spread out your food intake into smaller portions throughout the day.

Food sensitivities may fluctuate. Food that did not previously lead to indigestion may suddenly cause digestive issues. By contrast foods that you may have been previously sensitive to may suddenly become easier for you to ingest. This is because food allergies are often due to the reaction of the digestive system, rather than the food itself. Sure, it is important to read food labels, eat clean foods, and avoid eating a food beyond the expiration date. However, harmonizing the digestive system and balancing the energies of your body type are always the core focus of food allergy treatment, according to Sasang medicine.

General Tip #3: Adjust Your Food Temperature

Yin types benefit from consuming warmer-natured foods, while Yang types benefit from cooler-natured foods. If Yin types consume excessive amounts of very cold-natured foods, they may experience food allergies. If Yang types consume excessive amounts of very hot-natured foods, they too may experience food allergies. By eating according to our body type, we often avoid the onset of food allergies.

SKIN ALLERGIES (URTICARIA, CONTACT DERMATITIS, PSORIASIS, ECZEMA, COMMON RASHES, AND FIBROMYALGIA)

According to Eastern medicine, the lungs correspond to the skin. Healthy skin is a sign of healthy lungs. Skin-related allergies are commonly associated with lung issues, such as common colds, chronic sinusitis, asthma, or bronchitis. Children with asthma almost always have accompanying skin reactions, such as rashes or psoriasis. You may also notice that when you're fighting off a cold, suffering from asthma, and/or dealing with allergy symptoms your skin becomes more sensitive. Fibromyalgia, according to Sasang medicine, is another form of immune, or *wei-qi,* sensitivity in which the skin and surrounding tissue are very sensitive to even the slightest pressure. People who suffer from fibromyalgia do not necessarily experience allergy-related symptoms other than hypersensitivity to touch. In Sasang medicine fibromyalgia is often associated with weakened or blocked lung energy. Common factors, such as high stress, physical or emotional trauma, and/or issues relating to trust and acceptance, tend to affect the flow of lung energy. Thus, these factors may also contribute to the onset of fibromyalgia.

Skin allergies, like other allergies, are due to a sensitivity of the immune system. The immune system gets overwhelmed if the body is on high alert all the time. Some individuals with skin allergies eventually become sensitive to almost everything they touch. Others may notice a skin rash, boils, or skin inflammation from simply being too hot or cold, being around pets, or feeling stressed out. The immune system is controlled by phagocytes, or immune cells, that are constantly scavenging out our enemies. Nothing is more powerful than the influence of our mind, however, when it comes to the function of our body. According to Sasang medicine, a balanced mind is an essential component in the process of overcoming illness. Each body type has its own emotional tendencies. Balancing these emotional tendencies helps to promote a smooth flow of energy throughout the body, and this will help balance our immune system.

General Tip #1: Go Natural

Did you change shampoo, conditioner, or soap lately? If you experience skin or scalp allergies, try using a different type of shampoo, soap, and/or laundry detergent. Luckily, there are many products on the market made from organic or primarily natural ingredients. Products that contain larger amounts of alcohol or eucalyptus may cause dry skin. Just because a product is natural does not automatically exclude it from causing skin allergies. Keep on trying even if the shift to another shampoo or soap does not seem to make a difference.

General Tip #2: Keep Your Skin Moist

Dryness can exacerbate skin allergies and other conditions, such as psoriasis or eczema. The daily use of skin lotion may alleviate skin allergies and other skin problems. Try keeping your skin moist at all times to help it breathe and function better. The choice of which moisturizer to use is not easy. Oil-based products may help your skin feel moist longer but suffocate it in the process. Water- or wax-based products allow room for the skin to breathe but may offer only short-term moisture and need to be applied consistently throughout the day.

These quick tips may also be helpful:

- Try avoiding moisturizers made with difficult to pronounce chemicals to prevent your skin from feeling dry or more sensitive.
- Make sure to wash your skin before applying another layer of moisturizer. Applying a double layer of moisturizer before washing may lead to skin irritation because you may end up trapping sweat and dirt.
- Apply moisturizer lightly to prevent skin irritation.
- Using creamy soaps that are made with moisturizers may help prevent skin dryness for those who need to wash their hands often.

General Tip #3: Rub Instead of Scratching

Using your fingernails to scratch sensitive skin can lead to further irritation. If part of your skin is itchy, try using your palm or the pads of your fingers. Also, rubbing around the area causes less sensitivity than rubbing directly on it. Lastly, remember to wash your hands before rubbing! Tiny particles on your fingers and palms may trigger another allergic reaction.

TESTING FOR RESPIRATORY AND FOOD ALLERGIES

Allergy testing is becoming more and more common, due to the recent increase in allergy-related conditions. The most popular and readily available test, called a skin prick test, records the response to tiny pricks on a strip of paper placed on the skin. Allergies can also be tested using blood tests, such as the E95 Basic Food Panel, which is often performed by a naturopathic doctor. The results of these tests are helpful in some cases but debatable in others. They may help us determine whether or not the body is oversensitive to certain allergens. However, once the body reacts to a single allergen, it has a tendency to react quicker to other indicators on the same test. Before we know it, we may end up with false positive results for allergies in almost every category. Excess sensitivity is a key component of the allergy response.

THE SASANG APPROACH TO ALLERGIES

In the West allergy treatment often consists of using antihistamines, bronchodilators, immunosuppresants, or other pharmaceutical prescriptions based on your symptoms. Focus is also placed on avoiding certain foods and/or places that are believed to trigger allergic reactions. While avoidance may be beneficial in some cases, it fails to get to the root of the problem.

The Sasang medical approach focuses primarily on the person behind the symptom, rather than the symptom itself. The treatment of allergies is no exception. Like Western medicine, Sasang medicine acknowledges the importance of avoiding foods and/or places that may aggravate an allergic response. However, this is not of prime concern. Emphasis is placed on comforting and balancing the immune system, rather than suppressing it, by strengthening and supporting the function of each body type's weakest organ.

When an organ's energy is blocked or weakened, it sends an SOS signal to the rest of the body. The other organs then chip in to help out. For example, if you are having difficulty inhaling (a problem, that is, with the lungs), the heart beats faster or stronger to circulate as much oxygen as possible throughout your body. If an infection develops in your bladder, your kidneys will call for more urination. When our body is in harmony, this process occurs smoothly throughout every moment of our lives. When it doesn't the immune system kicks in to protect the body from invasion while the organs figure out what to do. This process may occur without our knowing what's happening. If the imbalance continues, the immune system will never have a chance to rest or replenish itself efficiently.

OVERALL ALLERGY TIPS

General Tip #1: Work on Acceptance and Trust

A continuously engaged immune system may cause hypersensitivity, which is not limited to food or pollen but also involves the emotions. Our stomach and/or sinuses will react to excessive stress and other emotional imbalances. In Eastern medicine the stomach is said to digest experience as well as food. Unpleasant experiences can lead to emotional indigestion, and this may trigger food allergies.

Try this quick and simple method, which is helpful in keeping your mind and body balanced throughout the day: Perform a health inventory every few hours by checking in to make sure everything is all right in your mind and body. You can do this by breathing in and out as deeply as you can. As you inhale take in your current situation and fully accept it. When exhaling imagine that you are releasing any tension or distress about the situation you are currently in. Repeat this as often as needed until it becomes a natural process.

General Tip #2: Avoid the Allergy Trigger

Is something in your environment clearly triggering an allergic response? Constant exposure to an allergy trigger may bring on nothing but misery. Your allergy symptoms could be prevented by avoiding the trigger or eliminating it from your immediate environment. Even when fighting, boxers need time to recoup between rounds. Giving your body a break from an allergen allows it to relax and heal more quickly. In some cases a little break is all your body needs to overcome an allergic response.

The process of avoiding an allergy trigger may require the cooperation of others around you. Say you have chemical sensitivities. If someone at your workplace consistently uses a potent perfume, this may set off a serious allergic reaction. In such cases you may need to request that others around you refrain from using strong perfumes. Mustering the courage to make this request and coming across respectfully is, in itself, an essential part of the healing process.

Simply avoiding an allergy trigger may not be enough for you to overcome allergies. When the stronger and weaker organs are balanced, your body should be able to deal with the allergy trigger without any problem. If you can remove and reintroduce a particular allergy trigger, then try to avoid the allergy trigger for a short period and reintroduce it back into your life slowly and in small doses. If you still get the same response, try again but give yourself more time away in between. In the process make an attempt to release stress through meditation, breathing, or other techniques. Ongoing chronic emotional stress can make it very difficult to overcome allergies. Also, try changing some old emotional or physical habits that you know may interfere with your well-being, such as a common fear, anger, or anxiety response triggered by situations in your daily life.

There are many situations in which the allergy trigger simply cannot be avoided. During the beautiful springtime in my hometown of Portland, Oregon, pollen covers everything in sight! Check out the next tip for more information about facing your allergies.

General Tip #3: Face Your Allergies

Most chronic allergic responses are a sign that our weaker organ is struggling. Avoiding the source of an allergy is not the only approach to overcoming it. Even if the allergy trigger is avoidable, try to address the reason why your system reacted to it. The Sasang medical approach focuses on strengthening your body type's weaker organ in order to overcome allergies. By paying attention to the weaker aspects of your body type, not only can you overcome allergy symptoms, but you can also improve your general health. This can be done by ingesting herbs, foods, and supplements that correspond to your body type and strengthen your weaker organ.

It is also important to keep your emotions in balance when you're suffering from allergies. Allergies have a tendency to bring on more stress, triggering excessive emotions, such as anger, sadness, and fear. These emotions also cause us to hold our breath, making it even more challenging for the lungs and immune system to deal with allergies.

ALLERGIES AND YIN TYPE A

Of all four body types, Yin Type A's are the most prone to allergies because of their weaker lungs. In Eastern medicine the lungs play a major role in regulating and balancing the immune system. Weaker lungs cause the immune system to become hypersensitive, leading to allergy-related symptoms, such as sneezing, itching, coughing, and wheezing. Yin Type A's are also born with an acute sense of smell, which makes them susceptible to hay fever, pet allergies, and other sensitivities. Supporting the lungs is always the core focus of treatment for Yin Type A's, even if they suffer from skin or digestion-related allergies.

It is also more common for Yin Type A's than for other body types to experience allergies to wheat, gluten, and milk. These foods have an abundant amount of Yin energy, which is moist and sticky, while Yang energy is dry and moving. Since Yin Type A's already have plenty of Yin, dairy products may cause sticky phlegm accumulation in the lungs. Wheat and gluten are also cold-natured foods. Cold-natured foods are beneficial for Yang types but can cause stagnation and indigestion in Yin types, who benefit from eating hot- or warm-natured foods. Dairy, wheat, and gluten may not produce immediately apparent symptoms. If you are a Yin Type A suffering from chronic headaches or indigestion, it may be a good idea to try eliminating wheat, dairy, and/or gluten from your diet to see if that alleviates your symptoms.

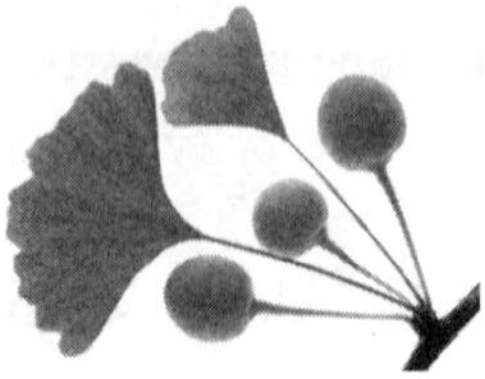

Ginkgo
(*Ginkgo Biloba*)

In Sasang medicine ginkgo is said to "melt" away the Yin Type A's phlegm by clearing congestion from the lungs and sinuses and stopping wheezing and coughing. As mentioned earlier there are two types of phlegm in the body: visible and invisible. Visible phlegm is usually expectorated when coughing or sneezing. Invisible phlegm sticks around and often goes undetected, but could lead to shortness of breath, asthma, or an audible rattle/wheeze when breathing. Ginkgo is commonly used to treat conditions involving both visible and invisible phlegm. The earliest recorded use of ginkgo as a remedy for allergies and asthma in China goes back to 2600 BCE. Modern research supports the use of ginkgo to boost memory by enhancing the circulation of blood to the brain.* In support of these findings, Sasang medicine holds that the lungs control the flow of energy to the brain. This is another example of how Eastern and Western medicine have reached the same conclusion by completely different means! Ginkgo leaves and nuts contain a substance called ginkgoloid, which has been known to promote blood circulation.

From the Clinic

I will never forget the day when Sandra brought her eight-year-old son Jake to our clinic. He was panting and completely out of breath. At first glance I thought he was suffering from respiratory arrest and was about to send him to the ER. To my surprise Sandra stated that his condition had been like this for several months. She had been to several allergy and asthma specialists who prescribed standard asthma medications that did not work. As a Yin Type A, Jake was born with very weak lungs. I immediately prescribed a Yin Type A formula that contained, among several other herbs, ginkgo and coltsfoot. Within days her son was breathing normally and a pink complexion had replaced the deep purple color on his face and the dark circles under his eyes. We were all filled with tears of joy.

---

*For example, see Sakatani, Kaoru, Masahiro Tanida, Naoyasu Hirao, and Naohiro Takemura, "*Ginkobiloba* Extract Improves Working Memory Performance in Middle-Aged Women: Role of Asymmetry of Prefrontal Cortex Activity During a Working Memory Task" *Advances in Experimental Medicine and Biology* 812 (2014): 295–301.

Common Uses of Ginkgo in Sasang Medicine

To alleviate asthma, wheezing, shortness of breath, allergies, common colds, coughing (dry or productive), and to boost memory

Sources of Ginkgo

Ginkgo extract is readily available online from companies such as Vitacost (vitacost.com) and Puritan's Pride (puritan.com) in pill form. Whole or preserved ginkgo nuts in airtight packages can be found at most Asian food markets.

Preparation and Dosage of Ginkgo

Follow manufacturer's dosage suggestions carefully when using ginkgo supplements. Ginkgo has a sweet and slightly acrid flavor when fried until golden brown. Consuming five fried ginkgo nuts a day can help prevent coughing and phlegm, while keeping the lungs clean and clear of bacteria.

Caution

Raw ginkgo nuts are poisonous and should not be consumed. Even cooked ginkgo nuts have been known to cause headaches, nausea, gastrointestinal upset, diarrhea, dizziness, and allergic skin reactions when consumed in excessive amounts. Do not take more than five whole ginkgo nuts a day. Make sure to fry the ginkgo nut until it turns yellowish brown before consuming it. When taking ginkgo in capsule form, follow the manufacturer's recommended dosage closely. Ginkgo intake is contraindicated during pregnancy. The circulation-enhancing properties of ginkgo make it unadvisable to consume if you're taking blood thinners or following an aspirin regimen. For more details about the side effects of ginkgo, do an online search of "Ginkgo Side Effects, National Institutes of Health."

Herbal Friends

Ginkgo is often used with coltsfoot to enhance its ability to stop coughing and clear the lungs and sinuses from congestion. Take one standard dose of ginkgo extract together with one standard dosage of coltsfoot, as directed by the manufacturer. Coltsfoot can be purchased from iherb.com or herbalextractsplus.com. Intake of coltsfoot is cautioned against when breast-feeding and if you have liver or kidney disease. As with other herbs with potential side effects, guidance from a Sasang medical profession is recommended.

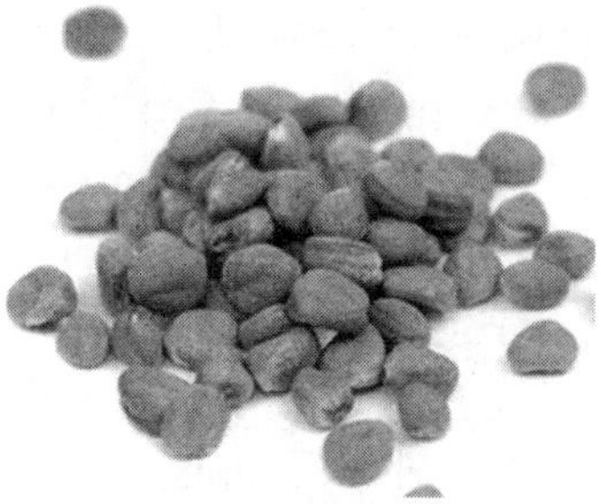

Daikon Radish Seeds (*Raphani Sativi*)

In Sasang medicine radish seeds are used to clear phlegm from the lungs and promote digestion. A sluggish digestive system contributes to the production of phlegm in the lungs. In Eastern medicine the digestive system is said to be the "mother" of the lungs. Therefore, digestive allergies may lead to phlegm accumulation in the lungs. Radish seeds can be used to treat phlegm accumulation in the lungs and/or sinuses due to a common cold or allergies. Radishes are rich in ascorbic acid (vitamin C) and folic acid (vitamin B_9). They also contain a substantial amount of potassium, vitamin B_6, riboflavin, magnesium, copper, and calcium.

Common Uses of Daikon Radish Seeds in Sasang Medicine

To alleviate indigestion (abdominal distention, bloating, fullness), digestive allergies, lung phlegm accumulation, coughing, sinus inflammation and congestion, weight gain

Sources of Daikon Radish Seeds

In the West daikon radish seeds are most often used for planting rather than eating, with the exception of a few gung-ho health food advocates who crave their zesty flavor in salads, soups, and meats. Since the seeds are hard as a rock, they need to be boiled or fried before use as a food. You will likely be able to purchase daikon radish seeds from a local Asian market. Daikon radish seeds can be ordered online from a seed distributor, such as sprouthouse.com or amazon.com by searching for "Radish Seed Sprouts."

Preparation and Dosage of Daikon Radish Seeds

As mentioned above radish seeds are way too hard to ingest in their raw form. In Asia they are commonly cooked with rice at a ratio of five (rice) to one (radish seed). Ginkgo nuts are often cooked with rice and radish seeds for added flavor and health benefits. Radish seeds can also be prepared separately by boiling 30 grams of seeds in two cups of water. Let simmer for five minutes or until the seeds become soft. Strain the seeds and store them in the refrigerator. Add softened radish seeds to salads, soups, and while cooking meat. Softened radish seeds can also be baked as part of your favorite granola recipe. Radish seeds can be sprouted and added to sandwiches and salads for a delicious, slightly spicy, and healthy salad or sandwich. In Sasang medicine radish seeds are made into a tea by boiling five cups of water with 30 grams of seed and simmered for thirty minutes on the lowest flame. Radish seed tea is consumed while still warm, up to three cups a day.

ALLERGIES AND YIN TYPE B

Born with a weaker digestive system, Yin Type B's are most prone to food-related allergies. A weakened digestive system causes the stomach to become hypersensitive to many different types of foods. It is common for Yin Type B's to limit their food intake because they fear the possibility of severe indigestion. Digestive issues may lead to respiratory allergies, since the digestive system is considered the "mother" of the lungs. The digestive system and lungs of Yin Type B's are often treated together, even if they have no signs of indigestion.

Yin Type B's also tend to be the most timid of the four body types. In Eastern medicine the stomach is said to digest experience as well as food. With their timid nature, Yin Type B's find it difficult to "digest" their experiences. Fear of rejection and lack of self-esteem often cause Yin Type B's to avoid interacting with others or going out in public. Being in such situations often leads to food stagnation and stomach-related issues for Yin Type B's. Balanced Yin Type B's challenge their own inner fears by making an effort to interact with others and getting involved in group activities. While this may be easier said than done, it is the only way to strengthen and balance the digestive system of Yin Type B's and is often a key component to overcoming allergies among Yin Type B's as well.

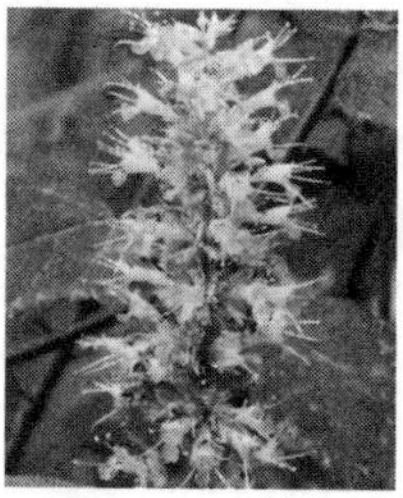

Patchouli Oil (*Agastaches Rugosa*)

In Eastern medicine patchouli is used as a tea to clear the sinuses and support the digestive system. Yin Type B's, in particular, benefit from this herb because its warm nature helps the stomach break down and assimilate foods while treating allergies, colds, and other respiratory issues. Recent studies have demonstrated the use of patchouli oil to prevent viral infections associated with influenza.* Another study suggests that the smell of essential oils, such as patchouli, helps to stimulate antioxidant and immune activity.† In Eastern medicine the sense of smell is governed by the energy of the lungs, which are in charge of regulating the immune system. Hence, the scent of patchouli may help

*For example, see Wu, Huaxing, Beili Li, Xue Wang, Mingyuan Jin, and Guonian Wang, "Inhibitory Effect and Possible Mechanism of Action of Patchouli Alcohol Against Influenza A (H2N2) Virus" *Molecules* 16, no. 8 (2011): 6489–501.

†For more on this, see Manoj, Godbole, Shiragambi Hanumantagouda Manohar, and Hosakatte Niranjana Murthy, "Chemical Constituents, Antioxidant and Antimicrobial Activity of Essential Oil of *Pogostemon paniculatus* (Willd.)" *Natural Product Research* 26, no. 22 (2012): 2152–54.

prevent allergies or colds by supporting the lung function. Patchouli has also been used for decades in the West as a fragrance and essential oil because of its highly aromatic properties. Remember that smell from your hippie days?

Common Uses of Patchouli in Sasang Medicine

To alleviate indigestion, allergies, common colds, congestion, coughing, shortness of breath, lack of appetite

Sources of Patchouli

Patchouli oil is available from manufacturers such as NOW Foods and Plantlife on amazon.com.

Preparation and Dosage of Patchouli

A few drops of patchouli oil may be dabbed onto a piece of cotton and rubbed underneath the nostrils up to three times a day. A few drops may also be applied to the abdomen and rubbed into the skin to promote digestion.

Caution

The application of essential oils directly onto the skin may produce localized skin sensitivity, such as rashes or redness. Try diluting the first few doses with small amounts of water to help your skin get used to it. If your skin is not irritated after a few doses, try applying it directly.

ALLERGIES AND YANG TYPE A

Yang Type A's are rarely prone to allergies, thanks to a stronger digestive system and lungs. Their stronger digestive system breaks down food so quickly that it does not have a chance to stick around and wreak havoc. Since the lungs of Yang Type A's are well developed, they can efficiently rid themselves of airborne allergic triggers. However, when the health of Yang Type A's is compromised, their immune system will become more sensitive. This situation can be compared to the need for heightened security around a palace if the king is ill. A sensitive immune system will attack whatever it comes in contact with, provoking the onset of allergy symptoms.

Each of the Sasang body types is affected in different ways by changes in temperature. Yang Type A's are sensitive to heat because Yang corresponds to heat. The excess Yang of Yang Type A's may cause them to sneeze when the sun is beating down on them. They may also be prone to skin sensitivities in the summertime or when they get overheated.

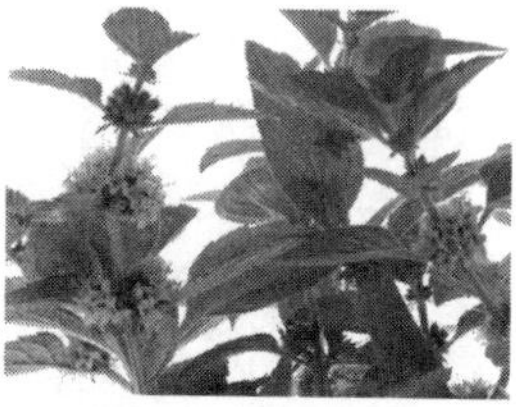

Field Mint (*Mentha Arvensis*)

Mint is an excellent herb for Yang Type A's; not only does it soothe the digestive system, but it also helps to clear the sinuses and eliminate phlegm from the lungs. Menthol, a component of mint, dilates the bronchial tubes, making it easier to breathe. Mint also has a cold nature, which helps to cool the excess Yang heat energy in Yang Type A's. Chilled mint tea is an effective way to keep Yang Type A's cool and healthy during the warmer months of the year.

Common Uses of Field Mint in Sasang Medicine

To address allergies, sinus congestion, sore throat, throat swelling, indigestion (gas, bloating, acid reflux), headaches

Sources of Field Mint

Organic mint tea can be purchased in tea bag form from Numi (luckyvitamin.com) and various other companies online.

Preparation and Dosage of Field Mint

If you are a Yang Type A who loves to garden, mint is the herb for you! It is easily cultivated and grows quickly from spring through summer. Plant it in the fall and you can enjoy it by late spring! While field mint has the strongest effect, other mint varieties can be used as a substitute.

Try drinking three to five cups of field mint tea a day if you have allergies. Otherwise two to three cups should be plenty. During the warmer months, chilled mint tea can be consumed throughout the day to keep the body feeling cool and healthy.

Herbal Friends

Field mint is often used in conjunction with qian hu (*Radix Peucedani*) in Sasang medicine to assist with stubborn sinus or lung phlegm issues. If you are a Yang Type A suffering from chronic coughing, stuffiness, or sneezing, the above combination may be the answer for you. Both these herbs have very strong sinus and lung clearing functions and are used together to treat allergies, long-term colds, coughing, and sinusitis. Qian hu, also known in the West as hog fennel root, can be purchased as a powder from 1st Chinese Herbs (1stchineseherbs.com). To prepare it place one tea bag of mint tea and one scoop of qian hu (a spoon is provided in the bottle) in hot water, stir and then steep for three minutes. Drink up to three times a day, either cool or lukewarm.

ALLERGIES AND YANG TYPE B

The lungs, which are the Yang Type B's strongest organ, correspond to the immune system and thus help prevent common colds and other immune-related disorders. Strength, however, is not always equated with health. As the strongest organ, the lungs may have a tendency to draw too much energy and fluid toward themselves and away from the other organs, resulting in chest and sinus congestion. The lungs need to use their strength to circulate energy throughout the body, rather than hoarding it all for themselves.

With such strong lungs, it is rare for Yang Type B's to suffer from allergies. If they experience signs and symptoms of allergies, however, it is a sure sign of failing health, since that means the strength of their strongest organ has been compromised. When treating the Yang Type B's allergies, it is necessary to promote the circulation of lung energy downward, toward their weaker liver by means of cool-natured, aromatic herbs that have an affinity for the lungs and liver.

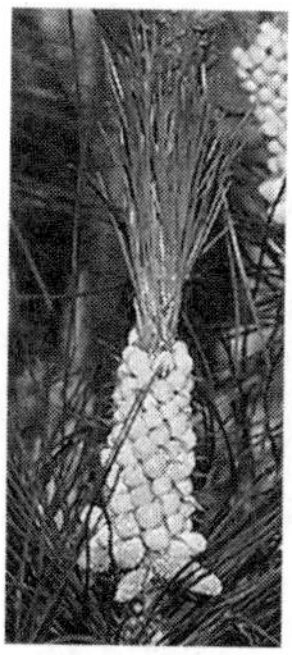

Chinese Red Pine/Masson Pine (*Lignum Pini Nodi*)

According to Sasang medicine, pine nodes, or the tiny part of the pine tree where the branch meets the prickly leaves, have numerous advantageous properties. They help prevent and soothe allergies and colds, alleviate pain due to swelling, and assist in the flow of lung energy. While other body types may benefit to some degree from this herb, it is especially suitable for Yang Type B's whose lung energy is prone to causing stagnation because it hoards energy from the other organs.

Most pine supplements utilize the entire bark of the pine tree, which contains the nodes. The bark and nodes of the Masson pine tree contain a flavonoid called pycnogenol; this has both anti-inflammatory and antioxidant properties. It is also believed to help support immune activity and strengthen the blood vessel walls. A recent study demonstrated that pine bark can also be effective in the treatment of melanoma, a life-threatening form of skin cancer.*

Common Uses of Chinese Red Pine/Masson Pine in Sasang Medicine

To alleviate allergies, common colds, water retention, joint pain, muscle and/or tendon pain

Sources of Chinese Red Pine/Masson Pine

Masson pine bark extract is available from Planetary Herbals (planetaryherbals.com) and from Puritan's Pride (puritan.com). Pine bark extract from other sources is often mixed with ingredients that are not suitable for Yang Type B's.

*For more on this, see Solovey, Matthew, "Pine Bark Substance Could Be Potent Melanoma Drug" (May 20 2014) http://news.psu.edu/story/316399/2014/05/20/research/pine-bark-substance-could-be-potent-melanoma-drug.

Preparation and Dosage of Chinese Red Pine/Masson Pine

Follow manufacturer's instructions for dosage.

Caution

Consult with a professional before using this supplement if you are pregnant, plan to become pregnant, are currently breast-feeding, or are taking any prescription drugs.

Herbal Friends

In Sasang medicine Masson pine bark is often mixed with devil's club to treat allergies and common colds by supporting the immune system and assisting with the flow of lung energy. Use two parts devil's club to one part pine bark extract (2:1 ratio). Follow the manufacturer's instructions to determine the recommended dosage range for each supplement.

Visual Challenges

Many of us would have trouble imagining life without vision, since we rely on this sense for just about everything we do. With the advent of televisions and computers, there has never been a time in history that demanded so much from our eyes. Did you know that approximately 61 percent (192 million) of all Americans require some form of vision correction? Even while writing this book, I can feel my eyes telling me to "Take a break!" With so much use, keeping our eyes happy can be a challenge for just about anyone.

GENETICS AND EYESIGHT

The strength of our vision depends, at least in part, on genetics. If you are prone to visual challenges, such as cataracts, nearsightedness, or farsightedness, your child may also have this tendency. In Sasang medicine our body type and genetic structure have significant effects on our physical and emotional tendencies. While there are genetic components to various vision problems, the onset is not necessarily related to our body type. Vision is also strongly dependent on how we use our eyes. This section provides several tips on how to keep your eyes healthy.

EARLY ONSET OF VISUAL IMPAIRMENT

Have you ever heard of the term "computer vision syndrome"? Even if you are not familiar with the name of this syndrome, its symptoms may be familiar: eyestrain, headaches, gritty eyes, and blurry vision after using the computer, watching TV up close, or reading a book for too long. Studies show that approximately 75 percent of American employees who use a computer and 25 percent of the total population will eventually suffer vision-related issues, such as nearsightedness.

Nearsightedness, also known as myopia, is the most common form of visual impairment in adolescents. When attempting to focus on an object, those with myopia may experience blurred vision, eyestrain, headaches, and fatigue. They will also notice issues with distal focus, since they are so used to focusing on objects closer to them. Children who glue themselves to textbooks or computers may also develop early onset of vision issues because their eyesight is still in the developing stages. After the age of thirty, when eyesight development is complete, myopia becomes less of a problem.

VISION AND AGING

As we age our eyes naturally experience wear and tear, which contribute to visual challenges. Thickening and stiffness of the lens in the eye make it difficult for us to focus on objects up close. Such conditions eventually lead to farsightedness, or presbyopia, which is characterized by difficulty focusing on objects that are near to us—a condition that affects most people after the age of fifty.

Another form of visual impairment that may occur as we age is cataracts, which come about from the clustering of protein on the retina. More than half of all Americans over sixty-five have either mild or severe cataract formation. Symptoms include blurred or dimmed vision, usually in the center of the visual field. Cataracts may result from other health problems, such as diabetes, or injection of corticosteroids.

Macular degeneration is another type of visual challenge of advanced age, mainly affecting the center of our visual field. The macula is a light-sensitive layer of tissue on the back of the eyeball that helps transform light into signals by means of which the brain interprets what we see. When these cells break down, the signal of vision to the brain may be hindered or cut off entirely. If left untreated, macular degeneration can lead to severe vision loss or blindness.

VISION AS A SECONDARY ISSUE

Visual challenges are not only caused by eyestrain or aging: they are occasionally a secondary issue resulting from other illnesses, such as diabetes or high blood pressure. In such cases it is important to treat the underlying cause of vision impairment, rather than simply addressing its symptoms. As with other vision-related issues, it is advisable to visit your ophthalmologist for a thorough evaluation.

THE SASANG APPROACH TO VISUAL CHALLENGES

So far in this section, we have introduced several types of visual impairment, each having its own etiology and treatment approach in Western medicine. Including separate treatment strategies for each of these disorders would make this section several hundred pages long! Luckily, addressing vision problems in Sasang medicine does not vary according to the disorder. Instead, it is based on supporting the flow of energy to the eyes from your constitutionally stronger organ. When the eyes do not receive a consistent flow of blood and energy, our vision is affected. When the eyes are bathed with fresh blood, there is little that can go wrong! Blood is a miraculous substance that is capable of healing just about everything in its path. Excessive use of the eyes and aging naturally cause a blockage and/or lack of blood flow to and through the eyes.

Each organ of the body has its own role in supporting our vision. The kidneys, for example, send essence (a concentrated mix of *qi* and essential nutrients) to the eyes. Without essence we could easily lose strength of vision. The liver sends blood to the eyes. Without blood the eyes become blurry and dry. The spleen offers clarity of vision. No matter how strong our vision is, without clarity, our brain has trouble interpreting what we see. Finally, the lungs send moisture to the eyes, without which the eyes dry out and feel itchy.

To cultivate our health the Sasang way, we must cater to the needs of our weaker organs. To support their vision, Yang Type A's benefit from foods and herbs that nourish the kidneys, their weakest organ. Supporting the liver would be the focus of Yang Type B's seeking to improve or sustain healthy vision. For Yin Type A's, supporting the lungs would help do the trick, and for Yin Type B's, keeping the kidneys happy would work.

MAINTAINING HEALTHY VISION

General Tip #1: Take Breaks

Do you find it difficult to take a break when you are in the midst of an important task? Most people do. Hence excessive focus is a primary factor in failing vision. Some experts argue that it is not the computer or TV screen that harms our vision, but the fact that we forget to blink when focusing on something for a prolonged period. A lack of blinking causes dryness of the eyes, impairing their function. Excess focus also causes strain of the eye muscles, leading to visual fatigue and eyestrain. Make an effort to blink regularly when you're focusing on a particular task for a protracted period.

General Tip #2: Massage the Occipital Lobe

The occipital lobe is an area located in the back of the head that controls our vision (see figure 4.3). Excessive demand on this part of the brain may cause tightness and/or occipital headaches in the back of the head. Massaging this area daily can help encourage blood and energy flow to the visual cortex.

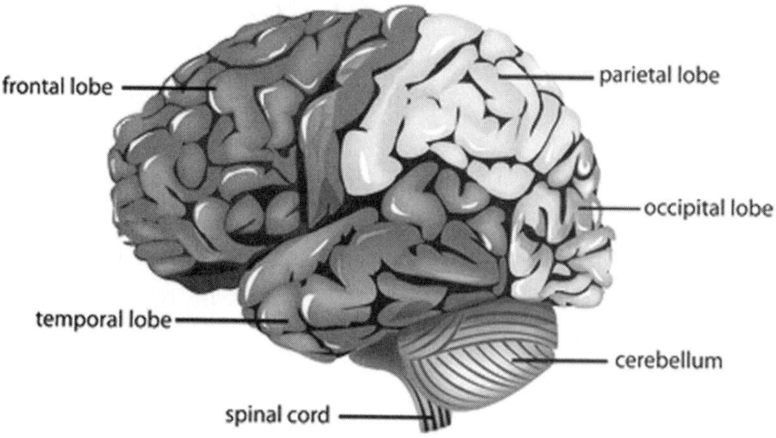

Figure 4.3. Parts of the human brain

HOW TO MASSAGE THE OCCIPITAL LOBE

* Apply light to heavy pressure with your thumb directly below both sides of your skull while slightly tilting your head forward (see figure 4.4).
* Rotate your thumbs in small circles, using your other fingers to stabilize the motion.
* Work your way up and down the base of the skull while continuing to rotate your thumbs.

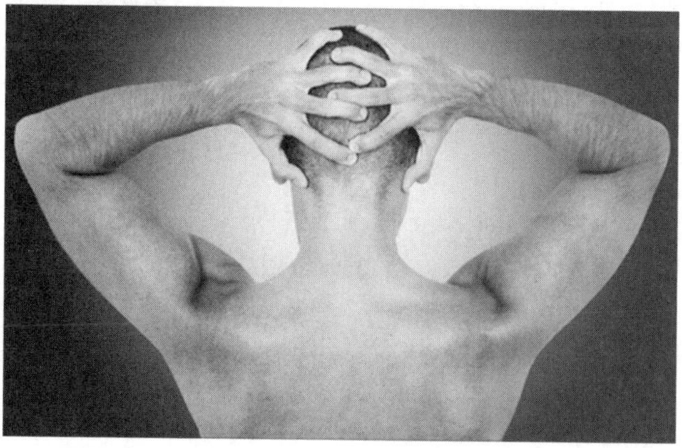

Figure 4.4. Hand position for massaging the occipital lobe

* Close your eyes, relax your shoulders, and breathe in and out slowly for added effect.
* This massage can be repeated as many times and as long as you like.

General Tip #3: Focus on Objects in the Distance

When using the computer, watching TV, or reading a book, try giving your eyes a break by taking a look at a distant object every twenty minutes or so. Shifting our focus from time to time helps relax the muscles of the eye and avoid strain.

General Tip #4: Enlarge Font Size

Most Internet and document writing programs offer font size viewing options. The zoom feature on Microsoft Word or Internet Explorer can save your eyes from getting fatigued and worn out. The use of computer glasses to magnify computer screen fonts is another option.

General Tip #5: Consume Food for Thought

A diet rich in eye-nourishing foods can help avoid and possibly slow down the progression of vision problems. In Sasang medicine foods that nourish the eyes also nourish the blood. Most dark green vegetables and darker fruits, such as blueberries, purple/red grapes, acai berries, goji berries, and raisins have this virtue.

Here are a few supplements that keep the eyes healthy:

Vitamins: C, E, and A (beta-carotene)
Minerals: Zinc, copper, iron
Other: Omega-3 fatty acids

See part 3, "Eating and Exercising Right for Your Yin Yang Body Type," for foods that contain the above supplements and are associated with your body type.

VISION AND YIN TYPE A

The eyesight of Yin Type A's depends on the health of their weakest organ, the lungs. When healthy the lungs send an ample amount of moisture and oxygen to the eyes. In Sasang medicine weaker lungs lead to a condition referred to as *pei jo,* or "lung dryness." The weaker the lungs get, the dryer and less elastic they become. If they can't expand and contract efficiently, the lungs cannot nourish the other upper-body organs and senses. Cardiovascular exercise, coupled with ample water consumption, is an excellent way to keep the lungs from drying out and to promote the circulation of moisture to the eyes.

The Yin Type A's strongest organ, the liver, sends blood to the eyes. Since blood is needed to repair and support vision, balancing liver function can be an effective way to promote healing of the eyes. One may think that having a strong liver is beneficial for Yin Type A's in such situations. In actuality a strong liver does not readily share its energy with the other organs and senses. Its ability to absorb often causes it to "soak up" energy from other parts of the body. Excessive stress and/or alcohol consumption will make matters worse, leading to failed vision due to liver stagnation and toxicity. Herbs that help promote the movement of liver energy toward the eyes are therefore used to help support the Yin Type A's vision.

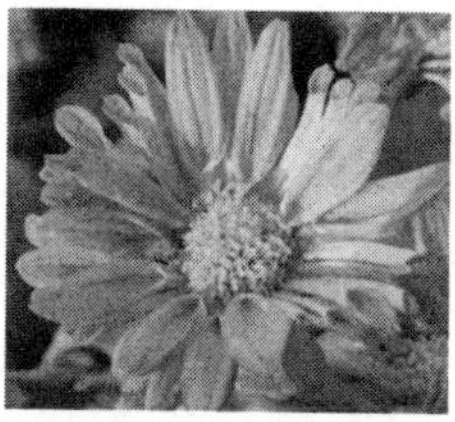

Chrysanthemum Tea (*Flos Chrysanthemi Morifolii*)

Chrysanthemum is often used in Sasang medicine for a variety of the Yin Type A's ailments. It was introduced on page 278 for its ability to alleviate occipital and sinus headaches, which are often due to excessive eyestrain. This is the herb of choice for the Yin Type A's vision problems because not only does it support the lung function, it also promotes the flow of energy from the liver to the eyes! Chrysanthemum is very useful in easing both eyestrain and chronic muscle inflammation. The chrysanthemum flower was traditionally thought to look like a glistening, wide-open human eye; hence it has been used for thousands of years to treat vision-related problems. Yin Type A's may benefit from daily consumption of chrysanthemum tea, not only to support vision, but also for their general health. The flower petals contain vitamins A and B_1, calcium, and phosphorus.

Common Uses of Chrysanthemum in Sasang Medicine

To alleviate headaches (occipital), vision disorders (blurry vision, cataracts, glaucoma, focal issues, itchy eyes, floaters, failing vision)

Sources of Chrysanthemum

Chrysanthemum tea can be purchased from manufacturers such as Mighty Leaf (mightyleaf.com) and Tea Spring (teaspring.com).

Preparation and Dosage of Chrysanthemum

Steep three to five flowers in one cup of hot water. Let sit for four minutes until the water turns light yellow. Drink warm. The leaves may also be chewed after finishing the tea to enhance its effect. Up to four cups a day may be consumed.

Caution

Chrysanthemum is a relatively safe herb when ingested. However, if you are taking this herb within the recommended dose range and experience indigestion or allergy-related symptoms (such as sinus inflammation, rash, or runny nose), it is likely that you may be allergic to chrysanthemum or that it does not correspond to your body type.

VISION AND YIN TYPE B

In Sasang medicine the kidneys are said to house the body's essence, which slowly decreases as we age. The kidneys also send essence to the eyes to support vision. The weakening of vision as we age is often a sign of waning essence. Born with stronger kidneys and plenty of essence, Yin Type B's tend to have vigorous visual strength, which tends to endure more than that of the other body types. Not all Yin Type B's have long-lasting healthy vision, however. Stronger organs have a tendency to absorb more than their share of energy. In doing so excessive energy and toxicity may accumulate in the Yin Type B's kidneys, causing overall health issues.

While the kidneys are in charge of visual strength, the spleen is the source of visual clarity. Unhealthy or aging Yin Type B's may still be able to see, but as their spleen gets weaker, so will the clarity of their vision. To support the Yin Type B's vision, we prescribe herbs that also support the function of the spleen.

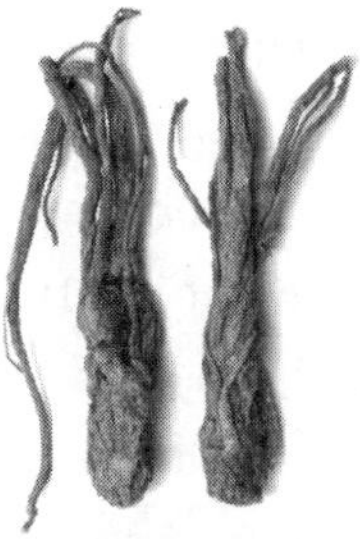

Dang Gui (aka Dong Quai) (*Angelica Sinensis*)

Dang gui is one of the most commonly used herbs for Yin Type B's because it has so many functions. To begin with it generates and circulates blood throughout the body, to enhance wound healing, address vascular issues, and alleviate anemic disorders, headaches, and menstrual cramps. Dang gui also supports the function of the spleen. Lastly, dang gui helps preserve the kidney essence and circulate it toward the eyes to support vision.

Dang gui looks like a dried squid, and emits an aromatic, earthy smell. If left sitting on a shelf, it will eventually cause the whole room to smell like an Eastern medical pharmacy! A small piece of dang gui placed inside the mouth will leave behind a tangy taste and sensation for hours. Try chewing on a little piece for a quick pick-me-up!

Common Uses of Dang Gui in Sasang Medicine

To alleviate circulatory issues (cold extremities, numbness of the extremities, heart palpitations), anemia, vision disorders (blurry vision, floaters, eyestrain), indigestion, insomnia, menstrual cramps, irregular menstruation (scanty, early, or late cycle), and to heal cuts and wounds

Sources of Dang Gui

An encapsulated form of dang gui root can be purchased from Nature's Way (naturesway.com). Liquid extract can be purchased from Nature's Answer (naturesanswer.com).

Preparation and Dosage of Dang Gui

Follow the dosage guidelines specified by the manufacturer.

Caution

Excessive intake of dang gui can lead to gas and bloating even for Yin Type B's. Start with smaller dosages and work your way up to the recommended dose. Volatile oil extracts of dang gui have been known to cause skin sensitivity to the sun, leading to a greater risk of skin cancer. The liquid extract sold by Nature's Answer (naturesanswer.com) and the capsule form sold by Nature's Way (naturesway.com) are not volatile oils and do not present this risk. Do not ingest dang gui if you are currently taking blood thinners, such as Warfarin, because it promotes circulation and could interfere with prescription-drug effects, causing excessive bleeding. Dang gui may cause bruising because of its potential blood-thinning effects.

There are several different species of angelica root that are native to North America. Most of these plants have high levels of toxicity and should not be ingested. Some sources say that dang gui should be avoided during pregnancy, nursing, or in case of breast cancer because it contains estrogenlike compounds. You can visit the Medline Plus website and type "Dong Quai" in the search engine to receive further information.

VISION AND YANG TYPE A

In Sasang medicine the spleen corresponds to the eyes. Since Yang Type A's are born with a stronger spleen, they inherit more acute eyesight than the other body types. Their "eagle" eyes not only contribute to clear vision, but also to a deeper insight that allows them to "see through" others. Yang Type A's, however, are not immune to eye disorders. Age, failing health, or excessive anger can contribute to weaker eyesight. Even in such cases, they rarely lose the power of insight. An elderly Yang Type A may lose most if not all of her eyesight, but still be keenly aware of what is going on around her. When I was a child, my Yang Type A grandmother with failing vision would always slap my hand as I reached for the cookie jar before dinner (I thought she would never notice!).

The kidneys, which are the weakest organ of Yang Type A's, also have a role to play in vision. Whereas the spleen is in charge of visual clarity, the kidneys are the source of visual strength. Here the spleen can be compared to windshield washer fluid, and the kidneys to windshield wipers. Both strength and clarity are needed to maintain healthy vision, just as both windshield wipers and windshield washer fluid are necessary to clean a windshield. Unhealthy Yang Type A's may still have clarity of vision, but as their kidneys get weaker, so will the strength of their vision. To support the Yang Type A's vision, it is therefore necessary to utilizes herbs that also support the function of the kidneys.

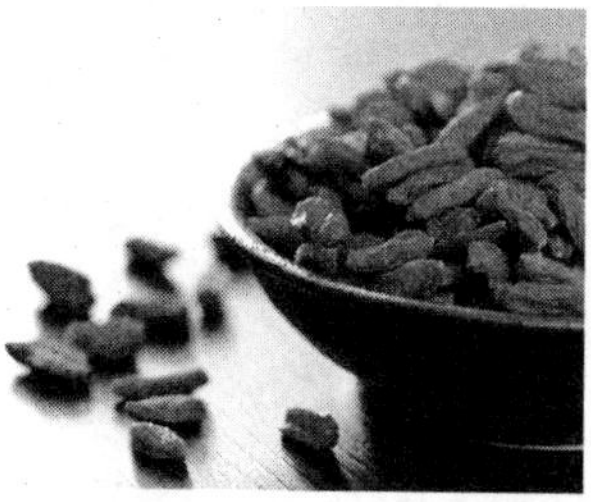

Chinese Wolfberry/Goji Berry (*Lycium Chinenses*)

Sound familiar? Wolfberry was introduced on page 303 as an herb effective in alleviating insomnia. Here it is worth mentioning again, this time as an herb to support eyesight. In Eastern medicine both insomnia and eyesight have one thing in common—a lack of energy and blood flow toward the head. As wolfberry helps support the flow of blood and energy upward from the kidneys, it supports eye and brain function. According to Eastern medicine, herbs that support the kidneys also strengthen the bones. Wolfberry can therefore also be used for bone-related issues in Yang Type A's. Several recent studies have reported positive effects of wolfberry in treating macular degeneration and glaucoma, cancer, and cardiovascular and inflammatory diseases.*

Common Uses of Wolfberry in Sasang Medicine

To treat insomnia, vision disorders (blurry vision, weak vision), fatigue, anxiety, osteoporosis/osteopenia

Sources of Wolfberry

Wolfberry (goji) in bulk form is available for purchase at most natural food stores. Wolfberry juice is available from healingnoni.com and dynamichealth.com.

Preparation and Dosage of Wolfberry

See page 304 for preparation and dosage of Wolfberry.

Caution

Diabetics should monitor sugar levels carefully when ingesting wolfberry, since it is a fruit and contains sugar. Wolfberry may interfere with the effects of Warfarin and other blood thinners. If you are taking a blood thinner, be sure to consult a medical professional before ingesting wolfberry.

Yang Type A's should not ingest wolfberry if they are experiencing heat-related symptoms, such as fever, sensitivity to heat, excessive appetite, or pounding (as opposed to dull) headaches, because this herb is slightly warm-natured.

---

*For example, see Gan, Lu, Sheng Hua Zhang, Xiang Liang Yang, and Hui Bi Xu, "Immunomodulation and Antitumor Activity by a Polysaccharide Protein Complex from *Lycium barbarum*" *International Immunopharmacology* 4, no. 4 (2004): 563–69; and Zhang, Min, Haixia Chen, Jin Huang, Zhong Li, Caiping Zhu, and Shenghua Zhang, "Effect of *Lycium barbarum* Polysaccharide on Human Hepatoma QGY7703 Cells: Inhibition of Proliferation and Induction of Apoptosis" *Life Sciences* 76, no. 18 (March 2005): 2115–24.

VISION AND YANG TYPE B

Both Yang types have a stronger upper body function, and, as a result, more acute eyesight. While the Yang Type B's eyesight may not be as clear as the Yang Type A's, it is still more acute than that of the Yin body types. Hearing, on the other hand, is their strongest sense. A combination of acute hearing and vision helps Yang Type B's become extremely aware of their surroundings, making them appear as if they are constantly focusing or preoccupied.

As discussed earlier each of the four major organs (lungs, spleen, liver, and kidneys) has a significant role to play in support of our vision. The liver is responsible for sending blood to the eyes. Without a consistent blood supply, the eyes cannot function. Born with a weaker liver, the unhealthy Yang Type B may suffer from dryness of the eyes, which eventually, if not addressed, leads to visual impairment. Herbs that benefit the liver therefore help to nourish the eyes of the Yang Type B.

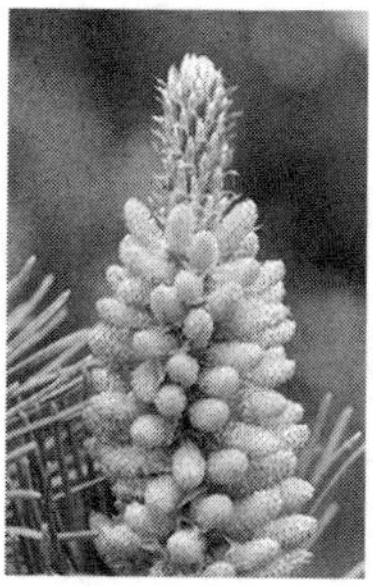

Pine Flower
(*Pinus sylvestris*)

In Eastern medicine there is an herbal concept of "Like treats like." So herbs that resemble part of the human body are frequently used in supporting that part's function. Flowers are said to resemble the eyes because they open during the day and close at night and have an overall roundish, eyeball-like appearance. For this reason flowers are often used for supporting vision.

Every part of the pine tree is beneficial for Yang Type B's because it supports their weaker liver. Pine nodes, for example, are used to alleviate joint pain, pine pollen to promote general circulation, and pine roots to address lower-body issues.

Common Uses of Pine Flower in Sasang Medicine

To remedy vision disorders (cataracts, glaucoma, blurry vision), dizziness, common colds and phlegm-related problems, chronic diarrhea

Sources of Pine Flower

Pine flower extract can be purchased at most natural food stores or from Bach Flower Essences (wildearthmarket.com).

Preparation and Dosage of Pine Flower

Refer to the manufacturer's instructions for appropriate dosage.

Caution

Bach Flower Essences cautions against using this herb during pregnancy or while nursing.

Useful Resources

The path toward discovering your Yin Yang Body Type is often as challenging as it is rewarding. Sasang medicine urges us to take a deep look within, to open our hearts and minds, and to explore hidden aspects of who we are. Even after reading this book, you may still have some lingering questions about your Yin Yang Body Type, which is often revealed only after persistent self-reflection and trial and error. While this book attempts to encompass all the basics of Sasang medicine, it cannot replace the expert advice of a qualified Sasang practitioner. Thus, if you wish to seek further guidance regarding your Yin Yang Body Type, consider trying one or more of the following options:

- Log onto sasangmedicine.com and visit our discussion forum, which covers various topics from discovering your Yin Yang Body Type to addressing specific health concerns. Simply click on "Sasang Discussion Forum" on the main menu to view the discussion. If you have a pressing question that is not already addressed in the forum, you may choose the option to log in and open a new discussion. There is no registration fee. My staff and I review this forum regularly and will post a response to your inquiry.
- Log onto sasangmedicine.com and click "Contact Us" to sign up for a direct consultation session with my team of Sasang professionals. This is a convenient way to seek assistance in discovering your Yin Yang Body Type and to receive one-on-one guidance regarding particular health conditions.

- Contact my clinic directly to make an appointment. Although, in most cases, your Yin Yang Body Type can be determined by the above methods, personal contact is the most accurate way for me to ascertain your body type. Along with the methods described in this book, Sasang practitioners also utilize a vast array of clinical diagnostic protocols, such as pulse-taking, skin texture analysis, and voice tone assessment to determine your body type. More information about our clinic can be found at harmonyclinics.com. We may be contacted at harmonyclinics.com or via the address and phone number below:

Harmony Acupuncture and Herbs
21730 Willamette Drive
West Linn, OR 97068
(503) 722–5224

Despite its firm establishment and popularity in Korea, Sasang medicine is still in its infancy in the West, with a limited amount of material available in English. Information regarding Sasang medicine that is currently scattered throughout the Internet can be located by typing the phrases *Sasang medicine, Four Constitutional Medicine, or Korean Constitutional Medicine* in any major search engine. Research in Sasang medicine has recently appeared in English-language journals. The pubmed.com website, hosted by the National Institutes of Health, provides one of the largest collections of published medical research worldwide; several Sasang medical studies translated into English can be found there.

All Sasang medical research so far has been conducted in Asia, with non-Caucasian populations. I have initiated the first Sasang medical study in the United States, a collaboration between the Korean Institute of Oriental Medicine in Daejeon, Korea, and the National College of Natural Medicine in Portland, Oregon. This study aims to develop a diagnostic tool for Yin Yang Body Type differentiation among individuals of European descent. Upon its conclusion the results of this study will be posted on sasangmedicine.com. For further information about this and other Sasang medicine studies in English, visit sasangmedicine.com and click "Sasang Research."

Even though the seed of Sasang medicine has but recently been planted in Western soil, it has already started to germinate. As time passes it will forge its way upward and reach fruition, with an expanding body of Sasang practitioners and sources of valuable material written in English. Meanwhile, I will do my best to keep you informed and updated about exciting new breakthroughs through my website and further publication.

Index

Page numbers in *italics* indicate illustrations.
Page numbers followed by *t* indicate tables.

abdominal breathing, 255–56
acupressure points, 310–11
addiction, 85–87, 218*t*
allergies
  airborne, 366–67
  food, 362–64
  overview, 360–61
  prevention and treatment, 368–70
  Sasang approach to, 367–68
  skin, 364–66
  testing for, 366–67
  Yang Type A and, 376–78
  Yang Type B and, 378–80
  Yin Type A and, 370–74
  Yin Type B and, 374–76
almond milk, 118, 131
aloe vera juice, 320–21
anger
  balanced versus unbalanced, 17*t*
  determining your body type and, 56
  spleen affected by, 23, 25, 42, 102
  Yang Type A and, 16, 18, 37, 56, 67, 101–2, 107
  Yin types and, 19
Appearance Test, Outward, 42–53
apple cider vinegar, 267–68, 334–36, 350–51
  See also vinegar
"arranging the home" (*go cho*), 90, 91
arthritis, 37, 346, 347, 351, 354
  See also joint pain
asthma, 35, 364, 371

barley tea, roasted, 261–62, 342–43
behavior modification, 28, 29–31
blackberries, 356–57
black cohosh tea, 277–78
blood pressure monitor, 264
  See also high blood pressure
body types
  energy cycles of, 206
  food energy and, 111–12
  four senses and, 19–22

four types, reason for, 22–23
nature versus nurture, 24–27
organ strength and, 14
population breakdown, 26
temperaments and, 14–19
traits of, 13, 40
See also determining your body type; tests, body type; *specific body types*

breakfast
eating light, 330
importance of, 309
yang types, 212–14
yin types, 208–10

breathing, 223, 255–56
buckwheat, 122, 142, 304–5

calcium, 166–67, 168, 171, 213, 215–16, 256–57
calories, 201–4
canker or coptis root, 283–84
carbohydrates, 198–99
cardiovascular exercise, 226, 227*t*, 231, 232–33, 332
cereals, seeds, and grains
Yang Type A, 159–60
Yang Type B, 176–77
Yin Type A, 120–23
Yin Type B, 141–43

chamomile, 257–58
cheerfulness, 84–85, 95–96
chestnuts, 315–16
chicken soup, 287
Chinese jujube, 301–2
Chinese quince fruit, 323–24, 358
Chinese red pine/Masson pine, 379–80
Chinese wolfberry/goji berry, 303–4
chin-up bar, hanging from, 349
chocolate, 11, 135, 326
cholesterol, 128–29, 167, 169, 176, 191–92, 263, 267, 334
chrysanthemum tea, 278–79, 387–88
cinnamon, 142, 152, 293, 340
cinnamon tea, 280–81, 354–55
coffee, 11, 212, 309
coltsfoot, 373
common colds
prevention and treatment, 10, 38, 286–88
Yang Type A and, 293–95
Yang Type B and, 296–97
Yin Type A and, 35, 127, 288–91
Yin Type B and, 291–93

compassion, 72, 76–77, 103–4, 105
complacency
effect of, 17*t*
liver and, 18, 24, 84–85
Yin Type A and, 16, 18, 33, 36, 37

Confucius, 72, 73, 74, 76, 88
constipation, 83, 121, 128, 218*t*, 333–34
cool/cold-natured food, 111–12, 113*t*, 307, 308*t*
coptis or canker root, 283–84
Cousins, Norman, 153
cravings, 21, 349
creative thinking, 82, 298

daikon radish seeds, 373–74
dairy. *See* meat and dairy
depression, 15, 17, 19
See also sorrow/sadness

dessert, 211
determining your body type
  Outward Appearance Test, 42–53
  overview, 40–41
  Yin Yang Body Type Test, 54–69
devil's club, 284–85, 296–97, 380
diabetes, 126, 218*t*, 339, 383
diakon radish seeds, 373–74
diet
  body type-specific foods, 110–11
  daily food intake, 206–8
  food as first line of defense, 248–49
  food energy and, 115–18
  food pyramid, 191–92
  how much to eat, 201–4
  importance of, 190
  what to eat, 192–201
  when to eat, 204–6
  yang types, 212–16
  yin types, 208–12
  See also foods, Yang Type A; foods, Yang Type B; foods, Yin Type A; foods, Yin Type B
digestive system
  listening to, 312
  red-light foods and, 117, 118
  spleen in charge of, 2–3
  Yin Type B and, 35, 38, 90–91, 141, 143
  See also food allergies; indigestion
dinner
  eating early, 330–31
  for yang types, 215–16
  for yin types, 211–12
echinacea tea, 289–90
Emerson, Ralph Waldo, 42
emotional tendencies
  overview, 72–75
  Yang Type A, 98–101
  Yang Type B, 105–8
  Yin Type A, 77–87
  Yin Type B, 89–96
  See also temperament
energy cycles, body type, 206
environment
  balanced response to, 29–31
  influence of, 27–28
  unbalanced response to, 32–34
  Yin Type B and, 91
exercise
  aerobic versus anaerobic, 222
  benefits of, 227*t*
  body types and, 227–28
  breathing during, 223
  calories burned during, 203*t*
  cardiovascular, 226, 227*t*, 231, 232–33, 332
  categories, 226–27
  health conditions improved by, 218*t*
  joint pain and, 224, 347–48
  music for, 227*t*
  for stress relief, 255
  stretching, 219–22, 227*t*, 348
  time for, 218–19, 224
  walking, 62, 348
  Yang Type A and, 237–41, 341
  Yang Type B and, 242–46
  Yin Type A and, 228–32
  Yin Type B and, 232–36
  See also meditation; weight lifting

faith and commitment, 79–80
fatigue
overcoming, 10–11, 38
red-light foods and, 117
Yang Type A and, 238–39
fear, 93–94
fennel root, hog, 378
fibromyalgia, 365
field mint, 282–83, 377–78
food allergies, 362–64
food energy
body types and, 112–13, 116
changing, 113–14
cool/cold-natured food, 111–12, 113*t*, 307, 308*t*
described, 111–12
determining the energy of, 114–15
diet and, 115–17
food allergies and, 364
green-light foods, 55, 115, 117–18, 192
red-light foods, 55, 117, 192
temperature guidelines, 113*t*
warm/hot-natured food, 111–12, 113*t*, 307, 308*t*, 338
yellow-light foods, 115–16, 117–18, 192
food pyramid, 191–92
foods, Yang Type A
cereals, seeds, and grains, 159–60
fruits and nuts, 163–65
meat and dairy, 165–68
overview, 157–58, 172–73
quick reference, 172–73*t*
supplements, 170–71
teas, 169–70
vegetables and spices, 160–63
foods, Yang Type B
cereals, seeds, and grains, 176–77
choosing, 176
fruits and nuts, 180–82
meat and dairy, 182–85
overview, 174–75
quick reference, 188–89*t*
supplements, 186–87
teas, 185–86
vegetables and spices, 177–80
foods, Yin Type A
avoiding in excess, 134–36
cereals, seeds, and grains, 120–23
choosing, 120
fruits and nuts, 126–29, 191–92
meat and dairy, 130–32
overview, 119
quick reference, 136–38*t*
supplements, 134
teas, 132–34
vegetables and spices, 123–26
foods, Yin Type B
cereals, seeds and grains, 141–43
choosing, 140–41
fruits and nuts, 146–49
meat and dairy, 149–51
overview, 139–40
quick reference, 155–56*t*
red-light foods, caution for, 117, 140
supplements, 153–54
teas, 152–53
vegetables and spices, 143–46
friendship, 68, 78–79

fruits and nuts
- Yang Type A, 163–65
- Yang Type B, 180–82
- Yin Type A, 126–29, 191–92
- Yin Type B, 146–49
- *See also specific types*

gardenia, 270–71
ginger
- cinnamon and, 281
- dried, 338–40
- tea, 235–36, 292–93
- for Yin Type B, 154, 318–20

ginkgo, 134, 370–73, 374
ginseng, 154
goji berry/Chinese wolfberry, 303–4
grains. *See* cereals, seeds, and grains
green-light foods, 55, 115, 117–18, 192
green tea, 211–12, 266–67

hands, strength of, 85
hawthorn berry, 269–70
headaches
- prevention and treatment, 274–76
- Yang Type A and, 25, 281–84
- Yang Type B and, 284–85
- Yin Type A and, 276–79
- Yin Type B and, 279–81

health
- food as first line of defense, 248–49
- maintenance, 8–10, 38–39
- organ strength and, 26–27, 34–35
- temperament and, 34–38

hearing, 22, 106
heart, polishing, 26–27, 72, 73
heart disease, 38, 218*t*
herbs, choosing, 3–4, 110
high blood pressure
- prevention and treatment, 38, 263–65, 334–35
- Yang Type A and, 270–71
- Yang Type B and, 271–73
- Yin Type A and, 265–68
- Yin Type B and, 268–69

hog fennel root (qian hu), 378
hospitality, 89–90
hot/warm-natured food, 111–12, 113*t*, 307, 308*t*, 338
humility, 97–98

indigestion
- prevention and treatment, 307–12
- Yang Type A and, 320–22
- Yang Type B and, 322–24
- Yin Type A and, 312–17
- Yin Type B and, 317–20
- *See also* digestive system; food allergies

"Inner Court" acupressure point, 311
insomnia
- prevention and treatment, 298–99
- Yang Type A and, 302–4
- Yang Type B and, 304–6
- Yin Type A and, 299–301
- Yin Type B and, 301–2
- *See also* sleep

Japanese honeysuckle, 294–95
Job's tears, 142, 317
joint pain
- prevention and treatment, 346–50
- Yang Type A and, 355–57

Yang Type B and, 357–59
Yin Type A and, 350–53
Yin Type B and, 354–55
joy, 17, 18, 24, 25
jujube, 300–302

kidneys
balanced energy of, 31
directing energy to, 240–41
fear associated with, 93–94
as "home" of the body's energy, 2, 91
joy and, 24, 25
satisfaction and, 18
sense of taste and, 20, 90
unbalanced energy of, 33
willpower and, 92
as Yang Type A's weaker organ, 67, 237–38, 240–41
as Yin Type B's stronger organ, 2, 23, 29–31, 35, 233, 234, 235
kiwi fruit, 272–73, 344–45
Korean shikye drink, 321–22
kudzu root, 313–15

leadership, 105
Lee Je-Ma, 7, 74, 106
limits, pushing beyond, 106–7
listening to your body, 363
liver
complacency and, 18, 24, 84–85
directing energy toward, 245–46
sensitivity to stress, 86
sweating and, 230
toxins absorbed by, 119, 229, 266, 313–14, 350
unbalanced energy of, 33
as Yang Type B's weaker organ, 24, 35, 68, 243, 344
as Yin organ, 12
as Yin Type A's stronger organ, 18, 23, 26, 29, 61–62, 76, 257, 312–13, 350
lower-back problems, 349
lower-body issues, 34–35, 37
lunch, 210–11, 214–15, 312
lungs
balanced energy of, 31
sorrow and, 17, 18–19, 23
strengthening, 228–29, 232
unbalanced energy of, 34
as Yang organ, 12
as Yang Type B's stronger organ, 23, 29–31, 103, 107, 242–43, 378
as Yin Type A's weaker organ, 35, 63, 78, 86, 257, 350, 370

magnesium, 256–57
meals
breakfast, 208–10, 212–14
dinner, 211–12, 215–16
drinking tea after, 210, 212, 301, 331
frequent and smaller, 309
lunch, 210–11, 214–15
when to eat, 204–6
meat and dairy
Yang Type A, 165–68
Yang Type B, 182–85
Yin Type A, 130–32
Yin Type B, 149–51
meditation
active and passive, 226

benefits of, 227*t*
directing energy to the kidneys, 240–41
directing energy to the liver, 245–46
exercise and, 223
"Meeting of the Valley" acupressure point, 310–11
memory, 28, 134, 371
Michelangelo, 80
mint tea, 215, 282–83
multitasking, 100–101
muscle ache/tightness, 8–9
music, 225

naps, 211, 312
nature versus nurture, 24–27
neck rotation, stretch, 220
nuts
chestnuts, 315–16
pine nuts, 353
as protein, 191–92
See also fruits and nuts

obesity, 325–27
obsession, 95–96
organic food, 192–93
organs
balancing the energy of, 27–31
four virtues correlated with, 74
illness and, 34–35, 38
role in health, 26–27, 34–35, 42
stronger versus weaker, 23–24, 263
temperament and, 16–17
as Yin or Yang, 12, 42
See also specific organs
osteoporosis, 150, 166, 171, 193, 218*t*, 353, 356
Outward Appearance Test, 42–53
oysters, 113

pain, ignoring, 358–59
pancreas, 3, 309
patchouli oil, 375–76
patience, cultivating, 100
perilla leaf, 260–61
pine nuts, 353
polishing one's heart (*su gi shin*), 26–27, 72–73
posture, lower-back and, 349
probiotics, 134
protein
nuts as, 191–92
sources, 199
for yang types, 213
Yin Type B and, 236
punctuality, 81–82

qian hu (hog fennel root), 378
quince fruit, Chinese, 323–24, 358

red-light foods, 55, 117, 192
relationships, 78–79
respiratory issues
airborne allergies, 366–67
Yin Type A's and, 35
See also common colds
rice milk, 118, 131, 150, 168
righteousness, 76–77

sadness. *See* sorrow/sadness
salt/sodium, 135

Sasang medicine
author's path toward, 2–4
central principle of, 3–4
focusing on the person, 10–11
four senses and, 19–22
four temperaments and, 14–19
healing with, 248–253
innate virtue, discovery of, 74
overview, 1, 6–10
Yin and Yang theory, 11–12
See also body types
satisfaction, 16, 17*t*, 18, 28, 238
schizandra fruit, 258–59
seasons, 199–200
seeds. *See* cereals, seeds, and grains
self-reflection, 27–28
senses, predominant
hearing, 22, 106
overview, 19–20
smell, 20, 80–81, 364–66
taste, 20, 90–91, 139–40
See also vision
shellfish, 65, 67, 118, 151, 166
skin allergies, 364–66
skullcap root, 290–91, 315
sleep, 82–83, 298–99
See also insomnia
smell, sense of, 20, 80–81
smoking, 6, 85, 86, 87, 218*t*
snacks, 205
social skills, 98–99
sorrow/sadness
anger and, 101–2
lungs and, 17, 18–19, 23
Yang Type B and, 16, 18–19, 69, 101, 107, 242–43
spices, yang types and, 200–201, 213
See also vegetables and spices
spleen
anger and, 18, 23, 25, 42, 102
balanced energy of, 31
digestive system ruled by, 2–3
as "heater" of the body, 233
strengthening, 232–33
unbalanced energy of, 34
vision and, 21
as Yang organ, 12
as Yang Type A's stronger organ, 23, 29–31, 98
as Yin Type B's weaker organ, 35, 63, 140, 233–35, 236
straightforwardness/rudeness, 99–100
stress
digestive issues from, 311–12
overview, 254
prevention and treatment, 255–57
weight gain and, 329
Yang Type A and, 261–62
Yin Type A and, 257–59, 334
Yin Type B and, 259–60
Yin Types and, 9
stretching, 219–22, 348
sugar, 126, 127, 134–35
supplements
body type and, 55
magnesium, 256–57
recommendations, 193–96
vitamins, 194
Yang Type A, 170–71
Yang Type B, 186–87

Yin Type A, 134
Yin Type B, 153–54
See also calcium
sweating
excessive, 236, 338
Yang Type A and, 238–39
Yin Type A and, 61–62, 230–31, 333
Yin Type B and, 338

tangerine peel tea, 279–80
taste, 20, 90–91, 139–40
teas
buckwheat, 304–5
drinking after meals, 210, 212, 301, 331
Yang Type A, 169–70, 261–62
Yang Type B, 185–86, 261–62
Yin Type A, 132–34
Yin Type B, 152–53
See also specific types
temperament
balanced, 29–31
effects of, 14–17*t*
illness and, 34–38
organ strength and, 16–17, 23–24
satisfaction, 16, 17*t*, 18, 28, 238
unbalanced, 32–34
See also anger; complacency; sorrow/sadness
temperature of food. *See* food energy
tests, body type
about, 40–42
Answer Key, 61–69
Outward Appearance, 42–53
Yin Yang Body Type, 54–69
trust issues, 78, 368
turmeric, 267, 352

vegetables and spices
Yang Type A, 160–63
Yang Type B, 177–80
Yin Type A, 123–26
Yin Type B, 143–46
vinegar
apple cider, 267–68, 334–36, 350–51
for boosting circulation, 209–10
Yin Type A and, 232, 350–51
virtues, innate
compassion, 72, 76–77, 103–4, 105
discovery of, 74
humility, 97–98
righteousness, 76–77
wisdom, 88–89, 104
vision
aging and, 382–83
early onset impairment, 382
genetics and, 381
maintaining health of, 384–86
Sasang approach to, 383–84
Yang Type A and, 20–21, 99, 390–92
Yin Type A and, 387–88
vitamins, 194–95*t*
See also supplements
voice of the heavens (*chon shi*), 103, 104, 106

walking, 62, 348
warm/hot-natured food, 111–12, 113*t*, 307, 308*t*, 338

water, drinking, 213–14, 215, 240
water retention, 238
weight gain
  obesity, 325–27
  prevention and treatment, 10–11, 327–32
  Yang Type A and, 340–43
  Yang Type B and, 343–45
  Yin Type A and, 82–83, 332–36
  Yin Type B and, 336–40
weight lifting
  excess, 226
  weight loss and, 331–32
  Yang Type A and, 239
  Yang Type B and, 244
  Yin Type A and, 232
  Yin Type B and, 234
  See also exercise
willpower, 92
wisdom, 88–89, 104

Yang body types
  breakfast for, 212–14
  diet guidelines, 212–16
  dinner for, 215–16
  spices and, 200–201, 213
  traits of, 13
Yang collapse, 236, 239
Yang Type A
  appearance, 42–43, *50–51*
  emotional tendencies, 98–101
  exercise and, 237–41, 341
  food energy for, 112–13
  key traits of, 97
  lower-body issues of, 34–35
  Question Group C, 59, 65–67
  sight/vision as strongest sense, 20–21, 99, 390–92
  temperament of (anger), 16, 18, 37, 56, 101–2, 107
  virtue of (humility), 97–98
  See also spleen
Yang Type B
  appearance, *52–53*, 343
  behavior modification and, 24–25
  emotional tendencies, 105–8
  hearing and, 22, 106
  key traits of, 103
  leadership abilities, 105
  masculine nature of, 107–8
  Question Group D, 60, 67–69
  temperament of (sorrow), 16, 18–19, 107
  virtue of (compassion), 72, 76–77, 103–4, 105
  yang energy of, 344
  See also liver; lungs
yellow-light foods, 115–16, 117–18, 192
Yin and Yang, 11–12, 13
Yin body types
  anger and, 19
  breakfast for, 208–10
  described, 13
  dinner for, 211–12
  lunch for, 210–11
  traits of, 9
Yin collapse, 239
Yin Type A
  appearance, *46–49*, 343
  desire to escape, 32–33
  emotional tendencies, 77–87

key traits of, 76
population breakdown, 26
Question Group A, 57, 61–63
smell as strongest sense, 20
Yin Yang Body Type Test, 57, 61–63
See also complacency; foods, Yin Type A; lungs
Yin Type B
appearance, *48–59*, 343
author as, 2–4, 35
emotional tendencies, 89–96
food temperature guidelines, 113
key traits of, 88
Question Group B, 58, 63–65
taste and, 20, 90–91, 139–40
temperament of (satisfaction), 18, 28, 36, 37–38
virtue of (wisdom), 88–89, 104
Yin Yang Body Type Test, 58, 63–65
See also foods, Yin Type B; kidneys; spleen
Yin Yang Body Type Test, 54–69